Cut the Guilt

Learn How
BIOLOGY & PSYCHOLOGY
Can EMPOWER You to
Take Control of Your Eating & Weight

By
Award Winning Authors

Dr. Kathleen Fuller & Dr. Jason P. Schwartz

http://www.drkathleenfuller.com
http://drkathleenfullereatingdisorders.blogspot.com/

ISBN-13: 978-1489531728
ISBN-10: 1489531726

TABLE OF CONTENTS

Cut the Guilt - Learn How Biology (Nature) Can Empower You to Take Control of Your Eating & Weight

A stark contrast exists between the way our bodies evolved over thousands of years and the way we live our lives today.

We are at an evolutionary new event where the ready availability of refined foods that are high in calories—but low in nutrition—keeps us craving more foods while rarely satiating our hunger.

Being healthy and looking healthy are not one in the same.

Let's explore the hormones and neurotransmitters that control our eating.

10 key solutions for achieving your healthy weight are introduced.

Modern-day imbalances of these essential fats sabotage many people's effort to achieve their healthy weight.

Wake up your body's power generators and emerge from the cellular semi-hibernation you may be stuck in.

Cut the Guilt - Learn How Psychology (Nurture) Can Empower You to Take Control of Your Eating & Weight

Introduction

How to Become the Amazing Woman You Are Without Guilt About Your Eating or Weight.

In *Cut the Guilt* you'll find out how to break through the traps and triggers of unhealthy eating and fully realize the amazing woman you are and how to finally—yes—finally accept your body. Free from guilt! How would it be to listen to yourself without judging, without blame?

As our understanding of the human body, mind, and emotions evolve, many of the previous *unknowns* are now falling into place. As they do an intricate and fascinating mosaic is emerging. What we once explained with hypotheses and theories now fit into a truly scientific model. But wait a moment, "What does this have to do with attaining and maintaining my healthy weight?" Everything!

The old debate of *nature* (biology) versus *nurture* (psychology) centers on the relative contributions these factors have in our lives. Yet, within that puzzle is the secret to your triumph over the common challenges of obesity and eating disorders.

So, what is the answer? Is biology (nature) or psychology (nurture), responsible for our modern day unhealthy eating patterns?

The answer is both. In the human body biology and psychology don't act separately.[1] Both dance together in such synchrony that trying to separate and teach only one partner a new set of dance steps is inviting frustration and failure.[2]

In the past, we drew an artificial distinction between our biology (nature), and psychology, our mind and emotions (nurture). Yet, medical science now reveals that every thought and emotion triggers a cascade of biochemical changes in the body. And our biochemicals—neurotransmitters and hormones—in turn direct every thought, mood, and emotion. These biochemicals also shape our personality, and modulate our experience of pleasure and pain. Neurotransmitters control our food experience of pleasure and pain. Neurotransmitters control our food cravings, appetite, energy levels, sex drive, and sleep. By understanding these triggers, you can tune-up your own neurotransmitters, giving you better health, balanced weight, and higher self-esteem. All this is revealed in *Cut the Guilt*.

When truly addressing the myriad of challenges to achieving and maintaining our healthy weight in today's modern society, we miss the mark unless both sides of the equation—biology and psychology—are discussed, and solutions presented.[3] Yet most of us, experts included, when discussing solutions for our unhealthy eating habits and weight, latch onto one side of the nature or nurture discussion. This common error can be the basis of our health stagnation.

So, how can you step beyond this obstacle? To empower your journey to better health, Dr. Kathleen Fuller and myself, Dr. Jason Schwartz, share with you the crucial tools to effectively balance both sides of our modern-day unhealthy weight predicament; biology and psychology.

By combining our expertise in *Cut the Guilt*, we have written a unique and empowering 'how to book' dedicated to your exciting, fulfilling journey to healthy eating behaviors and a healthy weight, thus awakening the amazing woman you are.

As experts in the fields of psychology and physiology (functioning of the body), Dr. Kathleen Fuller and Dr. Jason Schwartz, joined together to teach your mind, emotions and biochemistry to dance to a new rhythm of healthy eating.

Kathleen Fuller, Ph.D., is a leading eating disorder expert and author of the 1# Amazon Bestselling Book - *Not Your Mother's Diet—The CURE for Your Eating Issues*.

Dr. Jason Schwartz is a retired physician, professor of human anatomy and physiology and author of the contemporary book, *Fit Into Your Genes—Use Genetics to Achieve Your Healthy Weight*.

An Overview—Learn how Biology (Nature) can Empower You to Take Control of Your Eating & Weight

The failure to achieve and maintain a healthy weight can no longer be blamed on lack of willpower or weakness of character. We struggle to balance our abundance of food with the hunter-gather instincts that still exist within our genetic codes. Instead of helping us, the innate drives that once supported our species' survival are now quickly eroding our health and longevity.

Recently, medical science acknowledged this fact, yet for decades naive health advisers chanted the mantra of "calories-in/calories-out" as the answer to achieving and maintaining a healthy weight. These well-meaning, but ill-informed clinicians were certain that your excess weight was the result of too many calories consumed and too few burned. So, "eat less and exercise more" became their time-honored response. The *American Journal of Physiology—Regulatory, Integrative and Comparative Physiology* recently published an article summing up medicine's up-to-date overview:

"The current obesity epidemic is best explained as a mismatch between the modern environment/lifestyle and biological response patterns that evolved in a scarce environment. Biological traits like strong attraction to food and food cues, slow satiety mechanisms, and high metabolic efficiency, advantageous for survival in a scarce environment, seem now to be our worst enemies when it comes to resisting an abundance of food." [1]

Cut the Guilt presents easy to use, practical tools and enlightening insights, turning our dietary stumbling blocks into stepping stones to our healthy eating and healthy weight.

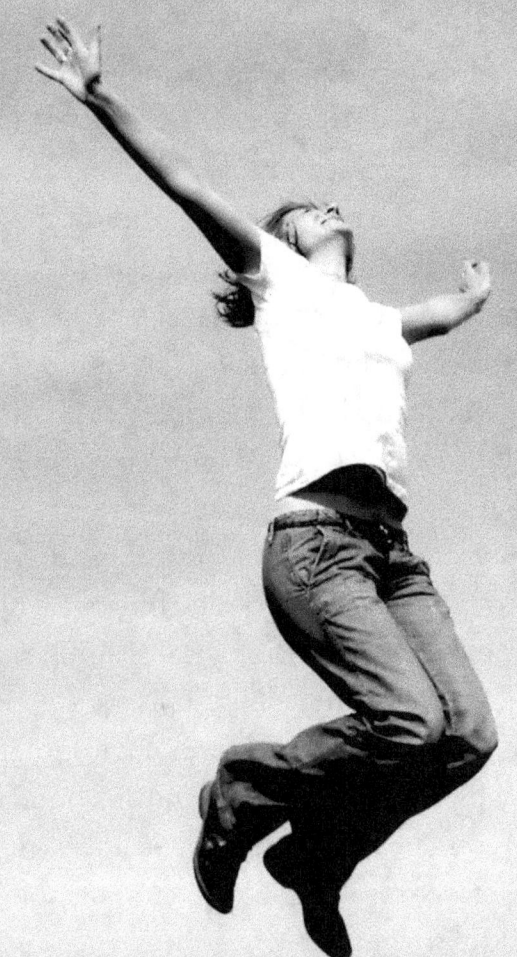

Section 1—Biology (Nature)

Comments by Dr. Jason P. Schwartz

The first section of *Cut the Guilt* is using *Biology* to change unhealthy eating patterns and achieve your healthy weight. Key insights on the nature—the biology—of our modern-day unhealthy eating predicament are shared to empower us to fit into our genes and cut the guilt! Throughout the first section of our book I use the term, "fit into your genes and cut the guilt" to describe adjusting our genetic survival responses to modern-day Western society.

A diverse readership, with much variance in educational backgrounds will read this important information. Some may read this section from beginning to end, while others will select chapters of interest. Others may use it as a reference, with specific topics being looked up as needed.

Analogies are used in many chapters to introduce complex concepts, in easily understandable ways. Many chapters also contain a glossary for readers less conversant with medical terminology.

Explaining a medical term or concept in one chapter and expecting most readers to recall that revelant information three chapters later, is a bit presumptuous. Therefore, essential key concepts and ideas are repeated in different chapters to familiarize the reader with important material.

Finally, a comment for our postgraduate readers; I ask you to appreciate the challenge of effectively sharing ideas with a diverse readership.

Acknowledgments

I am thankful to the many dedicated individuals whose help has contributed so greatly to this book. The scientists, researchers and clinicians that inspired me with their knowledge include, David Brownstein, M.D., Kathleen Fuller, Ph.D., Leo Galland, M.D., George J. Goodheart, Jr., D.C., Alan Hirsch, M.D., John R. Lee, M.D., William McKJefferies, M.D.,[*] Holly N. Schwartz, M.D., and David Zava, Ph.D.

Also I must thank the people that assisted me with editing including, Meghan Codd and Dianna Lorianni of Zuula Consulting, LLC, Suzy DiBartolo, Chris Meier and Wendy Wahlstedt.

Additionally, I am thankful for the support and inspiration provided to me by my family.

The encouragement I received from my wife Robin and my daughters Samantha and Holly empowered me. My son Adam was instrumental in my starting this book.

[*] William McKJefferies, M.D., author of *Safe Uses Of Cortisol*, Charles C. Thomas Publisher, LTD. 2004.

Section 1

Using Biology (Nature) to Empower You to Take Control of Your Eating & Weight

Chapter 1

Never Before—But Forever More

An Introduction

When was the last time you felt great? I don't mean not sick, but when was the last moment in your life that you truly felt healthy. Do you even remember or know what healthy feels like?

If you are like many people, today's modern lifestyle is taking a toll on your body, health and happiness. Perhaps you long for the vibrancy and energy you once experienced. Maybe years of searching for a cabbage soup, spicy lemonade, calorie-counting, low-carb diet that magically melts away extra pounds has only resulted in weight gain or unfulfilled goals. Or, like so many others going about their day-to-day lives, you do not feel bad, per se, but you certainly are not enjoying the vibrancy you could be, either.

Whatever the background reasons causing you to open the pages of *Cut the Guilt*, every reader has a similar starting point moving forward: You are yearning to create and enjoy a healthier lifestyle today, tomorrow and for the rest of your life.

Unlike many diet books focusing on lose-weight quick schemes, *Cut the Guilt* is here to show you how understanding your body's biological requirements—and the ways our current lifestyles conflict with these inherent needs—can help you discover vitality, health and a freedom from yo-yo dieting and exercise fads forever. With only a few simple changes to your perspective on health and your body, you can create a solid foundation on which to build a wiser, stronger and healthier approach to living.

Rather than ignoring your body's innate dietary and nutritional needs by imposing unnatural food restrictions or exercise programs, isn't it time you asked what you truly need to be healthy? With simple, down-to-earth tools and research-driven guidance, we have written this book so you can find your personalized solution for lifelong health. Are you ready to use biology to change your eating and weight, to *fit into your genes* and *cut the guilt?*

The Beginning: Where We Are Today

America is currently experiencing an epidemic. Coast-to-coast, obesity is on the rise, and today's children are the first generation whose life expectancies maybe lower than their parents. More and more people are experiencing serious health complications like diabetes and high blood pressure, and turning to prescription medications—rather than lifestyle changes—to right what has gone wrong in their bodies. As our collective health seems to spiral downward at an ever-increasing rate, it's natural to begin wondering what is happening to cause this epidemic?!

In my research and clinical experiences, one answer repeatedly presents itself: For one reason or another, a gulf exists between the way our bodies evolved over thousands of years and the way we live our lives today. In our species' earliest days, humans were a society of hunters and gatherers. We worked hard for our food, spent long hours observing the behaviors of our prey, hunting that prey, and learning how to eat what we killed. Likewise, through trial and error, we discovered the food options available around us: nuts, berries, and roots. Life as a hunter and gatherer meant relying on basic instincts to collect our food while using past experiences to find nutritionin the plants growing around us. Finding non-poisonous food sources in our immediate environment was a necessary skill to sustain life.

Survival also meant that our lifestyle encouraged and supported a fit body and healthy eating; gluttonous, wasteful dining habits matched with days sitting idle for hours on end simply were not an option in early society. Humans were more akin to other animals and in balance with the survival tactics inherent to our biological and genetic makeup.

With the development of agriculture, our nomadic, hunter-gatherer lifestyle changed significantly 10,000 years ago; however, the most drastic health transformations in developed nations have occurred over the past hundred years, greatly due to technological advances. With industrialization and the invention of the *food combine*, people are no longer directly tied to the land for their food. Add grain-fed livestock; and factories pumping out mass quantities of processed food, and our nutrition system has become so superficially efficient that the average individual does not need to have any direct involvement in the growth or production of their food.

In many ways, these advancements are a blessing. Starvation is rarely a threat. We have access to a blindingly diverse array of food to support various nutritional requirements. Our food diversity, then, enables us to easily craft a perfectly nutritious diet meeting every biological need.

Unfortunately, our advancements are also a curse. Humans now struggle to balance our food abundance with the hunter-gatherer instincts that still exist within our genetic codes. Instead of helping us, the innate drives that once supported our species' survival are now quickly eroding our health and longevity. Where once we craved sweets because fruit had dense nutritional offerings, we now have 24-hour access to processed cakes and cookies offering few nutritional benefits. The protein sources our ancestors skillfully hunted and ate moderately are now neatly packaged and consumed at every meal. Hunting for food has become an enjoyable sport, rather than a means for survival. Supermarkets are an overload on our basic gathering instincts—a visual assault of items that call to our most primitive needs.

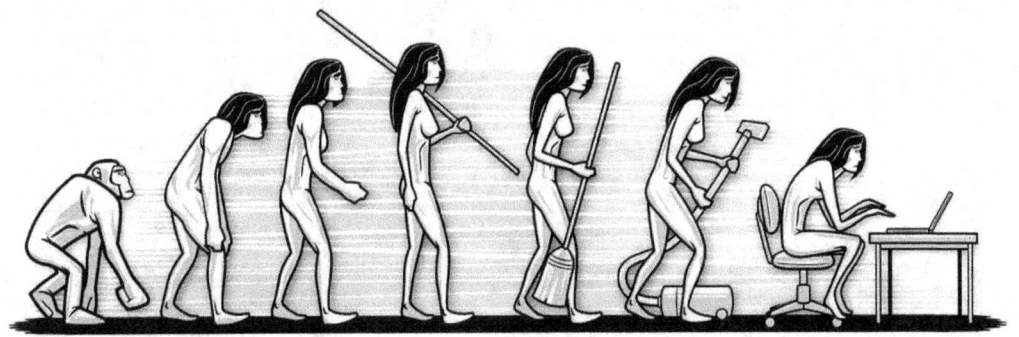

Yet, with knowledge and commitment, we can embrace opportunities presented with the evolution of technology and economics, and use these developments to support, rather than destroy, our long-term health.

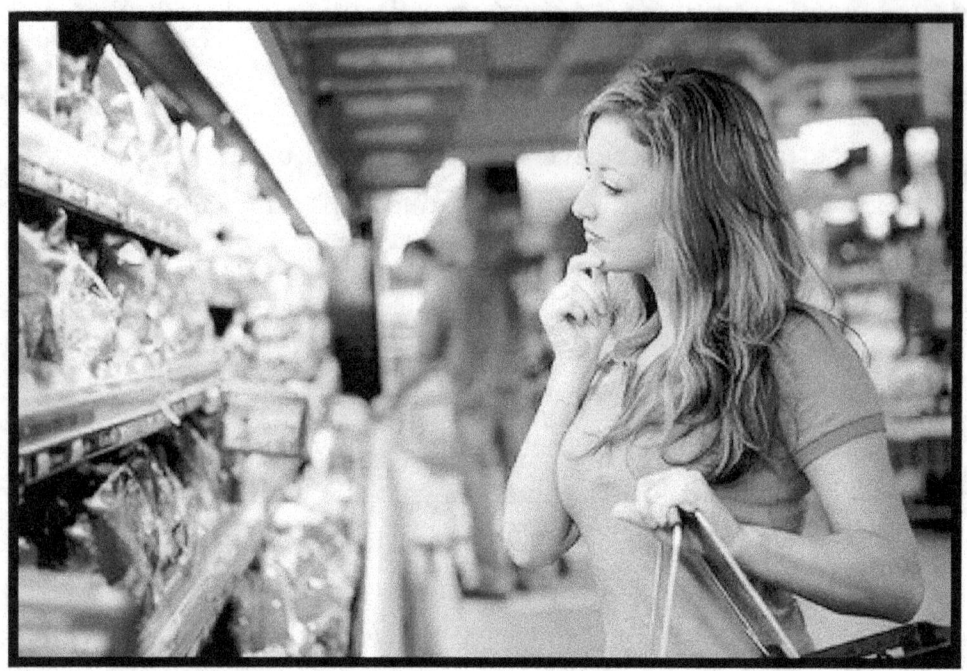

Supermarkets are an over-load on our basic hunter-gathering instincts—a visual assault of items that call to our most primitive needs.

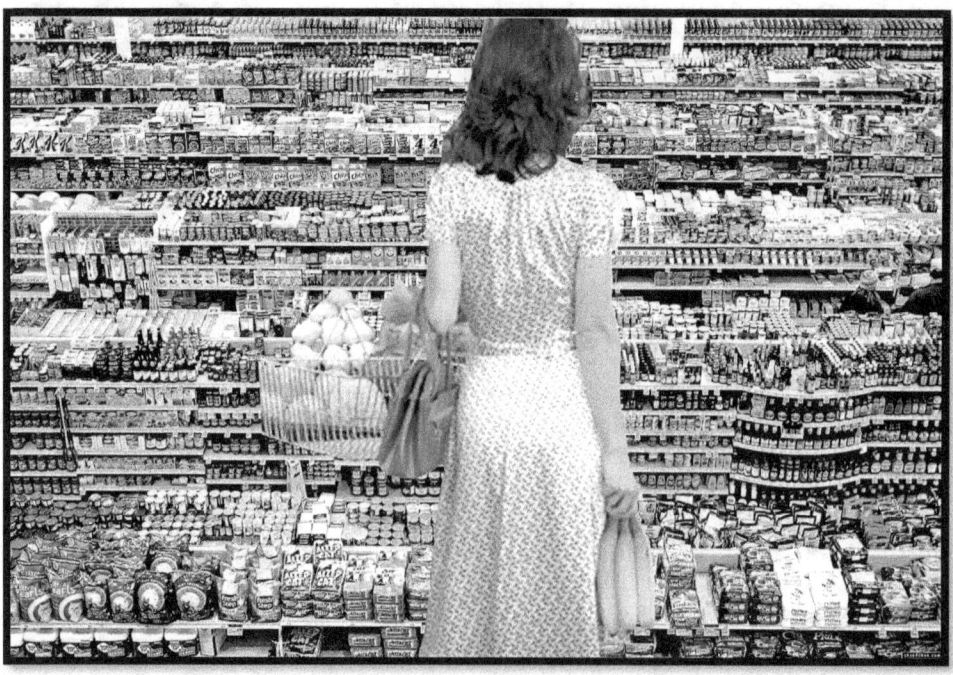

A Holistic Perspective

Just as the factors contributing to individual and societal health challenges are multifaceted and interconnected, your quest to achieve long-term health must also address the complex web of contributing influences. One of the first stumbling blocks many people encounter on their journey to a healthy weight is the temptation to latch onto one key point or approach as the answer to their overall health challenges. Humans are quick to find one solution and hope it can act as the end-all-be-all Band-Aid for all of our problems, but in reality, most of us have several factors contributing to our present health stagnation or quandary.

Think of your health this way—have you ever thrown your back out doing a simple task, such as leaning over to put on your socks? What really caused your lower back to go out when you reached down to put on your socks? How many times within that same week did you have no problem doing the same task? Bending down to put your socks on didn't make this happen, and more than likely, didn't cause the injury. You already had a problem with your back that perhaps you were unaware of. The act of putting on your socks was simply the proverbial, "final straw on the camel's back." And the pain is not the actual problem, but rather a symptom of more serious health issues. Because a myriad of contributing factors can allow even one relatively benign action to metaphorically "throw your back out," the root cause of your health challenges may not be immediately apparent.

Consequently, medical experts are commonly challenged to piece together the clues and reach an accurate assessment of the real cause or causes, almost as though they are playing "20 Questions" with your health. And if the doctors' detective work is done diligently and thoughtfully, they usually uncover a host of underlying factors that contribute to reaching a "critical mass," when the body exhibits easily recognized, classic signs and symptoms. To heal effectively, many positive factors and efforts may have to be combined before a breakthrough in your health occurs.

When dissecting a problem at work or in our relationships, we often do so until we feel satisfied that each item is examined and analyzed, and the proper solution is achieved. But when it comes to our health, on the other hand, we tend to experience tunnel vision and are quick to dismiss a solution if it does not automatically fit into our precategorized expectations. This tendency is common, but can prevent people from unlocking the answers to their health questions. So, throughout this section of the book, you may see an approach you've tried in the past and were unsuccessful with, and quickly disregard it; before doing so, I encourage you to revisit this particular method again. Challenge yourself to learn at least one new aspect about a tactic before dismissing it. With revised awareness and understanding of your health and the various factors contributing to it in your life, you are able to see new perspectives on even familiar topics. To really benefit from reading *Cut the Guilt*, I ask you to lay your preconceived notions to the side and prepare to consider, and reconsider, all of the perspectives, thoughts, angles, and attitudes presented to you; because more than likely, you will receive a wealth of information offered to you in entirely new, exciting ways.

Although some of the topics you discover here will have a greater impact in your life than others, examining everything discussed in this section of the book is imperative, as there are probably several aspects contributing to your ability to achieve and maintain your healthy weight. As you read about the factors, make a checklist for yourself. When exploring solutions to your personal challenges, ask: Does this answer fit my particular situation? When you come across an item that calls to you, I encourage you to write the topic or thought down, and rank on a scale of 1 to 10, how you believe your overall health is being affected by that component. Note the specific factors relating to your current situation, and evaluate how each can contribute to your challenges of maintaining a healthy weight.

As you read and categorize items, you will likely find that the dilemmas are greater than you expected. To enjoy a truly healthy, sustainable lifestyle, there is no one "quick fix" solution. By taking a holistic approach and honestly examining the complexity of your challenges, you will benefit from   1- A balanced, realistic perspective on your health,

2- A healthy, sustainable weight,

3- Increased energy and vitality,

4- Clarity of thought, and a centering of emotions.

Knowledge, coupled with action, should be the guiding compass on your path to achieving a healthy weight in today's modern world. Instead of fighting our bodies, let us look at how and why our body's systems work together, and discover the meaning of true well-being. I invite you to adapt and flourish. Do this for yourself, for those who love you, and those you love in return. Then, pass your newfound information to others. Empower your loved ones with the understanding needed to achieve a healthy weight with a new reality and a new you, who is no longer burdened by your preconceived notions of what healthy dieting truly means. By sharing the knowledge and inspiration gained from a refreshed, more wholesome lifestyle, you, your family, and future generations will be forever changed to live more fulfilled, uplifted, and aware in all that you do.

The Passé Past

Today, there are millions of people who believe the only way to control their weight is through starvation. Yet often, these individuals are plagued with multiple health challenges, not simply a problem with overeating. Fortunately, when empowered by knowledge, we can take the next evolutionary leap necessary to achieve a healthy weight through wise and informed eating decisions. In the many aspects of our modern Western lifestyle, a transition must occur from the old ways we used for survival of the fittest to the emerging new ways where we become more knowledgeable about how exercising, food choices, and our mental and emotional states ultimately affect our health. Trapping ourselves in "what did work" for our health is to be condemned by ingrained, obviously ineffective routines. And simply relinquishing responsibility for our health and well–being to health experts clearly isn't working. Perhaps our parents' or grandparents' generation felt so ignorant about health issues that believing the doctor was always right was rational. But today many are well informed patients and need to work in partnership with their clinicians in order to achieve their health goals.[1] Freeing ourselves individually from passé solutions to make room for modern answers is empowering and exciting. New paths to healthy living will be forged and created around who you are today and how you want to feel tomorrow. Often, what's necessary for truly improving our health is to take an honest, complete inventory of our emotional and historic connection to food and resultant eating habits—and then be open to implementing methods that establish new life patterns.

For example:

- Do you notice you tend to crave ice cream or other sweets when you are sad? If so, you may be feeding a hungry heart, not an empty stomach.

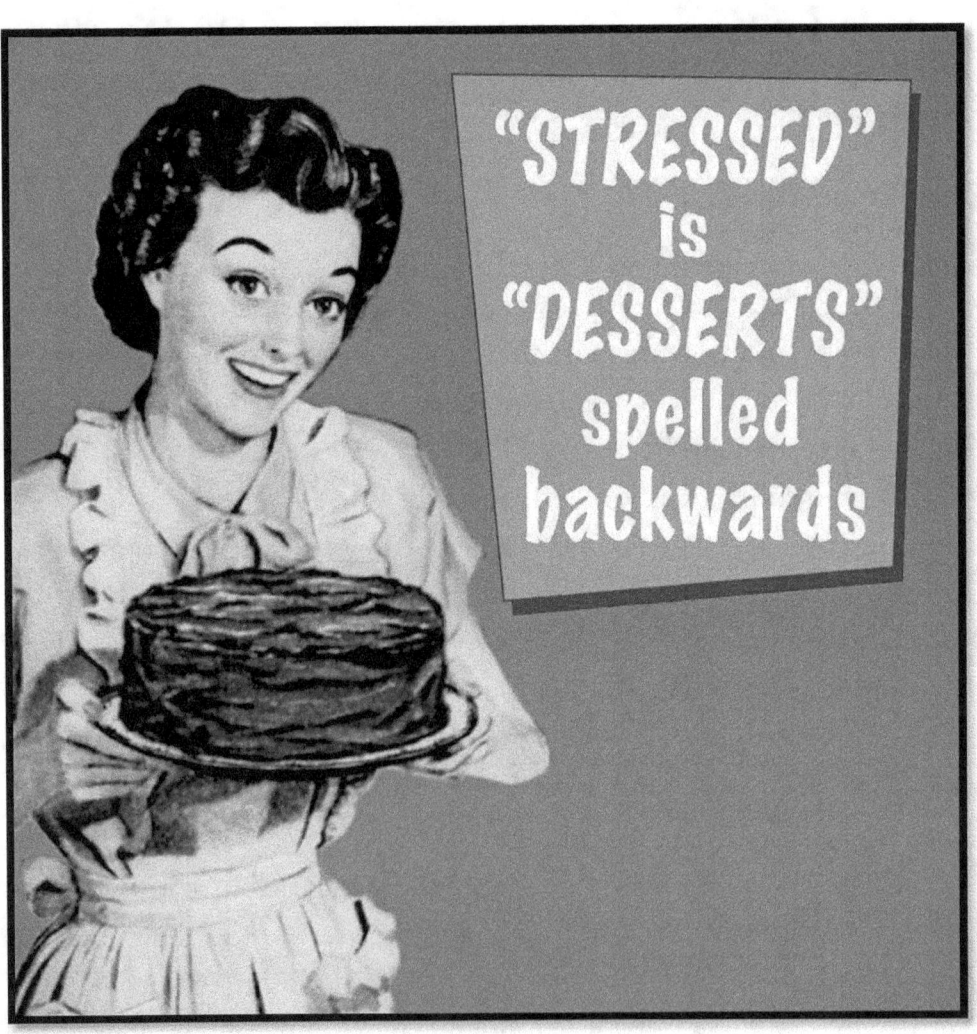

- Does your family have a longstanding tradition of enjoying Sunday feasts and refilling your plate over and over again? If so, reflect on these experiences now and try to separate your relationship with the meal and your loved ones to learn whether food, or family, is the true theme of the gathering.

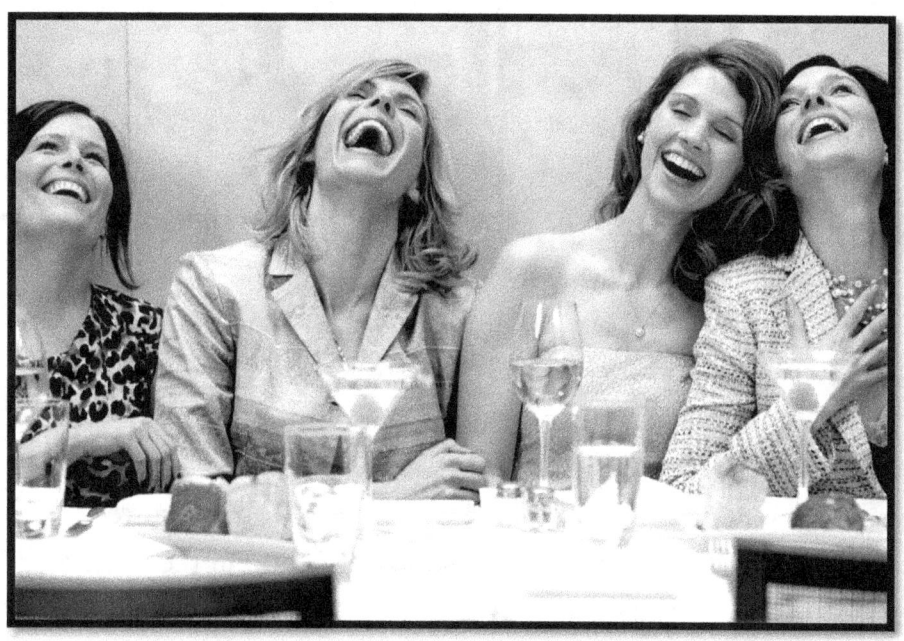

- Do you often sit down in front of your computer or TV with a snack? What is truly driving this consumption, hunger or boredom and habit?

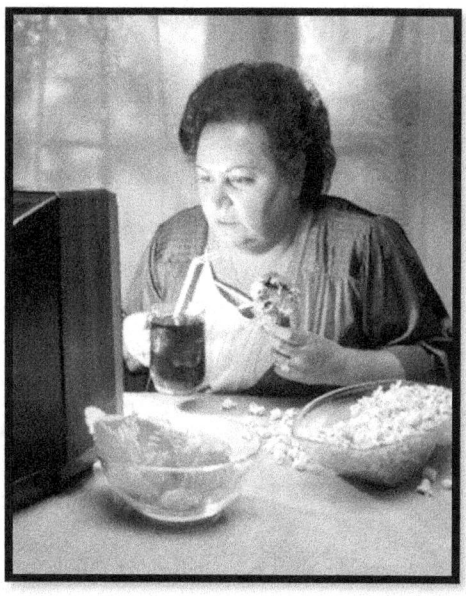

- How about your vehicle: Is it littered with empty food containers and bags? Why are you eating so often on the go? Are you not making time to enjoy meals or absentmindedly filling your stomach between meals while zoned out in the car?

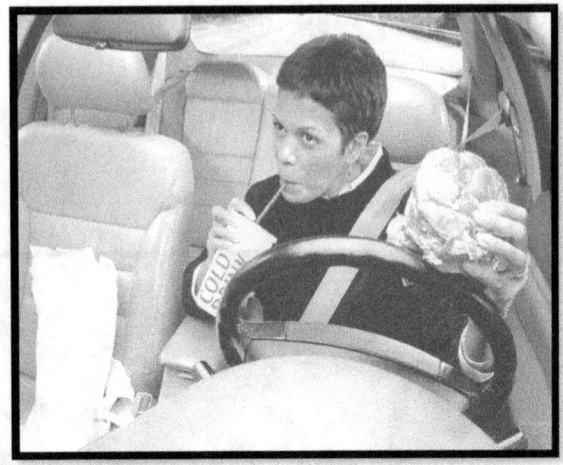

Take the time to recognize how you interact with your food and pay attention to the emotions experienced during your food audit. Recognizing the connections you have with food will often inform you of the patterns you need to change within your life to move forward and create a healthier you.

Food satisfies a multitude of cravings that go way beyond nourishing the body. Often, when we are upset, emotionally hurt, or tired, we pacify ourselves with food. You can teach yourself how to intercept these triggers and put an end to unhealthy eating patterns, and give yourself what you REALLY crave and deserve (such as pursuing a more fulfilling career or fulfilling hobbies to combat boredom) without ruining your health. And creating this healthier life for yourself begins with knowing and believing you don't need to rely on a piece of chocolate or a dish of ice cream to make it all better. I will show you your body is already prepared to overcome these cravings, and it all begins with awareness.

The circumstances affecting achieving a healthy weight have turned upside down in just a few generations. I invite you to set new health practices in place for yourself, your loved ones, and your future generations!

What this Book is About

Cut the Guilt takes an overview—a holistic view—of the latest information on health and weight loss, and explains what works through substantiated insights you can use to achieve and maintain your healthy weight.

Cut the Guilt was written to consider the health of the WHOLE you—your integrated being complete with a physical body, mind, and Soul. Science now reveals that our body's chemistry and hormonal levels are affected by our specific thoughts and feelings. For example, did you know that tears of joy are chemically different than tears of sorrow? Dr. William H. Frey, II, found that emotional tears contained a larger amount of stress hormones.[2]

Additionally, even your personality can modulate your body's chemistry to affect your hunger for certain types of food. Our sense of taste actually changes with our moods and varying personality types are drawn to different foods.[3] Obese people who lack assertiveness and are embittered, for example, tend to have a strong preference for the taste of sweets.[4-5] By taking a holistic approach and looking at how the individual parts relate to the sum, you will learn the fundamental causes of weight problems and how to permanently fix them. To truly tackle weight challenges, you need a balanced approach that integrates comprehensive health practices: correct thinking, exercise, new foods—and most importantly—a true understanding of the real, underlying causes of your weight issues. When you dig deeply, you may be surprised that your health problems are actually not what you believe them to be!

To start, achieving your healthy weight requires you to have a wider perspective on weight loss than most doctors can provide because they are usually focused on addressing specific weight challenges, rather than all of the underlying causes. When visiting a doctor, reception rooms are often full, schedules are hectic, insurance limits what procedures are covered, and malpractice claims place incredible pressures on our doctors. Instead of viewing weight gain as a holistic issue, doctors are expected to rush to identify the most obvious symptom of your health problems and make a diagnosis. Consequently, the typical Western trained physician can in turn, help if you are experiencing a medical crisis, such as diabetes, but they probably can't solve the weight problem that may be contributing to your diabetes. Why? From my perspective, medicine as commonly practiced today lacks the desire or diligence to troubleshoot and address the subtle, yet real factors often contributing to your unhealthy weight and eating.

In fact, 58% of obese individuals are not even encouraged to lose weight by their doctors, partly because many medical professionals view obesity as a chronic condition, rather than a health quandary that must be solved.[6] Remember, medical doctors may even ignore a weight gain of 20 pounds, but YOU cannot!

Cut the Guilt will educate you about the myriad of factors that should be considered to diligently address the challenges of achieving your healthy weight. For the average family physician to consider and evaluate a patient for all these contributing issues would require a very large investment in time and money. Additionally, a staff of medical specialists from a large spectrum of the health care community would have to be on the clinical team. That team might include an exercise physiologist, physiatrist, endocrinologist, clinical nutritionist, dietitian, psychologist, and a psychiatrist.

Don't be discouraged. *Cut the Guilt* will give you the information and clues you need to chart a course to achieving your healthy weight. You may enlist the help of medical professionals as part of that course, but your knowledge will help narrow and streamline the focus and shorten the journey.

Living overweight or obese can cause an array of debilitating health problems, such as high blood pressure, chronic back and knee pain, fatigue, high blood sugar, high cholesterol, stroke, coronary heart disease, gall-bladder disease, osteoarthritis, sleep apnea, and a higher incidence of breast, colorectal, endometrial and kidney cancers, as well as a poor self-image. We all know that excess pounds are not healthy, but when you take this perspective a step farther, you learn to recognize that the unwanted weight is actually trying to tell us something is definitely wrong with our lifestyle! *It's time we all recognize that when we're overweight or obese that means our body is out of balance, and definitely needs a physiological tune-up.* And more than likely, our mental and emotional well-being are part of the mix.

Now, if all of these health connections sound heavy and complicated, take a deep breath and relax. Surprisingly, our hidden health issues aren't as bewilderingly complex as we might believe them to be. Unearthing and identifying the core reasons for your weight dilemma is possible, and your health can be reclaimed more easily than you might think. Doing so begins with learning and understanding that the secret to long-term weight loss is hiding in your genetics—your body's computer programming.

The following quote, taken from the *Merck Manual of Diagnosis and Therapy,* (a source commonly used by physicians) illustrates medical science's acknowledgement of how genetics influences obesity and weight control:

"All of the metabolic factors that modulate and control the biochemical pathways and efficiency of energy metabolism are poorly understood. Genetic factors may be involved, since some persons do not gain any appreciable amount of weight regardless of food intake. This phenomenon is poorly understood, but it suggests that some people are able, through an unknown mechanism, to turn on or off certain energy-wasting biochemical pathways as a defense against excessive fat storage. If such metabolic sequences could be defined it might be possible to control body weight without a special diet." [7]

Believe it or not, this fact was written in the 1977 edition of that medical book, and I'll bet that your doctor or monthly health and fitness magazine, or any of the other websites and studies you may have read, barely mention a genetic influence on our weight.

To be fair, research demonstrating the genetic correlation to today's overweight epidemic is recent and still emerging. Many clinicians are just not up to date on this new thinking about contributing factors to their patients' overweight health issues.

But why cheat yourself out of balanced wellness and a healthy physique while waiting for your doctors to mention genetic correlations? Achieving your ideal weight may be a matter of changing your thoughts, emotional cravings, foods, or metabolism. In fact, you may have to adjust all of these factors. But your body is wise; it will help you find the appropriate tools. Remember to read with an open mind and take care not to dismiss a method simply because you think you've heard it before. The path to creating a healthier you begins today.

Do you want to recapture your health?

We can get there by working together. By following the guidance provided within this book, you will start to see the pounds come off while your health and wellness reach long-forgotten (or never-known) heights.

With your new found health awakening, you will more than likely feel better than you have in years. Your toolbox for fighting excess fat will include up-to-date knowledge about how the body functions (physiology), as well as discussions about nutritional supplementation, dietary factors, importance of attitude and life style changes, keys to effective exercising, and ways these factors work together to sustain a healthier lifestyle.

Cut the Guilt will also discuss the most effective approaches for counterbalancing each of the primary causes of weight gain. Arming yourself with wide ranging and substantial information is the first step to a healthier weight. Many of the outlined approaches will be safe to try on your own; others may require the help of a healthcare professional. As a physician, I believe all the suggested treatments would be best administered under the care of a health practitioner, and I encourage you to open a dialogue with your clinician. By diving deeply into the information and analyzing how these factors might affect you, you'll start recognizing which of these insights best applies to your life. Trust yourself as you read this book. The information may be new to you, but now is the time to allow your body and intuition to help guide you as you begin a new journey of healthy, natural choices in your life. Whether you tackle your problem alone or with an army of doctors, achieving optimal well-being and health is ultimately up to you.

What This Book is *Not*:

More than likely, you already know about many weight-loss programs that haven't worked for you. From extreme fasting to low-carb dieting, the yo-yo results of unsuccessful weight-loss attempts plague Western societies. In fact, about 80% of people who lose weight through dieting gain every pound back, regardless of the type of diet used. Can you believe that? Eight out of ten Americans who diet will not sustainably lose a single pound. And they may end up even heavier than when they began.[8]

So, are you sick of the short-term fixes? *Cut the Guilt* is here to end the yo-yo madness, but, this is not your stereotypical dieting book.

Cut the Guilt is Not: A book about fad diets and gimmicks

You will not learn new tips to feed the "one more diet syndrome." The latest "grapefruit-seaweed-bird-nest-diet" in the magazine last month has no hidden, magical cures; neither does the new liquid slim-trim "whip it into a mousse dessert diet." Besides the fact these diets offer no long-term weight loss solutions, they can also send your health into a dangerous tailspin when they are your sole means for weight loss and control.

Actually, fad diets have been hawked since the 1800's. Advertising, from the late 19th and early 20th century pushed everything from "sanitized tapeworms" to lard diets as the new miracle way to help women maintain a slim figure.

A 1903 advertisement for La Parle Obesity Soap, that "never fails to reduce flesh" and was selling at a pricey-for-then $1.00 a bar.

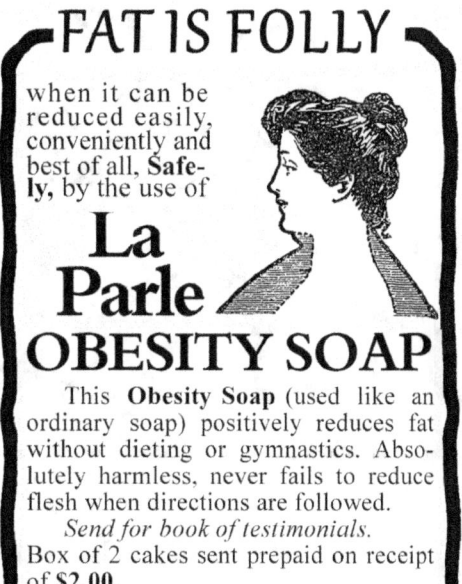

FAT IS FOLLY

when it can be reduced easily, conveniently and best of all, **Safe-ly,** by the use of

La Parle

OBESITY SOAP

This **Obesity Soap** (used like an ordinary soap) positively reduces fat without dieting or gymnastics. Absolutely harmless, never fails to reduce flesh when directions are followed.
Send for book of testimonials.
Box of 2 cakes sent prepaid on receipt of **$2.00.**

AP Photo–The Advertising Archives via
Library of Congress

In the early 1900's weight loss diets with
'sanitized tapeworms' were advertised.

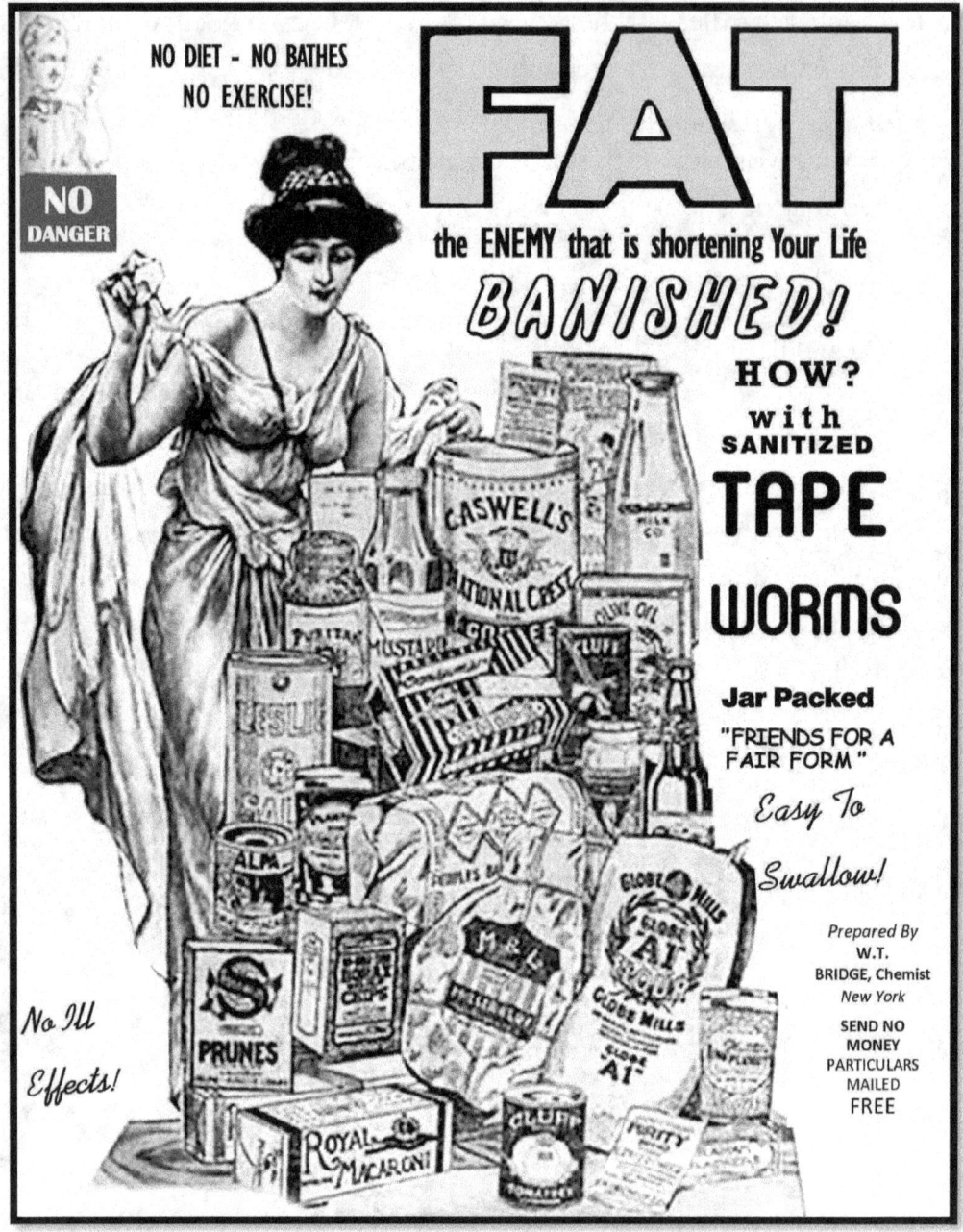

Diabetes and Obesity, Bloomgarden, Z. *Diabetes Care*,Vol. 23,
No. 1, Jan. 2000, p. 123.

Cut the Guilt is **Not: Another "exercise your troubles away" approach**

Our society already has a subculture of workout addicts. For many, their goal is not a healthy aerobic workout or muscle toning and strengthening. Instead, they focus on burning up those "nasty" calories. They can be seen in the health clubs bobbing up and down on stair-step machines or frantically pedaling exercise bicycles; others log countless miles of running or devote entire rooms at home to their calorie-burning apparatuses. *If they burn a few hundred calories while exercising, then they can indulge in dessert tonight.* Right? Wrong! Exercise can be part of the road to health, but very few will shed their extra 30 to 50 pounds or more by focusing on burning calories on the treadmill alone.

Cut the Guilt is **Not: A "calorie-counting training" manual**

Counting calories makes you conscious of what and how much you are eating, but it rarely offers long-term dieting solutions. For a few lucky dieters, once the caloric content of their favorite foods is discovered, and a change in diet choices ensues, their problem is easily resolved. But, for the rest of us, counting calories isn't the path to sustained weight loss; rather, we must seek out and identify the lifestyle changes and the imbalances in our bodies that are needed for true weight loss to occur.

In Western society, many of us were raised with dietary ignorance and a poor understanding of healthy food choices. Consider the fact that a hamburger, French fries, and soda pop are frequently considered an acceptable meal for a child. With the plethora of fast food joints that abound and cheaply processed food products available in grocery stores and convenience marts, our concept of balanced meals is completely skewed. We focus our eating habits on putting *food* into the body, rather than nourishing our bodies. As a result, when trying to gain control of a diet that is causing weight gain, the answer becomes to just cut out the calories, rather than replace the calories with more nutritious choices.

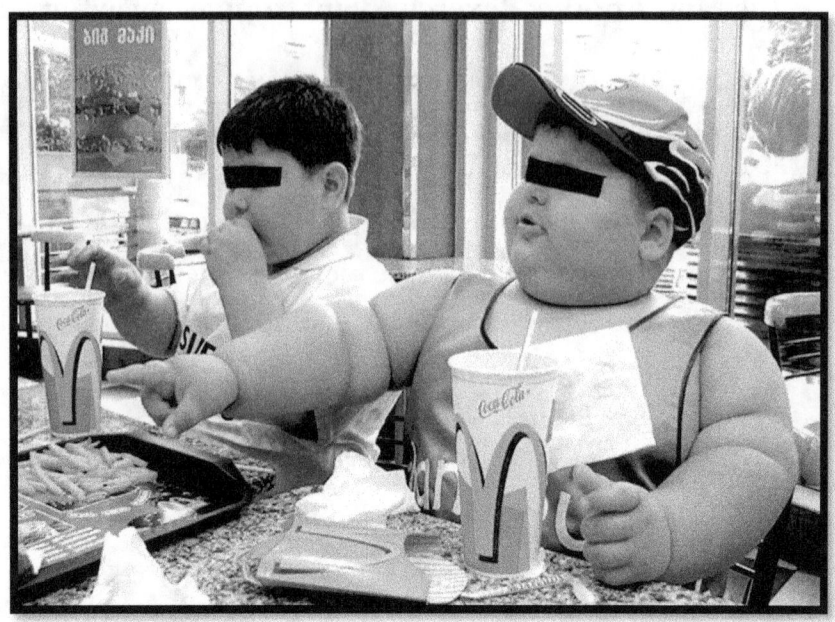

One in Five Preschoolers–2 to 5 year olds–is Overweight or Obese
Report: *Fight Fat Even in Toddlers, Preschoolers*   *AP*, June 23, 2011

The time has arrived to abandon the "calories-in/calories-out" obesity myth.

For decades, naive health advisers chanted the mantra of "calories-in/calories-out" as the answer to achieving and maintaining a healthy weight. These well-meaning, but ill-informed clinicians were certain that your excess weight was the result of too many calories consumed and too few burned. So, "eat less and exercise more" became their time-honored response. This simplistic reasoning was even used in the *New England Journal of Medicine* as recently as February 2009, when the researchers concluded that the key to losing weight boiled down to the same basic calories-in versus calories-out equation. Yet, the article's authors admitted that in their study very little weight was actually lost: After two years the average weight loss was only nine pounds. [9]

Nine pounds of weight loss after two years does not solve anyone's healthy weight management problems. While the calories-in/calories-out formula may make sense on a rudimentary level, its dangerous simplicity diverts our focus from the real causes of uncontrollable weight gain: most people fail to properly manage their weight.

By only focusing on calories, doctors and dieters rush to make a diagnosis and trouble shoot only a small piece of the puzzle, thereby missing the entire picture.

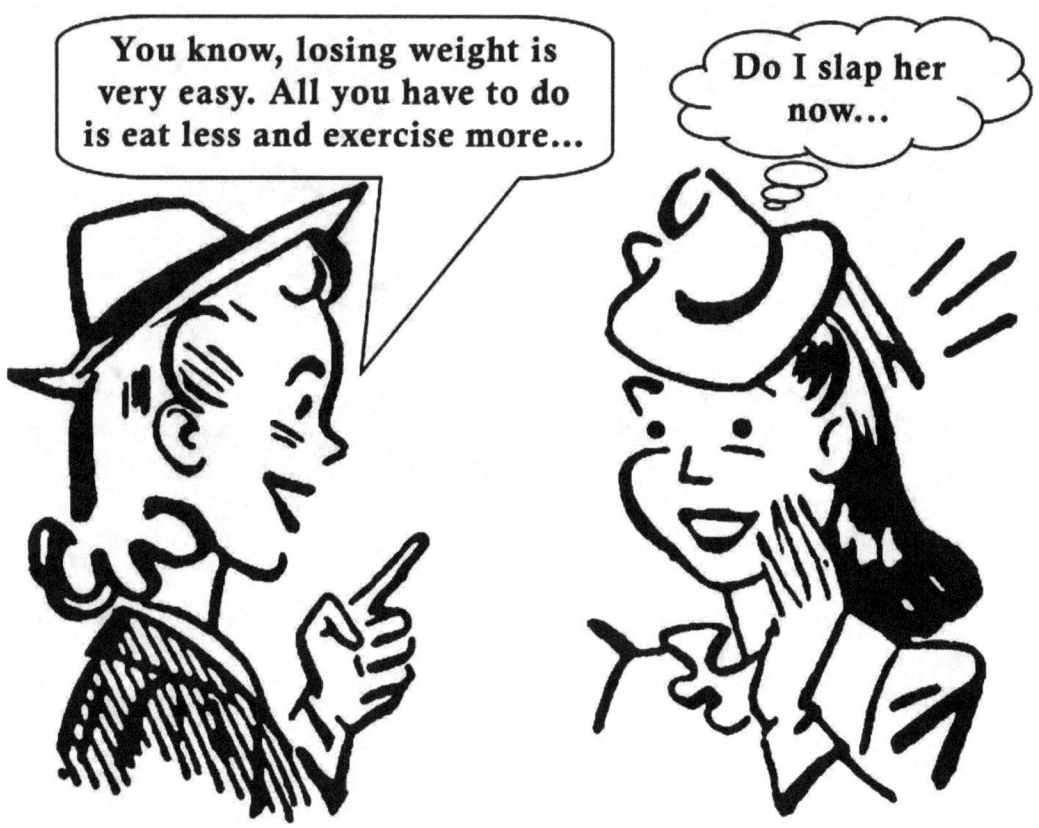

It's time to abandon the "calories- in/calories-out" obesity myth.

Studies show that women who eat junk food while pregnant or breast-feeding, give birth to "junk food junkies". [11]

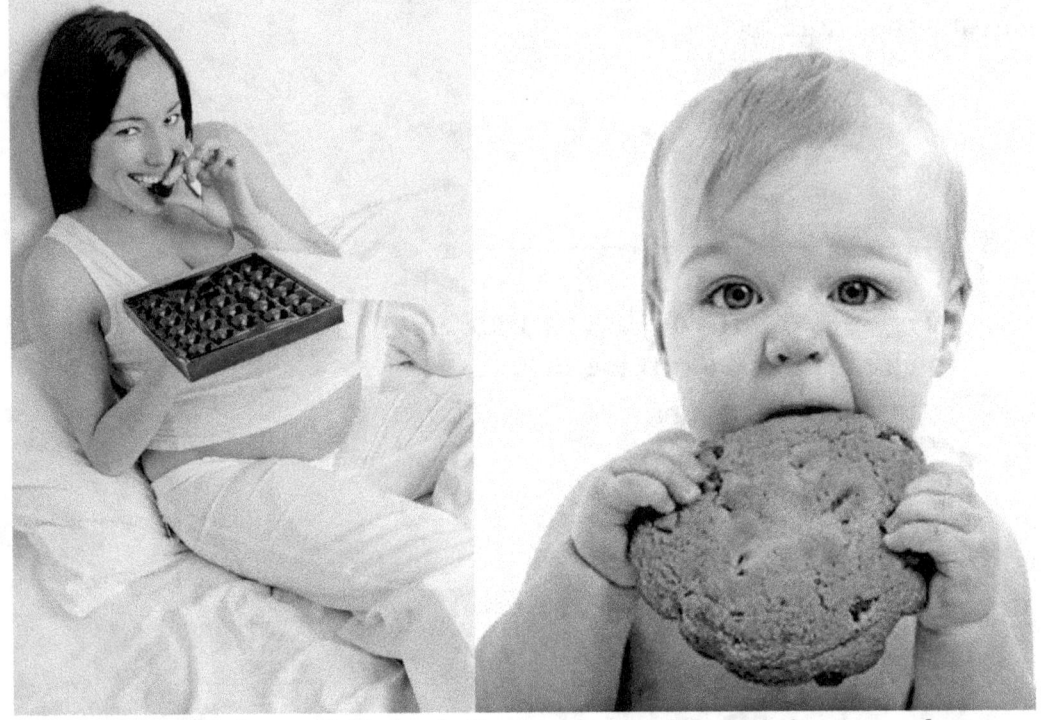

(In the second part of this book, Dr. Kathleen Fuller can help you cut free from any guilt feelings you may have about this medical information.)

Chapter 2

Where We Are Today and How We Got Here

A third of Americans are obese and another third are overweight, as defined by the U.S. federal government.

Here is a secret: failure to achieve and maintain a healthy weight can no longer naively be blamed on lack of willpower or weakness of character. Since the mid-twentieth century, our society's diet, lifestyle, and environment have changed so dramatically and rapidly that our bodies' genetics and ingrained responses to such lifestyles have not yet adapted.

The obstacles most people face on the road to achieving their healthy weight are rooted in biochemical and physiological causes. And when these systems fail to work properly, an individual may be unable to feel satiated ("I'm full") and struggle to avoid overindulging.

When it comes to eating behavior and body chemistry, we are genetically programmed to survive scarceness, remain active during the day, and spend time outdoors. However, most people's lives don't mirror our instinctual needs:

- We no longer live a hunter-gatherer lifestyle (details in chapter 1).
- Food is now available to most Americans, 24/7, 365 days per year (details in chapter 4).
- Our food chain has shifted, effecting every cell in our bodies, as well as our hormones and brain chemistry (details in chapter 6).
- Many of us live a relatively sedentary life when compared to our ancestors (details in chapter 7).

Is it any surprise these drastic changes are having drastic effects on our health?! Today in America, about 34% of adults are medically classified as obese (30% or more above their healthy weight), whereas, in 1985, 17% of Americans were medically obese.[1]

So, in roughly 25 years, the number of adults struggling with obesity in our society has doubled to about one in three Americans. [2]

Think about that for a second.

For every three people surrounding you in a park, sitting beside you at a sporting event, or perhaps even members of your own family, one of these individuals is likely clinically obese.

Now, add the overweight Americans into the mix (those whose weight is 10% higher than their healthy weight), and we arrive at the frightening figure that approximately *two-thirds of adults in the United States are medically classified with serious weight problems*. Or in other words, 100 million Americans are overweight or obese—three in five men and half of all women.

Startling numbers, aren't they?

Between 1989 and 2009, the average American's daily food intake increased by 250 calories and was 23 pounds overweight! And consequently, obesity-related health spending reached $147 billion in 2008, about double that of just a decade before. [3]

If this frightening trend continues, *half of all U.S. adults will be obese and about 90% will be overweight by 2030*. At the same time, health care costs are projected to double every decade, to nearly $1 trillion per year.[4]

Prevalence of Obesity in the Adult US Population (%)

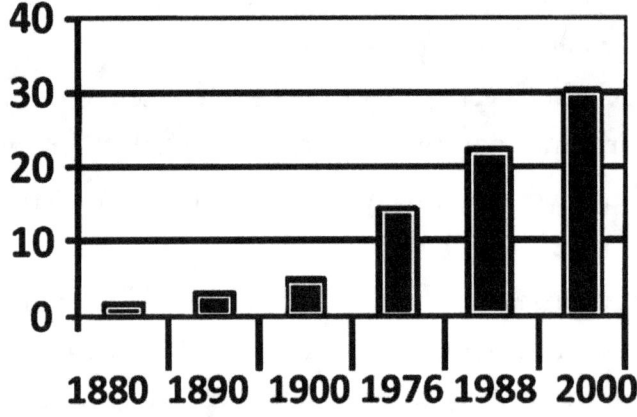

Endocrine Reviews 30 (1): 96-116. Richard J. Johnson, Santos E. Perez-Pozo. Hypothes is:
Could Excessive Fructose Intake and Uric Acid Cause Type 2 Diabetes?

Truly, America is experiencing an epidemic. So don't feel alone. We are at an evolutionary new event, where the ready availability of refined foods that are high in calories—but low in nutrition—keeps us craving more foods while rarely satiating our hunger making over-consumption inevitable. Though many people share a challenging, confusing path to a healthy weight, you can find the health destination you desire. The key is understanding the genetic and lifestyle factors that make long-term weight loss and true health a challenge; discovering which factors most affect your own experiences, and implementing changes to create an individualized approach.

The Rotund Rationale

In America today, we are obsessed with thinness. We seek out diet trends, exercise fads, and surgical assistance to help create/attain that thin body type glorified as acceptable and attractive.

People who don't gain weight easily after eating a reasonable amount of calories are envied. Our ancestors, on the other hand, could not survive if their genetically determined body type allowed them to eat an average amount of food and stay thinner than their peers. In hunter-gatherer societies, the less fat (fuel reserves) an individual stored, the more likely they would perish in periods of food scarcity. Ironically, that "naturally thin" genetic trait that so many of us wish we could have today, would have brought about our ancestors' demise. In just a handful of decades, we have gone from being a society of people who see 'fat on the bones' as healthy and necessary for survival to a society of people who immediately judge excess weight as unattractive and unhealthy. We have transitioned our thinking and perspectives on what "being fat" means to our health.

Survival once depended on the ability to maintain adequate body fat, and historically, heavy people were considered the most attractive because they represented health and vitality. Slender people were viewed as frail or sickly. And men sought voluptuous mates, because women need about 7% more body fat than men to support healthy reproduction. For thousands of years, if a woman wanted to attract a mate, she'd better eat up!

Our genetics even encourage women to maintain higher body fat. Women tend to have more taste buds than men and, as a result, are often better at tasting. They are also more accurate than men in identifying odors. In general a person's gustatory awareness (the ability to taste) increases in proportion to the number of taste buds present and according to the acuteness of their sense of smell. Additionally, a woman's brain is more stimulated by food and cannot suppress hunger as easily as a man's can.[6]

When added up, women generally get more pleasure from foods than men do! Nature intended women to have this increased drive for food in order to better prepare for pregnancy, as well as feeding and raising their offspring.

If you are a woman who has wondered why your male partner seems to eat and eat and never gain weight, and you feel like you could gain a pound just by smelling a donut, you may have your genes to blame!

The Abuse of Abundance

To survive throughout history, humans had to eat the "See Food Diet," that is, see food and eat it. Living in our close-knit tribal communities with very little communication from outside that tribe, no one was sure when more wild game would be found or if natural disasters might strike. So, we ate when food was available, and sought out high-calorie, high-fat nourishment that would sustain us until our next meal.

Our genetics contain our human survival programming, and reflect our long history of food scarcity. In many ways, our bodies are now at war with our lifestyles. As far back as 1962, geneticist, J.V. Neel recognized a "thrifty gene" that prepared our bodies for the nutritional ebb and flow that our diets once included. But, the thrifty gene that once protected us from starvation now sets the stage for obesity in our bodies, according to Neel.[7] Our body's automatic weight homeostasis system is still genetically set to protect against weight loss, not to save us from unhealthy weight gain.[8]

In other words, we are genetically predisposed to hold onto fat stores. Although our bodies are extremely well prepared to handle fluctuating food supplies, they are ill equipped to handle abundance.

For the first time in the history of humanity, the masses the face challenges of what I term "the abuse of abundance." This concept actually applies to many challenges of modern Western society: In our hyper-industrialized, fast food society, never before has the populace been able to eat as much as they want, 24 hours per day, seven days per week, in the manner we can today.

In fact, the U.S. produces so much food that it can supply 3,800 calories per day to each man, woman, and child in our country (and we now have over 300 million people!).[9] When the average person needs only 2,200 calories per day for or a healthy diet, we clearly produce—and consume—more food than is needed to meet our daily requirements. Surrounded by so many calorie sources, the average person does not stop their caloric consumption at daily requirement levels.

Simply put—we have food in abundance and we're abusing the system. Next time you walk through your local grocery store, I challenge you to stop and take a detailed look at the individuals surrounding you. More than likely, you will see the direct results of our abused abundance in the obese patrons strolling through the aisles. Or, look at the vast array of food products presented to you on the shelves. Pick one of the items and review the labels. What are the ingredients? How many of those ingredients do you recognize? And when you return home, check out the products you normally buy, and measure an actual serving of cereal or ice cream suggested on the nutritional label. Does the serving size look like the same amount you normally consume? Chances are you may be eating much more than what the package recommends.

When overcoming society's abuse of abundance, we must sensibly engage in new attitudes and approaches to our relationship with food and health. We must reacquaint ourselves with how to eat for our genetics and for nourishment, rather than how to satiate our unhealthy cravings and lifestyles.

The Human Sweet Tooth

Our primitive survival instincts have turned into a plague in these modern times. Historically, the taste for sweets was a survival instinct, a matter of life and death.[11] When our ancestors foraged for foods in the fields and woodlands, they actively sought sweet tastes because fruit is most nutritious—and sweetest—when it is ripe. They also avoided bitter substances, as toxic plants often have a bitter taste. Thus, we are genetically programmed to prefer sweet foods and are hesitant to consume bitter foods, because of what they represent in nature: high-density calories and potential poison, respectively. Only in the past hundred or so years has our instinctive taste for the sweeter things in life caused health problems.

Why?

Today, the sweet truth is a bitter pill to swallow. Those candies and cookies we are scarfing down at our desks everyday don't just taste good, they are actually tricking our basic survival instincts by mimicking the tastes of necessary calories. In the meantime, our bodies desperately seek absorption of real nutrition. While the sweets we crave taste lovely to the tongue, consumption of fructose or high fructose corn syrup (HFCS) activates our hunger signals while depressing those internal triggers that tell us we are full. So, by eating the unnecessary sugar calories, our bodies are rigged to feel that if we keep eating the sweets, then the real nutrition will soon arrive. Without a signal that our nutritional needs have been satisfied, we continue eating and eating these tasty foods, consuming much more than our caloric needs. With more calories in, and no increase of physical activities to burn the excess off, weight gain is inevitable.[12]

In simple terms, since one function of fat is to act as stored energy, if we consume more energy (calories) in our diet than we expend, pounds of fat will accumulate. This is known as a "positive energy balance." The reverse of this can apply too. If we take in less energy than we burn, the fat will be broken down to make up the difference, a "negative energy balance." Thus the calories-in/calories-out paradigm means eating less and moving more. Unfortunately, our body is not quite so simple and that is why this basic formula is not enough; you must combine diet, exercise and an understanding of your body's systems in order to truly fit into your genes and cut the guilt.

In addition to weight gain, our intake of refined carbohydrates (white flour and white sugar) causes devastating results for our brain. We expend neurochemicals and bodily functions in a vain attempt to extract fuel from refined carbohydrates. But because most of the sugars we consume aren't the raw, natural types found in food like fruits, the processed sugars and chemicals, such as high fructose corn syrup, that we do consume are stored as fat in the body. Unsure whether to rid itself of these processed sugars or keep them as fuel reserves, the body holds on to them—causing weight gain in the process.

Hormones and Weight Gain

Even today, humans would die if their brain did not naturally trigger hunger when their nutritional supplies and energy were depleted. But, problems arise when one of the key hormones that helps control these hunger signals, leptin, is not in proper balance.

The word *leptin* comes from the Greek word "leptos," meaning thin. Leptin is produced by fat cells, shuts down our appetite for food, and is thought to be a short-term appetite-balancing hormone. Because fat (adipose) cells make and release leptin, the more fat we have, the more leptin we have. And since lepin also reduces our appetite, its presence ought to keep us from gaining excess weight. Logic tells us that obese individuals, whose higher percentage of fat (adipose tissue) results in higher quantities of leptin, would have greatly reduced appetites. But for most obese people, their leptin checks-and-balances system is not working sufficiently.

Why?

Sustained high levels of leptin created from large amounts of fat tissue result in leptin desensitization, also known as "leptin-resistance." So, obese individuals who carry excess fat for long durations (years!), we now know become leptin-resistant. The causes of leptin-resistance are thought to be a combination of genetic factors; regardless of an individual's specific cause, however, obese individuals experience an absence of appetite control and fail to receive the appropriate satiety signals to tell the brain they are full.

In short, leptin-resistant individuals will continue eating past the point of feeling full. As we continue to see the connection between leptin-resistance and obesity, pharmaceutical research is now focusing on medications that can reverse or attenuate this imbalance, so leptin is able to properly curb our appetites.[13]

Hunger—Friend or Foe?

Hunger is as hunger does.

Seems fitting doesn't it?

The actual feeling of hunger can be difficult to gauge and may be hoodwinked by aberrant appetite and satiety chemistry. In today's society, many people experience a love-hate relationship with hunger. We need our appetite to survive, but we also don't necessarily need to give into it every time we hear its voice whispering to eat more.

One common example is the kitchen cabal. Instead of working for hours to prepare every meal, modern kitchen technology coupled with food technology enables us to skip the preparatory steps and indulge in "impulse meals." Simply put—we crave a food, and we are immediately able to eat the object of our desires.

Craving chicken teriyaki? No problem, just microwave a box!

Have a desire for potatoes? Why not settle for the family-sized bag potato chips! Or pop those pre-made, triple-stuffed potatoes into the oven, instead.

Whatever we want to eat is immediately available to us in a variety of conveniences. A pitfall of this instant gratification lies in our body's genetically determined ability to regulate our appetites. We were not designed to function properly under today's express-eating conditions. Before we can even breakdown and process our foods, and feel full, our hunter-gatherer instincts are driving us to search for the next food source.

And while these conditions are not doing wonders for our health, they have done wonders for the food industry's pockets. Over the past several decades, the food industry has consciously capitalized on manufacturing culinary concoctions that stimulate the brain's pleasure/ reward center and carry almost drug-like effects. Creating foods that trigger the release of the "feel good" neurotransmitter dopamine, these foods also trick our brain to ignore the "I am full" signals other parts of the brain are sending.

According to a report published in 2009, Dr. David Kessler, former FDA Director (Food and Drug Administration) and Dean of medical programs at Yale and the University of California, says the food industry has figured out what combinations of ingredients trigger the release of the "feel good" brain chemicals and are flooding the market with these addicting foods. He states they are, "layered and loaded" with combinations of fat, sugar, and salt and often are so processed that you almost do not even have to chew. Dr. Kessler also reported on neuroscientists' research that confirmed the fact that fat-and-sugar combinations, in particular, light up the brain's dopamine pathway—its pleasure sensing spot—the same pathway that conditions people to alcohol or drugs. [14]

The food industry has used the concept of food addiction in their advertisements: suggesting that "I bet you can't eat just one." High sugar foods and high fat foods as well as chocolate are the foods that stand out as having addictive effects on the human brain.

Why does this happen?

Certain combinations of sugar, fat, and salt "hyperstimulate" the brain's pleasure center, thereby *turning off our appetite control switch*. And unfortunately, this extremely common addictive mixture is present in an array of inexpensive "junk foods." So, in addition to overeating, the consumer also insults their chemistry with artificial colors and flavors, trans-fatty acids, as well as a plethora of other complex substances only a food scientist could explain. The bottom line with these unnatural additives and adulterated phony fats is the body does not process these substances as foods, but instead these chemical agents have drug-like effects on our systems.

Sadly 10,000 new processed foods are introduced to the market-place annually.[15] That is an unbelievable number of unhealthy foods on the market for you to consume! Dr. Kessler claims the food industry is intentionally using these "addictive food" recipes to move Americans to eat even when they are not really *hungry*. As a result, our food purchases may not be driven by true appetite, but rather an addiction to ingredients purposefully added into our food for the sole purpose of making us buy more. And unfortunately, in the USA, about 90% of money spent on food is for processed food.[16]

Where Do We Go From Here?

To thrive in a food-abundant society, we must use new tools and techniques, and a fresh mindset, to avoid the now destructive survival reflex to "see food and eat it." Because the majority of us have the financial means to buy and eat food whenever we are hungry, we no longer need to rely on the instinctual *eat-as-much-as-you-can-now-because-I-don't-know-the-next-time-I'll-have-food* mentality.

But I want to eat snacks between my meals! And my large tub of popcorn and monster-sized soft drink is how I enjoy watching movies, even if I'm not hungry! This is my lifestyle, and I can eat however I wish!

Sound familiar?

"Be careful what you wish for" comes to mind, for what you *wish* or *desire* to do is often times not what you *should* be doing (or eating) for yourself or your body type. So, perhaps a more fitting statement would be: Be ready to *handle* what you wish for.

It is important to realize that many of our *wishes* are affected by the ingrained, genetically programmed instincts and drives for survival left over from our hunter-gatherer days and are no longer utilitarian or appropriate. Yet these instincts are "prewired" into our brain's physiology and governed by DNA and the nucleotide sequences of our genes.

And believe it or not, our family upbringing does not override our brains' hardwired genetic marching orders. The eating and exercising habits passed down to us by our parents and guardians cannot change or alter our body's inherent, genetic ability to process/crave the foods we eat. While discipline and social restraint may control a minor command from the brain (wanting to eat that third brownie but choosing not to), our basic instincts (like eating carbohydrates and fat to safeguard against starvation) are not as easily ignored. Human survival instincts and drives use our body's nervous system and chemicals to command us. Imagine disregarding the urge to swim to the surface of the pool for a gulp of air or choosing not to drink water when you are dehydrated. When neurochemical signals trigger a serious survival message, we have evolved to heed the calls, no matter the circumstances. Ignoring those impulses demands more than self-control. It is time to outgrow the childish feeling of guilt for following your body's eating commands

Remember, it's not your *fault* but it is your *responsibility*.

You are responsible to educate yourself and then initiate the changes needed to achieve your healthy weight. Our bodies naturally crave foods high in protein, carbohydrates and fat because the dense energy (calories) and nutrition found in such foods substantially fuels our bodies. And when we were hunter-gatherers foraging in the forests all day, unsure how soon we might find our next meal, we needed lasting endurance and energy. But when you transfer these cravings into today's lifestyles, our high-fat, high-carbohydrate, high-protein desires are not as necessary, since many of us spend our days inside at a desk, exerting very little physical energy all day long. Additionally, in Western societies, we rarely are left unable to find our next meal. Consequently, those cravings very often lead us to eating when we aren't even hungry, indulging in unhealthy, fatty, and high-caloric foods, such as chips and cookies. What we *wish* to eat, then, is not what we *need* to eat at all!

To achieve lasting health, we must reevaluate and adjust the way we manifest our bodies' genetically determined survival signals. In other words, we must choose to translate our cravings into food choices that make sense for us today and provide the nutritional value we need, not just what we desire. We must find our balance within "the abuse of abundance." We must fit into our genes and cut the guilt.

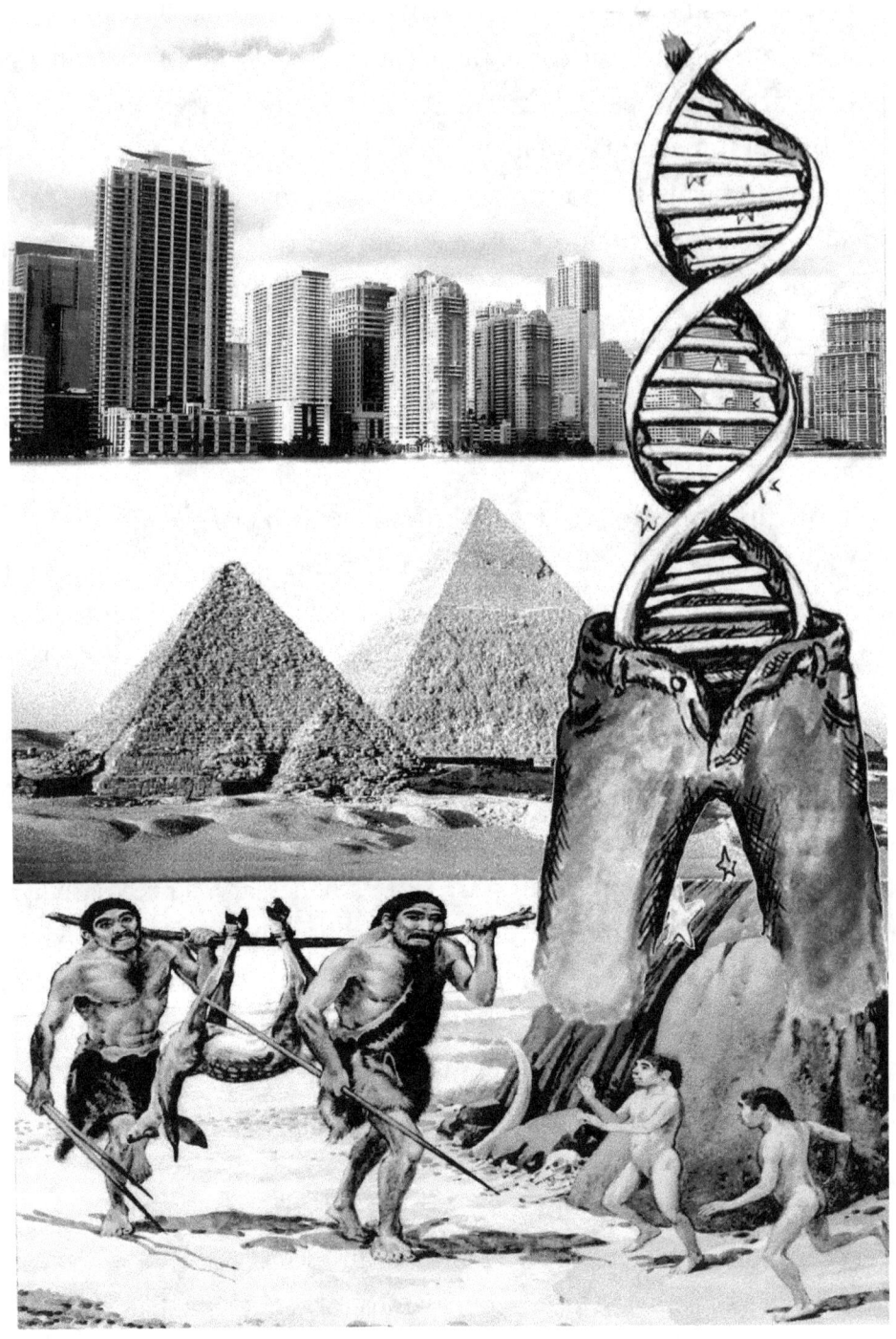

Since the mid-twentieth century, our society's diet, lifestyle, and environment have changed so dramatically and rapidly that our bodies' genetics and ingrained responses to such lifestyles have not yet adapted.

Chapter 3

A Healthy Look at Health: Real Health and True Beauty

"Health is a state of complete physical, mental and social well-being and not merely the absence of disease or infirmity." – World Health Organization [1]

What does it mean to be disease free?

What does it mean to be healthy?

If you are disease free, does that mean you are healthy too?

Not necessarily.

You may not be suffering from an overt disease, but subtle health imbalances can sabotage your attainment of an optimum weight, and in turn, living healthfully. And too often, these health issues are overlooked.

When addressing the nuances that cause us to be truly healthy versus just disease free, the missing pieces to the health puzzle frequently include common hormonal imbalances, such as:

1. Estrogen dominance or progesterone deficiency,

2. Overworked or exhausted adrenal glands, and

3. An underactive thyroid gland or improperly managed thyroid condition.

Unfortunately, many of these nuanced issues about how the body functions in relation to weight gain are often lost in the clinicians' peripheral vision. When we have a medical system that is not holistically approaching weight problems, neglecting these factors perpetuates the cycle of weight management failure and frustration.

Adding to the weight management frustration is the fact that too many clinicians naively define health as "being disease free." The danger of such an assumption is that it enables physicians to continue ignoring effective therapies and techniques that can dramatically improve our health with the goal of achieving optimal wellness not just lack of disease.

Disease Free Does *Not* Equal Health
Disease Care Does *Not* Equal Health Care

Today, many clinicians can diagnose and treat diseases, but few can diagnose and treat the absence of health or the lack of wellness. This distinction between an expertise in diagnosing and treating diseases versus finding health imbalances is crucial for troubleshooting the root causes of poor weight management.

As an example, when looking for liver problems, most physicians consider a blood test an important part of a preliminary evaluation along with checking for other classic signs and symptoms. Generally, these blood tests check for liver enzymes that are normally found within the cells of the liver. If the liver is diseased, liver cells die at an abnormally high rate. As a result, the liver enzymes from inside the liver cells spill into the blood, causing elevated liver enzyme levels. And when a person shows elevated liver enzymes, a medical diagnosis of liver disease is commonly agreed upon; whereas, liver enzymes within the normal range assumingly rules out liver disease.

But wait a minute! Is it really that black and white?

While the liver test example is standard medical protocol, let's take a closer look at the scenario.

Have you ever known someone who was not healthy by any stretch of the imagination, yet was also not dead? Of course you have. A large percentage of our population may be dismissed as "disease free" and find themselves in a medical *Twilight Zone*, as members of the "walking wounded" club. Just because these individuals do not have a disease diagnosis, does not mean they are healthy: Reading between the lines is absolutely critical for forming a holistic or comprehensive view of lasting health.

Consequently, to simply declare that the liver is "healthy" because the body count of dead liver cells is not abnormally high, does not make sense, and is an unfair diagnosis. Isn't there a middle ground between an optimally functioning liver and one that is horribly diseased?

The liver is actually a great example of underdiagnosed health issues. Unfortunately, abuse of the liver is widespread in industrialized countries. There are no pain receptors within the liver itself, thus, if we beat the organ up, the pain and destruction often goes unnoticed. Meanwhile, the liver is the body's largest gland and one of the most complex. More than 500 functions have been identified and linked to the liver, and the medical community suspects there are hundreds more. The liver breaks down the drugs we take, as well as the pollutants and chemicals in air, water and food; alcoholic beverages also stress the liver. If the liver did have pain receptors, we would diligently avoid chemical pollution, most of our medications, and alcohol.

Without pain receptors, we often do not uncover suboptimal liver function until it becomes truly diseased. Fortunately, a new type of laboratory test has evolved to check the liver's *functional* efficiency. The test is used to identify patients whose livers are technically "disease free," but not functioning up to par. Often, these patients have a diverse and confusing set of complaints, such as being sensitive to the smell of household cleaning chemicals or perfumes. Sufferers of environmental illnesses commonly have impaired liver function. If the liver is not functioning optimally, it will lead to symptoms throughout the body due to the presence of toxins in the blood and increased oxidative stress.

Of the various tests that assess liver function, the most widely used is probably the challenge test. In this test, patients are given a number of challenge substances, typically caffeine, acetaminophen (Tylenol®), and salicylate (aspirin). To handle each of these substances within the body, the liver uses different processes; consequently, we are able to receive an overall picture of how effectively the liver is breaking down these chemicals. And after a certain period of time, urine and saliva samples are collected and tested for metabolites of the challenge substances to see how well the liver detoxified them.

Again, a whole array of health care modalities exists in the peripheral vision of many clinicians. Diagnoses and treatment options are often overlooked if they exist in the gray area between health or wellness and frank disease.

Consequently, to simply declare that the liver is "healthy" because the body count of dead liver cells is not abnormally high, does not make sense, and is an unfair diagnosis.

Imagination versus Willpower

Imagination is Stronger than Willpower !

Surprisingly, most people do not know that our imagination is much stronger than our willpower.

So, quickly, let's revisit all those times you have told yourself: Tomorrow, I'll start eating healthier, or, I'll get into my workout routine starting on Monday.

And the times when you have had these conversations with yourself, how many of the imagined goals were left unfulfilled? If you are like many individuals, chances are, your *thoughts* about the goals were much stronger than the *actions* you took supporting it.

If these scenarios are familiar to you, I encourage you to avoid these discussions with yourself. You'll only feel guilty and defeated.

Changing just your thoughts may not slim your body. On the other hand, changing your IMAGINATION can lead you to a whole new approach to weight management.

For example, when addressing your dietary rut, you might actually be in an imaginary rut concerning the role of food in your life. Because our mind is a powerful tool, it can warp normal instinctual drives, such as sex and eating, and blow our relationships to them completely out of proportion. Our minds can "groove" thoughts into a predetermined sense of need and resultant self-indulgence, and not turn you loose. So, in order to harness the root causes, you need to start with your imagination of a situation, to change your true thoughts and feelings toward it.

Are you eating because you are hungry or is this a social occasion? Is your selection of foods for your meal based on habits or are you making healthy conscious choices? The information and understanding you will gain from *Cut the Guilt* will empower you to break old eating habits and adopt a new, healthier diet in your everyday world.

Another example of the power of imagination is seen with the belief that pregnant women have a greater number of food cravings. Surprisingly, studies show that despite the myth, pregnant women do *not* crave food more frequently per day than women who aren't pregnant. Instead, they give into their cravings much more readily, since Western society says it's socially acceptable to yield to cravings and gain weight when you are pregnant and "eating for two." [2]

Perhaps the significance of this surprising fact is that mental discipline does have a role in attaining your healthy weight. Consider the following story from Dr. David Sobel, a placebo specialist at Kaiser Hospital, in California, about an asthma patient who was having an unusually difficult time keeping his bronchial tubes open:

The doctor ordered a sample of a potent new experimental medicine from a pharmaceutical company and gave it to the man. Within minutes, the man showed a spectacular improvement and breathed more easily.

However, the next time he had an attack, the doctor decided to see what would happen if he gave the man a placebo. [A placebo is a preparation containing no active ingredients, given to a patient participating in a clinical trial in order to assess the performance of a new drug.]

This time, the man complained that there must be something wrong with the prescription because it didn't completely eliminate his breathing difficulty. This convinced the doctor that the sample drug was indeed a potent new asthma medication until he received a letter from the pharmaceutical company informing him that instead of the new drug, they had accidentally sent him all placebos! Apparently it was the doctor's unwitting enthusiasm for the first placebo, and not the second, that accounted for the discrepancy. [3]

Does the above scenario surprise you?

Are you moved to ask yourself, how many drugs, surgeries, medical procedures, and therapies have worked or not worked because of the attitude the doctors, nurses, and staff conveyed while administering them?

In this true story given as an example, it is the power of the imagination, not the administered *drug,* providing medical relief for the patient. The enthusiasm supporting the first "medicine" successfully convinced the imaginations of both the doctor and patient that the drug worked, even though there was no real drug administered at all!

Now, look to your health and weight, apply this thinking toward your success or failure of achieving your health goals. Are you using the *power of the imagination, mind, and attitude* to achieve your healthy weight? If not, start doing this today!

Remember, our imaginations are more powerful than our willpower. So the sooner you rally your imagination behind the cause: *I enjoy eating fruits and vegetables!* the better able you'll be to drive your willpower to stand behind you and help create the change you desire!

True Beauty

True Beauty is Eternal

Do you know the saying, "True beauty comes from within?"

While this popular phrase is typically used in reference to an individual's personality or the "person" on the inside, it can also apply to how an individual's health affects their beauty.

Now, I'm not referring to a certain body image or look. Skinny, trim, "pumped," and "cut," for example, are all contemporary—yet temporary— body styles and preferences. Today these looks may be desirable to many in Western societies, but these preferences are only a recent cultural phenomenon and not an objective, physical-medical health status. Actually, *being healthy and looking healthy* are not one in the same. In fact, looking healthy is subjective and tremendously influenced by society and culture, because the body's specific, nuanced signs of unbalanced health systems, such as blood sugar imbalances or digestive problems, may not be visable to the naked eye.

Styles change with the times and culture. Your attraction to the opposite sex is heavily filtered by society's whims and, of course, our perceptions of those whims' reality. Instead of focusing on achieving a transitory body style that is a sign of beauty today, let us focus on achieving a healthy body that is timeless in the beauty of its wisdom and function.

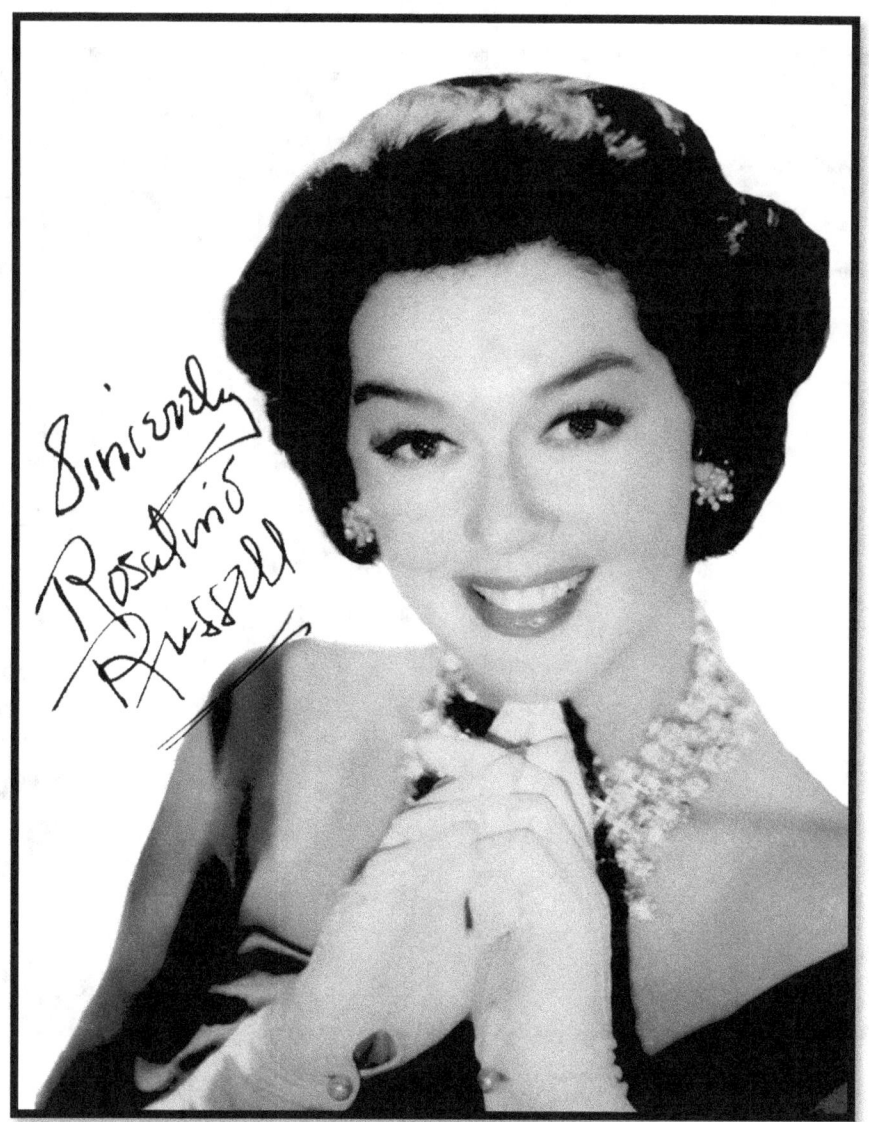

"Taking joy in living is a women's best cosmetic."
Rosalind Russel, American actor of stage and screen.

The *ideal* female figure, as painted by Rubens in the 17th century.

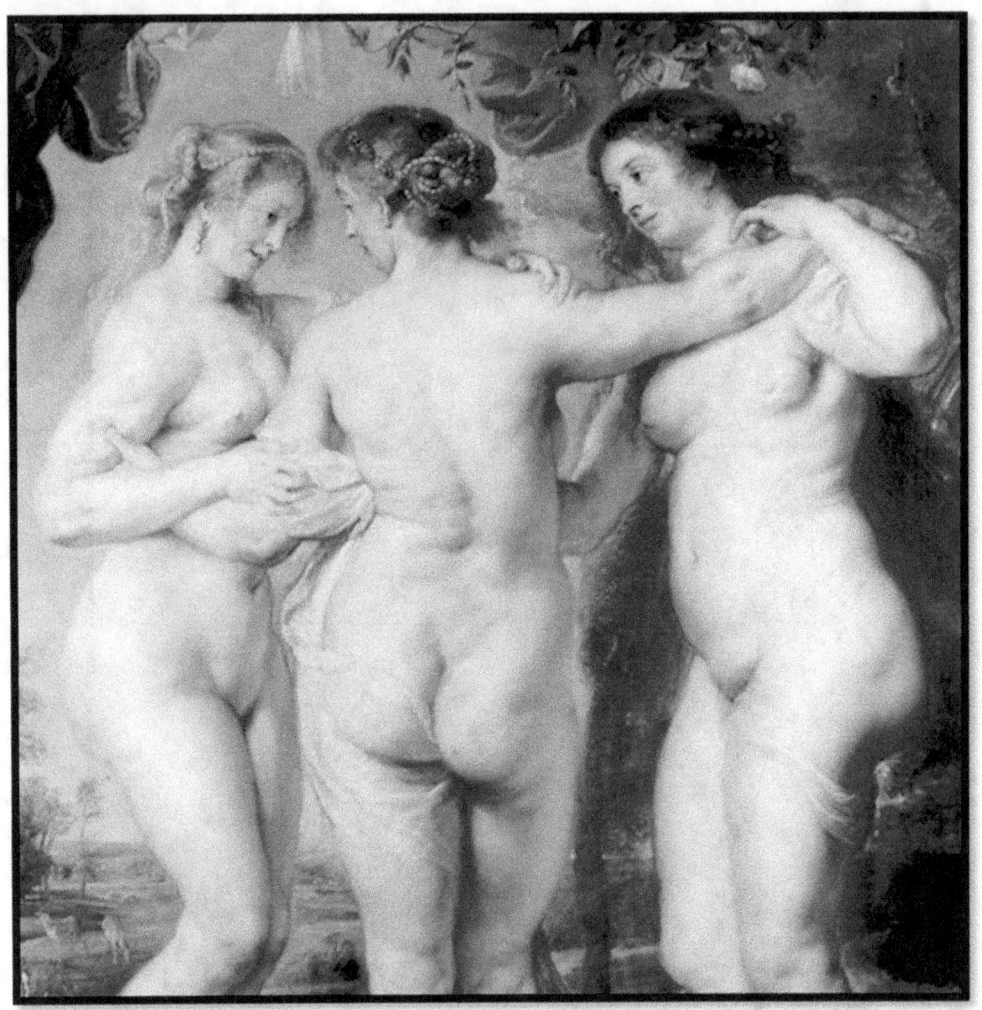

The Three Graces by Peter Paul Rubens—1635.

Chapter 4

Eat to Live, Don't Live to Eat

You know the saying, "You are what you eat?"

The statement can be translated in various ways in reference to health. When it comes to achieving our healthy weight, the core message all boils down to your relationship with food and your body's ability to satiate your appetite.

The temptation to oversimplify your body's response to hunger is understandable. When viewed superficially, our appetites are a black and white case of hungry versus full; we eat when we experience hunger and stop when we feel full.

Oh, but if only hunger were this simple who would struggle with weight, right?!

In reality, our appetites, thereby our relationships with food are complex and difficult to truly decipher and control. Anyone who has found themselves eating when they know they aren't hungry or reaching for food with little nutritional value understands the difficulties that arise when gauging and controlling the appetite. Because many processes, hormones, and neurotransmitters contribute to our appetites (and eating is not as simple as saying, "Hungry. Food."), ensuring these factors are properly balanced is essential. When they are off-kilter, controlling when and how much we eat becomes difficult, making weight gain inevitable.

Appetite versus Hunger

Understanding the difference between hunger and appetite is the first step in learning to *eat to live* rather than *live to eat*. Many people believe these two feelings are synonymous, but "appetite" and "hunger" actually represent different needs.

Appetite is a set of positive sensations that make us aware we want to eat something tasty. Appetite whispers stealthily in our ears:

Wouldn't a cheeseburger be delicious right now? Mmm-maybe even with bacon and avocado. Ooh and some fries, too.

Hunger, on the other hand, is a set of unpleasant sensations, which will drive us to hunt, forage or do just about anything to get some food. Hunger is not as subtle or specifically suggestive as appetite. Hunger communicates the ravenous feeling that nourishment is desperately needed: *Blood sugar is low! Energy is fading! You need to eat something. Immediately!*

Now, when deciphering between hunger and appetite, you can imagine the type of problems that arise when our creative, imaginative, complicated brains tell us we want to eat, rather than our digestive system. When our appetite takes over, we do not just look for foods that meet our nutritional needs, but instead seek foods that satisfy our brain's pleasure center. The pleasure center is behind those intense cravings and elated feelings we experience when we indulge in so-called comfort foods: sugary, chocolaty, or salt laden snacks full of empty calories, refined carbohydrates, and processed ingredients.

After eating junk comfort foods, our brains are quickly flooded with serotonin and dopamine, the brain chemicals that satisfy our pleasure sensors and we initially feel full. With a full belly and satisfied brain, we feel good all over. Our fulfilled feelings, however, are short-lived, creating only a short-term appetite fix. A series of biological reactions cause dopamine and serotonin levels to drop rapidly after eating comfort foods, and once they do, we are left yearning to recover those happy moods. And because many individuals develop a relationship between food and happiness, before we know it, we're reaching for a big plate of macaroni and cheese; our favorite chips; or those chocolate-covered, multi-colored candies, instead of preparing a salad balanced by a complete protein or snacking on fruits and vegetables.

We have unintentionally created a false happiness-appetite cycle where we subconsciously link comfort foods and the fulfillment of our emotional needs, rather than of our nutritional needs. Now, take this perspective and look at our society's relationship with food, where widespread junk food availability is the norm and not the exception.

When we live in a society that promotes quick-food fixes and processed food choices in a virtual 24/7 buffet, achieving a healthy weight by chanting the "just say no" mantra is, then unrealistic.[1] Choosing to eat to live rather than live to eat becomes extremely difficult, especially when you lack the knowledge or willpower to make better food choices.

So, how do we avoid triggering these appetite reflexes?

Simply put, we should never allow ourselves to become hungry in the first place! To do so, most of us must overlook the standard "three meals a day" adage and instead, eat scheduled meals and snacks (nutritionally based foods, of course!) throughout the day to maintain our body's blood sugar levels.

Have you ever known someone who maintains a healthy weight by enjoying six small meals a day, or another person who regularly snacks in order to starve off hunger pangs? These people probably seem to eat constantly, yet never struggle with real weight gain. While many of us eat three meals per day and snack as well, we often find ourselves exclaiming, "I'm starving!"

Why is this happening?

If we have gone only a few hours between meals or snacks, why are we hungry?

The solution isn't only to change how often we are eating, but *what* and *why* we are eating.

Were we to consume enough calories and nutrients to optimally function—meaning we achieve the complete nutrient balance necessary for energy output—we would not experience hunger pangs so acutely nor would our appetites focus on unhealthy foods for a quick fix. When we give our bodies the actual nourishment required to be and feel healthy, we no longer base our diet on over-consumed "comfort foods" to pacify hunger pangs. In fact, hunger pangs will no longer be a driving force in our diets. Balanced nutrition supports balanced chemical messages within the brain and body, which encourages a balanced lifestyle.

Understanding the Importance of Properly Balanced Hormones and Brain Chemistry

The human body is unbelievably complex. There are approximately 100 billion cells in the brain and spinal cord that communicate with each other and all parts of the body to make our bodies function. Furthermore, the brain processes 100 trillion instructions every second! These rapid-fire instructions are done through communication nerve cells called neurons. At any given moment, the brain has 14 billion neurons firing at speeds of up to 450 miles per hour. These neurons rely on chemicals called neurotransmitters to speak to each other, and over 100 different variations of neurotransmitters have been identified that regulate appetite, mood mental function, sleep, memory, and all of our body's movement.

When you think about the number and speed of these lightning-quick exchanges, it's easy to understand how just a few 'misfires' can cause a breakdown in communication.

Consider the transmission of the "I'm full. Stop eating!" message.

As infants and young children, we begin our lives obeying the *stop-eating-when-full message* our brains send. As adults, however, we rarely stop eating because we have a full stomach. Instead, we'll continue eating way past our full point, sometimes simply because the food tastes so good. Ultimately, our brain calls the shots. Our responses to hunger have variations and nuances, but basically we eat when our brain tells us we are *hungry.* Now remember, being hungry and having an appetite are not the same. Consequently, when eating, we rely on our brain to communicate messages from the belly that we are full. To do so, a series of chemical reactions take place that stimulate the brain's *satiety center,* and only then do we feel full.

So the act of being full is actually associated with the ability to "feel" full.

Sigmund Freud, the founder of psychoanalysis, proposed that our actions are fundamentally motivated by seeking pleasure and avoiding pain.[2] While Freud's views are specifically addressing human behavior, his analysis can also be applied to our eating patterns and passion for food.

In keeping with Freud's view, our hunger and appetite are greatly determined by our innate desire to seek pleasure and avoid pain. Each day, as we go about our lives, a cascade of biochemicals sent to the brain push and pull on three levers:

1. On (hungry)

2. Off (satiated)

3. Pleasure response (our appetite's powerful *oomph*)

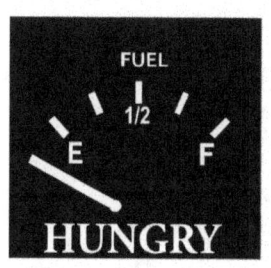

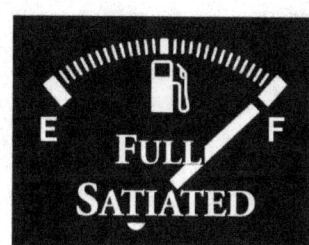

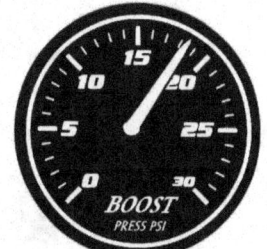

TURBOCHARGED
that **OOMPH**

We may eat well beyond the point where our actual hunger has been satiated, simply because our neurotransmitters can create a pleasure response from food. We are eating for enjoyment, rather than nourishment. Thus, the pleasure drive may push us to consume more food than is necessary to meet our caloric and basic nutrient needs. That extra push, that extra driving force to our eating is why I use the term "oomph" to signify the energy or enthusiasm behind this aspect of our appetite.

When breaking down the hunger pangs we experience, not feeling hungry isn't as simple as having an adequate amount of food in your stomach or digestive tract. Instead, satiety actually requires the proper balance between the hormones and brain chemicals that turn hunger on and off. In fact, humans have two distinct chemical groupings for *hungry* (pain) and *full* (pleasure). While one group of these chemicals triggers the brain to tell us we are hungry, another group signals the brain to let us know we are satisfied and can now stop eating.

But, unfortunately, these chemicals do not always perform as intended.

People who overeat often have a problem with the satiety part of their brain receiving sufficient stimulation. Many times, they are not consciously eating more than is healthy; instead, their on/off switches (appetite, satiety, and pleasure centers) are not functioning properly.

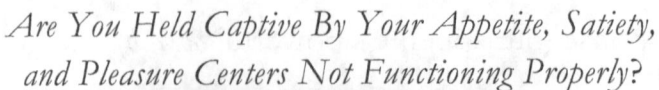

Are You Held Captive By Your Appetite, Satiety,
and Pleasure Centers Not Functioning Properly?

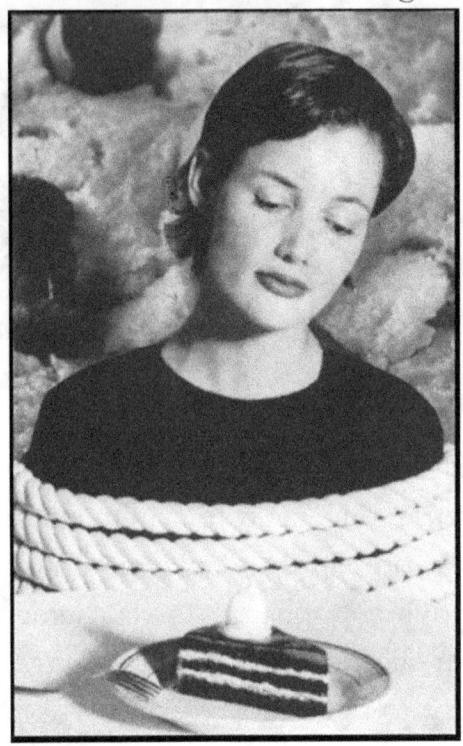

Why?

One of the signals that informs the brain you are becoming full, for example, is a rise in blood sugar (glucose) levels. And, studies now reveal that the time it takes for the brain to recognize a glucose signal is not the same for all people. People who eat a healthy amount for their body type take an average of **12 minutes** for their systems to recognize the rise in glucose. People, who routinely overeat, on the other hand, require over **20 minutes** to process the identical signal. [3]

So, generally, overweight or obese individuals who frequently overeat are not receiving the "I feel full" signal until a minimum of 8 minutes after the norm. In other words, *overweight people may be eating for almost twice as long before they feel full!*

Think about the amount of food you can eat in eight minutes: Depending on how hungry or rushed you might be, you could easily eat more than enough food to sustain you for the next few hours. And that's the amount consumed *after* they are physically full.

So, if an overeater receives their *full* signal late, are they consciously overindulging? Not necessarily. The overweight eater is simply reacting to the body's commands as they come to them, just as the thinner person does. The eater only becomes gluttonous when they eat past the signal's message.

At the other end of the 'mixed-up signal' spectrum are people who emaciate themselves. They often have an imbalance with either an under stimulation of the appetite center or an over stimulation of the satiety center.

Considering our bodies' complexity, is the key to controlling our hunger really as simple as understanding the chemical forces that drive our eating behaviors?

Surprisingly—yes! The answer is that simple.

Medical science now concludes that obesity, anorexia, and bulimia are all associated with a wide variety of neurological, endocrine, and metabolic abnormalities initiated in the brain. Fortunately, the satiety center of the brain requires just a little fine-tuning in order to work properly; our genetics have already programmed our brains for optimal functionality. Of course, psychological challenges can play a part in eating disorders, as well. But, for many individuals struggling with unhealthy eating behaviors, living and eating healthfully may simply be a matter of flipping the right hormonal or neurotransmitter switches.

The Dairy Dilemma

There is a common food group that breaks the rules and often snafus our healthy eating goals: dairy. Dr. Alan Hirsch is a neurologist, a psychiatrist and a leading expert on smell and taste physiology. He states, "The odor of food usually stimulates the 'I am full' signal in the brain but there is one important exception—milk. In infancy, milk is our primary food, and it promotes rapid growth in the first year of life. It appears that this is a permanent mechanism; it doesn't change with age. As adults, we can eat large amounts of dairy products without getting the, 'I am full, message'. It's not unusual for one person to eat up to half a pound of cheese without a hint of fullness. The same is true for ice cream." [4]

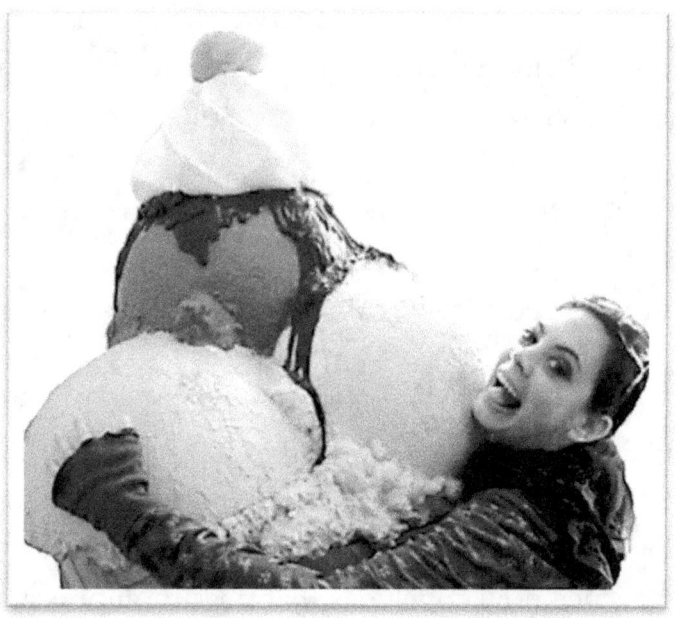

Over Consumption of Dairy Products is Common, Since Dairy Does Not Stimulates the 'I Am Full' Signals in the Brain.

Taste is a Nerve Impulse

Just as our bodies are complex, so too is our ability to taste. In short, the human brain reacts to food as a pleasurable experience:

I know those little, chocolate covered, processed cake-snacks aren't nutritious, but they taste so good!

While wheat pasta with marinara and baked chicken is fulfilling, but greasy pizza is so much more exciting.

While you may know the difference between healthy and unhealthy foods, recognizing the role our taste plays in the eating experience will enable you to make logic-driven, sound food choices.

In general, sweet and fatty foods excite the pleasure or reward part of the brain, since throughout human history rich-tasting foods were high in nutritional value. Inherent to human nature then, is the drive to eat good-tasting foods, which prompts our brain to release dopamine, the "feel good" neurotransmitter. When dopamine is released, designated receptors in the brain absorb the chemical, thereby causing the brain to react and trigger the emotion that we call "pleasure."

So, our ability to enjoy the taste of the food we eat is dependent on our ability to properly release and absorb dopamine. Consequently, when you eat more than you probably should because something tastes so good, it is likely your dopamine levels are high and encouraging you to continue the pleasure. As we previously discussed, women generally have more taste buds than men and are more accurate in identifying odors. As a result, women often are more gustatorily stimulated than men and therefore may get greater pleasure from foods than men do! A study commissioned by *Weight Watchers* showed that while 58% of women surveyed think about sex at least 10 times a day, some 70% admitted to having far more regular fantasies about food. Nature intended women to have this increased drive for food in order to have the necessary fat stores to prepare for pregnancy and carry and raise the offspring.

It's Not Your Fault, But it is Your Responsibility

As we begin moving away from living to eat and start eating to live, thus far we have learned that we must:

- Know the difference between our appetite and true hunger pangs,

- Eat nutritionally rich foods that support our bodies' proper chemical balance,

- Recognize the relationship between satiating hunger and experiencing pleasure.

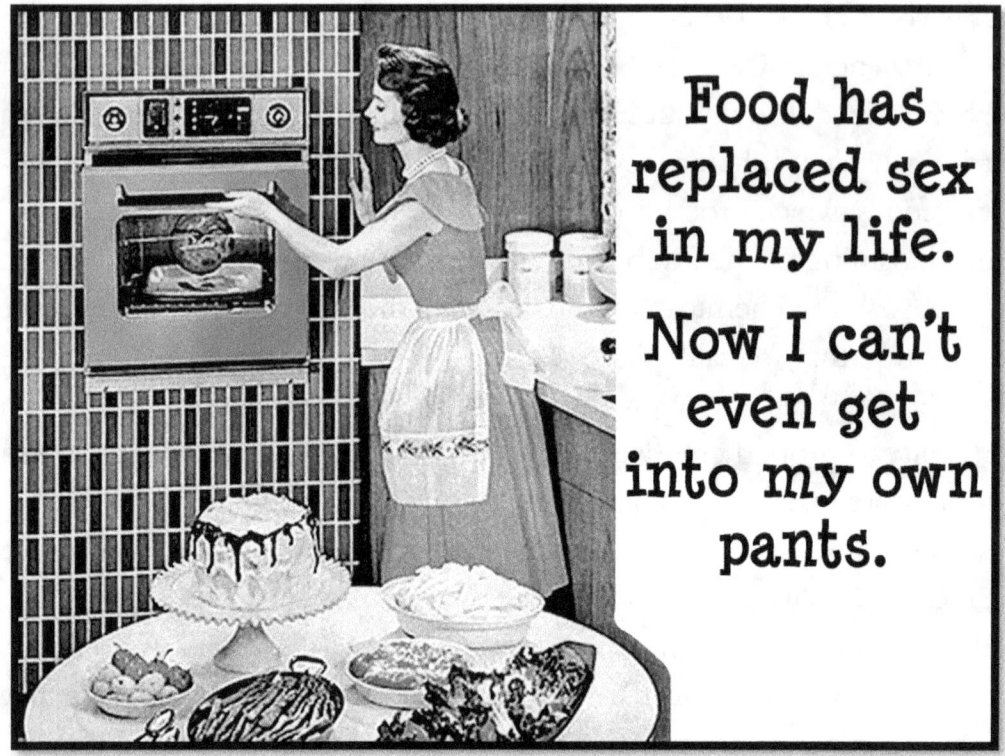

From glucose triggers in the brain to innately strong taste receptors, physiology, genetics, and your environment all contribute to health challenges and an individual's ability to overcome their overeating or unhealthy eating habits. Consequently, the old idea that only lazy or gluttonous people are overweight is inaccurate, as is the illusion that your weight issues are entirely your fault!

Did you hear that? *Your weight issues are not all your fault!* You are not solely to blame.

How does it feel to read that statement?

How does it feel to have someone tell you, you no longer have to bear all the guilt?

Instead of overgeneralizing weight difficulties, we must use our scientific understanding to replace unnecessary guilt with the empowerment and control that come from knowledge. Your responsibility is to learn everything reasonable about the causes and contributory factors preventing you from achieving your healthy weight. Then—get going!

Part of 'cutting the guilt' may be realizing you unconsciously expect perfection of yourself.

Does this sound familiar?

Many people unfairly expect perfection of themselves, yet such feelings do very little except immediately create unattainable standards. "Perfection" will not allow for life's inevitable setbacks or other challenges without placing judgment. And with judgment, you unwittingly set yourself up for disappointment when you achieve less than your idea of perfection. While striving for excellence is ideal, striving for perfection is self-defeating and impossible to realize.

Just as expecting perfection in life is unrealistic, so is underestimating the enormous influence neurochemical imbalances have on our eating patterns. Tweaking your body's neurotransmitters and adjusting your hormonal responses takes patience, self-awareness, and understanding the body as explained in *Cut the Guilt*. As you move forward reading *Cut the Guilt* and begin the journey to achieving lasting health, remember to listen closely to your body and resist the urge to judge yourself.

Go for improvement.

Strive for excellence.

Learn to appreciate every positive step on the path.

NewScientist

The global science and technology weekly | 1 February 2003-Issue 2380

ALL-AMERICAN
HIGH

CAN FAST FOOD ALTER
YOUR BRAIN IN THE
SAME WAY AS TOBACCO
AND HEROIN?

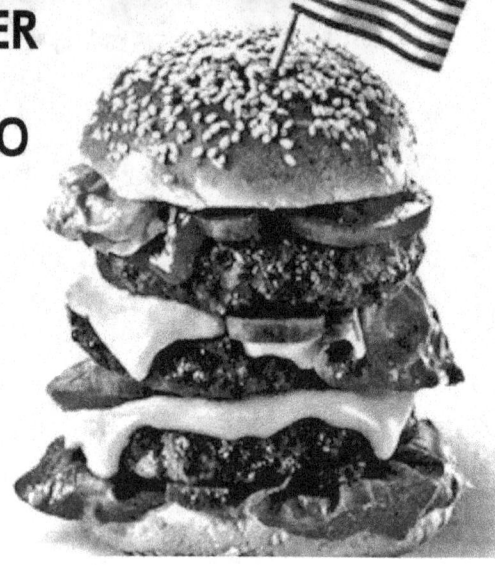

Chapter 5

A Brief Overview of the Topics in the Biology (Nature) Section of *Cut the Guilt*

Building Upon the Four Pillars

Ancient Roman structures still standing today have depended on strong, solid pillars to support their weight over hundreds of years. Together, the pillars withstand immense pressure, but if one were to fall, the entire building's stability would be compromised. Just as these ancient structures' endurance relies on stable, unified support, so too does your long-term health. Building a successful and sustainable lifestyle—and achieving your long-term weight-management goals—depends on four wellness pillars:

1. **Establishing the proper ratio of omega-3 to omega-6 essential fatty acids**

2. **Maximizing your body's ability to sustain healthy cells that efficiently burn fuel to generate energy**

3. **Balancing and fine-tuning your hormonal system to diminish food cravings and boost energy**

4. **Balancing and fine-tuning your appetite chemistry to diminish excessive food cravings**

Coupled with a balanced mindset and the emotional well-being necessary to make healthy food choices, anyone can build a solid, lasting, healthy lifestyle by using these four essential pillars.

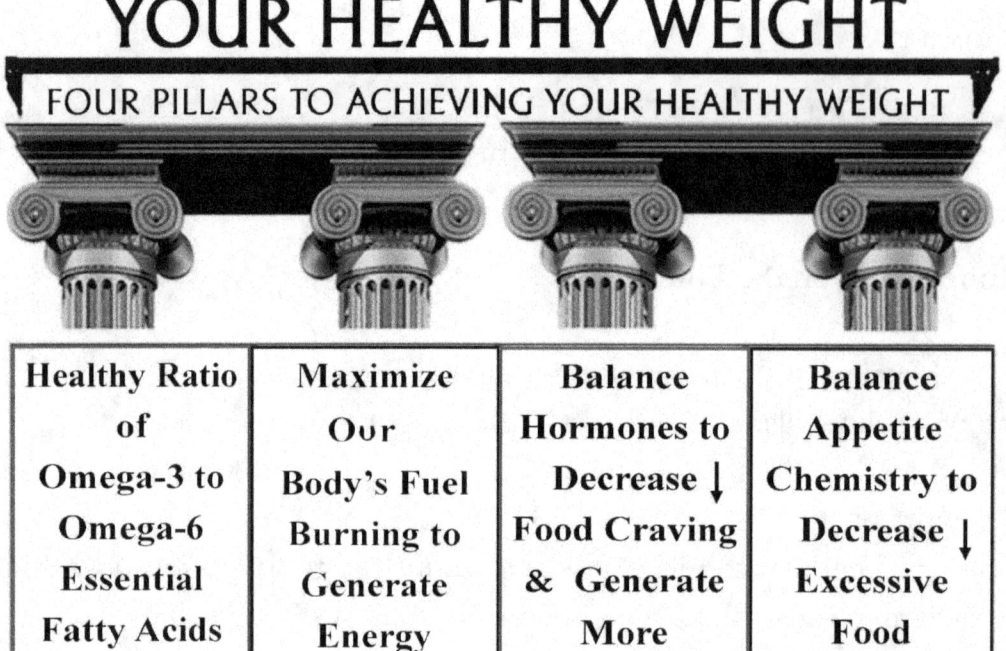

YOUR HEALTHY WEIGHT

FOUR PILLARS TO ACHIEVING YOUR HEALTHY WEIGHT

Healthy Ratio of Omega-3 to Omega-6 Essential Fatty Acids	Maximize Our Body's Fuel Burning to Generate Energy	Balance Hormones to Decrease ↓ Food Craving & Generate More Energy ↑	Balance Appetite Chemistry to Decrease ↓ Excessive Food Cravings

As you read further, *Cut the Guilt* will discuss many scientific and health based topics that may be unfamiliar. So, to help you better understand any newfound information and apply the guidance within each chapter, the following is a brief overview of the information you will encounter in the chapters that follow. Relax, no one expects you to fully understand or remember all of this information the first time you read it, so key points will be explained several times, in multiple chapters.

The four pillars of achieving your healthy weight are built on a foundation of the following 10 topics:

1. Serotonin

Adequate levels of serotonin turn off our appetite.
Low serotonin levels trigger carbohydrate cravings.

Serotonin is a neurotransmitter that imparts a feeling of well-being and satiates our food appetite. *Carbohydrates, especially sweets and white starches, raise serotonin levels.* Eating carbohydrates also triggers the release of insulin, which normally should satiate our appetite. Serotonin is made in the body from tryptophan, an amino acid, which is absorbed after the insulin response is triggered. Interestingly, simply chewing or crunching on food also boosts our serotonin levels.

Daily life stresses, on the other hand, often reduce our serotonin supplies. Many researchers now believe the average American's increasingly busy, multitasking, stressful life is directly responsible for the too commonly found suboptimal levels of serotonin in the United States. [1]

Low serotonin levels trigger the brain to send powerful survival-level signals for us to eat carbohydrates (*Boost my levels, now!*). Try to deny your brain the object of its desire, and you may not be a happy camper. Consequently, if a strong will or unavailability of carbohydrates stops you from eating the desired foods, and instead you eat protein, you may become irritable and restless. If you substitute fatty foods for carbohydrates, you might fall asleep overcome by fatigue and apathy.

Women make about seven times less serotonin in their brains then men do and this may explain why women crave sweets more than men. One reason may be the fact that the female body has a lower percentage of muscle mass and therefore can make and store less serotonin than the male body. [2]

As you will discover in *Cut the Guilt*, many cravings and unhealthy eating behaviors are actually caused by serotonin imbalances. Properly managing this neurotransmitter can support your long-term weight loss goals.

2. Dopamine

> *Dopamine turns on the pleasure response from foods.*
> *Low dopamine levels increase our appetite.*

Dopamine is a neurotransmitter that creates the euphoria associated with sex, eating certain foods, and even shopping. Hyper-elevated levels of dopamine are also connected with addictive substances such as cocaine and nicotine that produce a feeling of elated mood by increasing dopamine levels in the brain above the physiological norm.

Low levels of dopamine affect us by impairing our ability to focus on tasks. When both serotonin and dopamine are low, the manifestations often are appetite and eating disorders, compulsive disorders, fatigue, and seasonal affective disorder (SAD).

The "got to have it" impulse effect of dopamine is normally balanced by adequate levels of the neurotransmitter serotonin. So, in most instances, the problem driving addictions such as craving certain foods, compulsive shopping, gambling, and over preoccupation on sex, is not too much dopamine, but instead a lack of adequate serotonin.

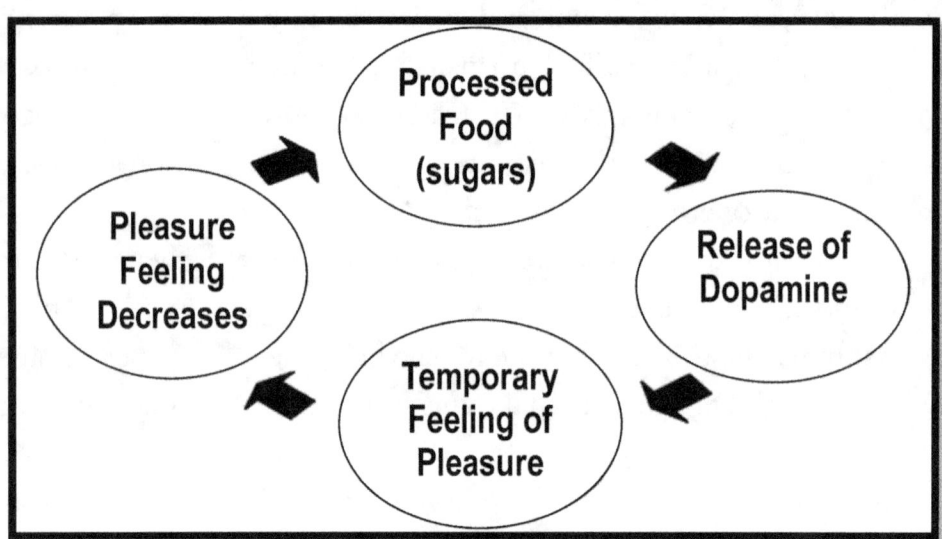

3. Omega-3 vs. Omega-6 Essential Fatty Acids

> *Excess omega-6 EFAs cause the body's fuel to 'bounce off'*
> *our cells' membranes and become deposited as fat.*

Essential fatty acids (EFAs) are vital nutrients our bodies need for health and daily functioning, and can be divided into two main types: omega-3 and omega-6. Because essential fatty acids are the fatty acids our bodies can't produce, we have to obtain them from food.

A healthy diet should consist of roughly one to four times more omega-6 fatty acids than omega-3 fatty acids. The typical American diet today, however, contains 11 to 30 times more omega-6 than omega-3 essential fatty acids. When essential fatty acid consumption is unbalanced, you can experience a number of health problems, including weight gain.

One serious stumbling block presented by excessive omega-6 essential fatty acids in our diet is the hampering of our cells' ability to burn fuel, glucose (blood sugar), causing the glucose to "bounce off" our cells' membranes and become deposited as fat. [3]

Additionally, inadequate intake of omega-3s inhibit dopamine and serotonin,[4] triggering food addictions and cravings, in particular, the desire for sweets, chocolate, fatty, and salty foods. [See Chapter 6]

4. Mitochondria

> *The sedentary lifestyle many of us lead today causes the number of the power generators in our cells to decrease, triggering low energy, and excess fat accumulation.*

Mitochondria are organelles (little organs) within our body's cells that function as our body's power generating factories. A crucial fact is, they have the ability to reproduce and increase in number, and the more mitochondria you have, the more food you can burn and energy you can generate.

The sedentary lifestyle many of us lead today causes the number of these power generators in our cells to decrease, triggering low energy, and excess fat accumulation. By doing just 2 to 4 hours per week of a specific type of exercise (that we'll discuss in Chapter 7), we can dramatically increase the number of mitochondria so we have more energy and store less fat.

5. Underactive Thyroids

> *Thyroid experts believe 50% of the population in the United States may have underactive thyroids.* [5]

Metabolism is the term used for the process by which food is converted into energy—and your thyroid gland is the master controller of your body's metabolism. A sluggish thyroid (hypothyroid) can slow your metabolism, causing you to burn approximately 600 fewer calories per day as compared to someone whose thyroid is functioning normally. Besides slowing down our metabolism, another way a sluggish thyroid causes eating challenges is to "numb" the body's receptors for adrenaline (epinephrine), dopamine and other neurotransmitters, which can trigger a sweet tooth.

Symptoms of an underactive, or hypoactive thyroid gland can include weight gain, fatigue, and depression.

Thyroid expert, David Brownstein, M.D., believes 50% of the population in the U. S. may have underactive thyroids. [5] [See Chapter 8]

6. Adrenal Glands

The stress hormone produced by the adrenals triggers the accumulation of belly fat and sugar cravings.

The two adrenal glands each sit atop a kidney and produce several hormones that influence our eating habits and fat accumulation. One of the adrenal hormones, cortisol, has been called the *stress hormone*. Under modern life's chronic stresses, cortisol triggers the accumulation of belly fat and sugar cravings, as well as slowing down our thyroid function, which controls our metabolism.

By balancing your adrenal hormones, which is doable, you can experience greater energy and a healthier weight. [See Chapter 9]

7. Vitamin B12

Forty percent of us have suboptimal B12 levels, triggering excessive food cravings and low energy. [6]

Vitamin B12 is needed for the metabolism of every cell of the body and also is involved in fat and carbohydrate metabolism. According to USDA research, about 40% of Americans have low levels of vitamin B12. [6]

A leading medical journal suggests that when pondering, "to B12 or not to B12," assume you have a suboptimal level of vitamin B12 until proven differently! [7]

Low levels of vitamin B12 can affect your healthy weight in a multitude of ways, including excessive food cravings due to low dopamine and serotonin levels and a sluggish metabolism due to low thyroid hormone function.

But, in Chapter 10, I'll show you how a $5.00 per month *special vitamin* can solve this common problem.

8. Progesterone

Progesterone turns fat into energy, helps avoid depression and reduces the risk of breast cancer by 80%. By age 35, half of the women in the United States have low levels of progesterone.

Progesterone is a natural hormone that turns fat into energy and must be kept in balance with estrogen for women to maintain a healthy weight, prevent breast cancer and avoid depression. The problem is that by age thirty-five, 50% of the women in the United States have low levels of progesterone. Also, be aware that birth control pills suppress your body's production of this fat-burning hormone.

The great news is that once you become knowledgeable about this remarkable hormone, you will be able to fine tune your own levels. And natural, bioidentical, progesterone is available over-the-counter (OTC) and by medical prescription. [See Chapter 11]

9. Hypoglycemia–Low Blood Sugar

There is nothing sweet about a "sweet tooth" as it is a sure sign that your body's chemistry is out of balance.

Many people today consume large quantities of refined carbohydrates, such as sugars and white-flour based foods, which trigger an over-release of insulin. Insulin is a hormone produced in the pancreas that carries your blood sugar (fuel for your cells) across the cell membrane so it can be burned for energy. Yet, refined carbohydrates, such as white flour and white sugar, are much too quickly converted in the body to glucose. This rapid increase in glucose triggers the pancreas to over respond and release a flood of insulin. The flood of insulin in turn, transports too much glucose from the blood into the body's tissue cells. The result is a lower than desired blood sugar level, which causes the brain to command us to eat sweets again.

This cycle of refined "carbs" triggering a drop in blood sugar, and that drop sending us looking for our next snack of sweets is how many struggle for decades. But with knowledge, we can break this cycle without having to suffer. [See Chapter 12]

10. Seasonal Affective Disorder

> *This "semi-hibernation" mode is a genetic survival mechanism triggering carbohydrate cravings and a lower metabolism to conserve fuel reserves during the darker months of winter.*

Seasonal affective disorder (SAD), also known as winter depression, is a condition characterized by mental and emotional depression in the fall and winter months. This "semi-hibernation" mode is a genetic survival mechanism triggering carbohydrate cravings and a lower metabolism to conserve fuel reserves during the darker months of winter. People with seasonal affective disorder therefore commonly crave carbohydrates and gain weight during the months of the year when less exposure to sunlight lowers levels of the neurotransmitters serotonin, norepinephrine and dopamine.

This upset in brain chemistry can be treated by nutrients, medications, or exposure to full spectrum lighting for brief morning periods weekly. [See Chapter 13]

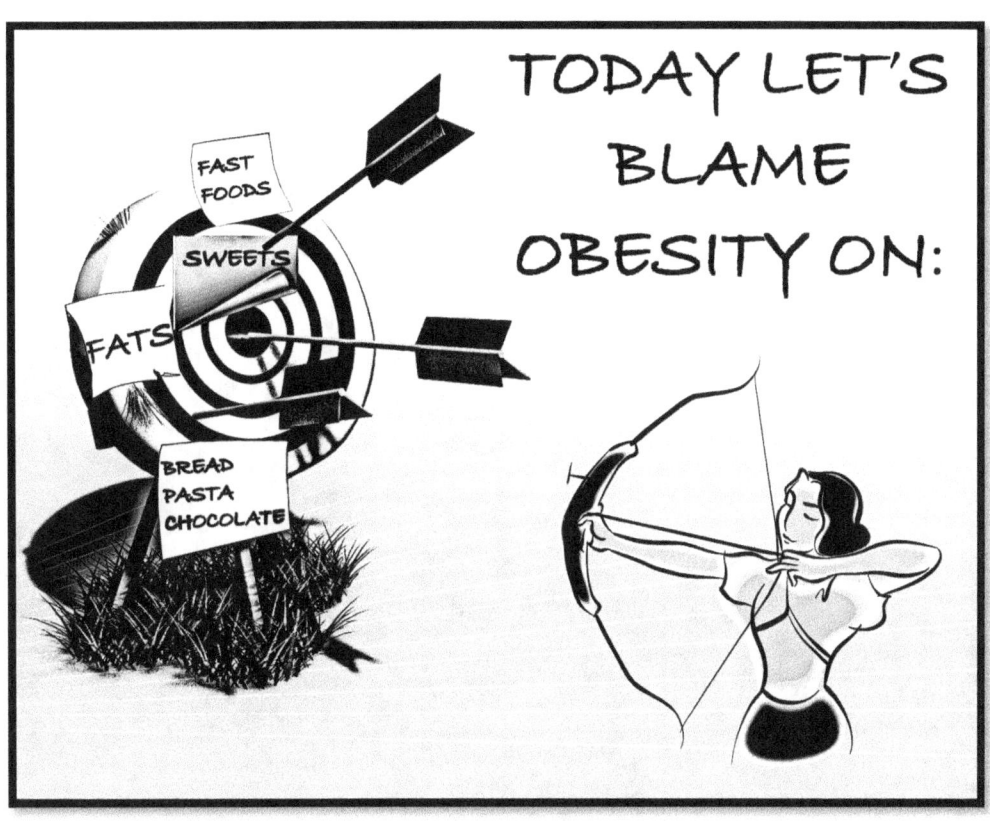

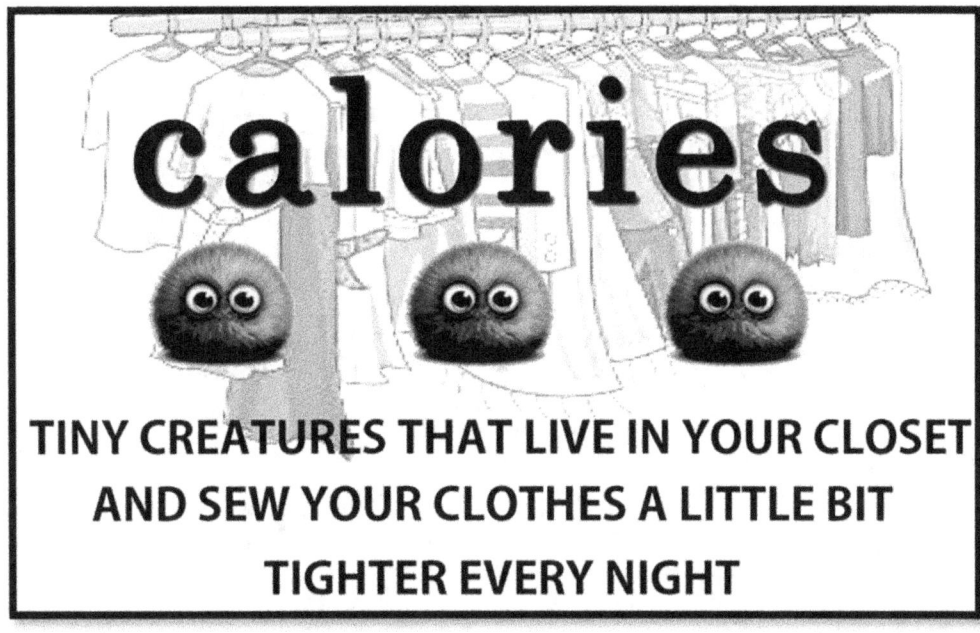

Chapter 6

Balancing Omega-3 and Omega-6 Essential Fatty Acids

Imagine a fuel truck transporting 9,000 gallons of diesel fuel. En route, the truck runs out of diesel fuel for its engine and is stranded on the side of the highway. Seems ironic that a truck transporting fuel should run out of fuel doesn't it?

Actually, not quite.

Just because the truck is transporting fuel, does not mean the vehicle has the ability to *use* that stored fuel. Though its freight would provide the very diesel fuel the vehicle needs to keep going, the engine's systems cannot access the fuel in the tanker. So the truck is stuck, overloaded with cargo that could provide the energy it needs, if only it could burn that fuel.

For many people who struggle with weight, their bodies have become like this truck: they have plenty of fuel, but no way to access it.

Simply put, your body is designed to use its stored fuel—your fat— for energy; however, just because you are built to store and access fat doesn't necessarily mean your body is using the fuel as intended.

Why?

If you carry more fat than is considered healthy (remember, an obese individual is 20% over their healthy weight), an inability to access the body's stored fat is frequently occurring. When your energy level is consistently low—despite excess fat—some obstacle is preventing your engine from using your fuel. Even though, superficially, it seems you have more than enough energy reserves, your body is struggling to access the fuel it needs.

Over the past 75 years, the types of fats in our diet have dramatically changed. From processed foods, to grain-fed beef, critical ratios of the essential fatty acids (EFAs) in our cuisine have been unnaturally skewed, and therefore, so has the chemistry and functioning of our cells and brain.

The result?

Our bodies' ability to turn fuel, blood glucose, into energy is hampered, and an ever greater percentage of the population finds themselves like the truck, stuck on the side of the road: with plenty of fuel, but no way to burn it.

Essential Fatty Acids:
The Key to Unlocking Your Stored Energy [2-3]

Essential fatty acids (EFAs)—see the word "fat" in there? Believe it or not, "fat" doesn't necessarily have to be a dirty word. In fact, the human body is designed to consume, break down, and absorb specific types of fat that help provide the essential nutrients and energy we need for a healthy life.

Essential fatty acids are fatty acids the human body can't create, so we must rely on our diet to provide them. Omega-3 and omega-6 are the two main types of essential fatty acids, and their proper balanceis crucial to our bodies' efficient functioning. These fatty acids maintain the cell membranes' fluidity and ability to produce energy; aid in the healthy development and functioning of the nervous system; and play a key role in the body's immune functions, hormonal responses, and inflammatory processes.

Omega-3 essential fatty acids:

- Are anti-inflammatory (decreases production of inflammatory prostaglandins) [4-5]

- Make the cell (plasma) membrane more fluid, facilitating the cell's ability to transform glucose into energy [6]

- "Thin the blood" (inhibit platelet aggregation)

- Support healthy brain function

- Can be an antidepressant as potent as *Prozac*® [7-17]

Omega-6 essential fatty acids:

- "Thicken the blood"

- Promote the inflammatory process

- Make the cell (plasma) membrane more rigid

Our ancestor's diets were much different than what is common today. For countless generations our bodies adapted to diets lower in calories but higher in fiber, and filled with fruits, vegetables, lean meats, and fish.

Historically, this diet contained approximately equal amounts of omega-3 and omega-6 essential fatty acids: between a 1:1 ratio (equal amounts) and a 2:1 ratio (twice as much) of omega-6 to omega-3. [18] This historic ratio however, has changed over the past century. Fast forward to today, and the American diet typically contains about 20 to 30 times more omega-6 fats than omega-3 fats.

The bottom line is we are missing adequate amounts of omega-3, an essential fat our bodies cannot manufacture. And we have an over-abundance of the counter-balancing essential fatty acid, omega-6.

The contemporary imbalance of the omega-3 to omega-6 essential fatty acid ratio in our food chain is sabotaging many people's healthy weight attainment goals.

When essential fatty acid ratios are unbalanced we are hit with a one-two punch:

1) hindering utilization of glucose (blood sugar) for energy, and

2) triggering brain chemistry that makes us crave sweets, fatty foods and salty foods. This vicious cycle contributes to the unprecedented obesity rates. But with simple changes to the essential fatty acids eaten, we can achieve an optimization of *food energy,* and a balanced brain chemistry.

In addition to weight gain, lack of healthy amounts of omega-3 essential fatty acids in our diets contributes to a long list of ailments endemic in our population today, including:

- Fatigue
- Mood swings or depression [19]
- Arthritis
- Weight gain
- Poor memory
- Dementia [20]

- Immune weakness
- Impaired language, learning, and focusing skills in infants and children [21]
- Dry skin, eczema, psoriasis, and hair loss
- Dry eye syndrome
- Poor circulation [22]
- Heart problems [23]
- Reproductive problems, for both men and women
- Cancer
- Aggression and anger
- Diabetes
- Prostate problems
- Ulcerative colitis
- Vision problems
- Asthma
- Compromised infant development (brain, eyes, immune and nervous systems) [24]

How Did We Get Into this 'Big Fat Mess'?

To say America's eating habits and skewed relationship with fat happened because of one specific cause would drastically understate the situation; however, we can pinpoint a major factor contributing to the change in the fats we are eating: An increase in the amount of grains we consume, both in our own diets and the diets of the animals we eat.

While our genes have not changed significantly over the past 100,000 years—our diets have. Today, much of what we think of as an essential part of good nutrition, such as breads, cereals, and dairy products, are new additions to the human diet.

For most of our species' history, we did not consume refined grains, bread, and pasta. The human digestive system is designed to thrive on a diet of low-fat protein, low-density carbohydrate fruits, and fiber-rich vegetables. Until modern times, grains were a minor farm crop. The increase in their production and consumption, however, caused a far-reaching change in our population's nutrition.

In their paper, *Back To Our Ancestor's Diet A Healthy Move*, my colleagues, Dr. Ken Edwards and Dr. William J. Rice, explain these rapid changes: "To put this into another perspective, 100,000 generations of people were hunter-gatherers, 500 generations have depended on agriculture, 10 generations have lived since the start of the industrial age, and only two generations have grown up with highly processed fast foods.

The problem is that our genes don't know it. They are programming us today in much the same way they have been programming humans for at least 40,000 years. Genetically, our bodies now are virtually the same as they were then." [25]

Today's Grains Yield Tomorrow's Gains

In 1939, the yearly per capita consumption in the U.S. of corn was about 17.5 bushels and 4.1 bushels of wheat. By 2000, our consumption had risen to 35.3 bushels of corn and 8 bushels of wheat a year, per capita. The typical American diet now has double the quantity of corn and wheat as compared to just 60 years ago. And in the same time frame, the population of obese American adults has grown by 50%. [26]

Our Love Affair with Grains and the Breakfast of Champions

Cold milk. Crunchy grains. Perhaps even a spoonful of sugar. And do not forget the friendly cartoon characters and catchy jingles.

Breakfast cereal is ingrained in our culture.

This classic American meal was actually developed in the 1800's by the Seventh-Day Adventists, strict vegetarians who manufactured and sold grain cereals as a meat-free breakfast option.

While working at the Adventists' Battle Creek Sanitarium (hospital) in 1894, a scientist named Will Keith (W.K.) Kellogg was tinkering with the hospital patients' vegetarian diets. He was researching bread substitutes with an experiment that involved boiling wheat. In a truly serendipitous moment, Kellogg became distracted and forgot about the boiling pot. By the time he remembered the boiling experiment, the wheat had softened. Hoping to save his product, Kellogg tried to dry the softened wheat by rolling the dough. As the over-cooked, rolled wheat dried, each grain was transformed into a thin flake.

And much to his surprise, the flakes turned out deliciously, and breakfast cereals were instantly born.

Realizing his discovery's commercial potential, W.K. wanted to keep the flakes a secret. But his brother John, who ran the hospital, allowed anyone into the hospital to observe the flaking process.

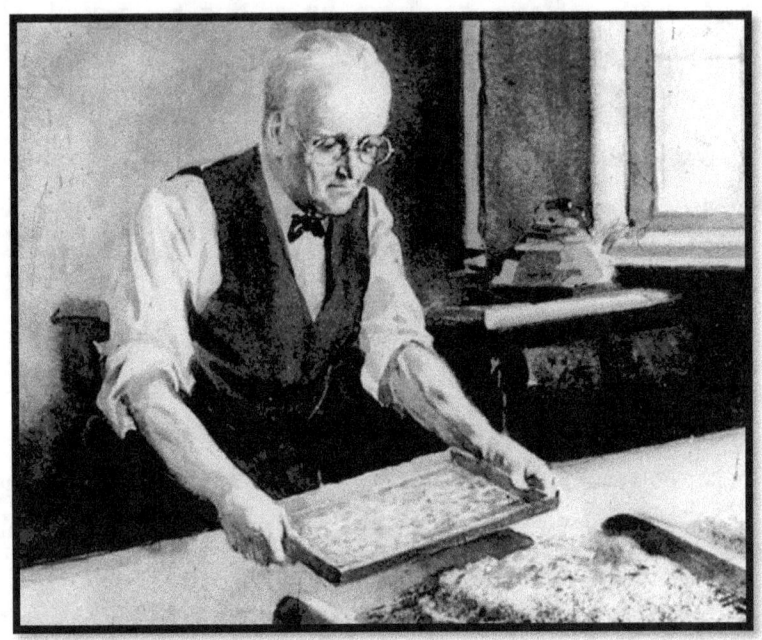

One particular guest named C.W. Post saw the potential of the new food and decided to copy the process and start his own company. Upset over his secret's discovery, W.K. Kellogg immediately left the hospital to start a business and in 1895 introduced *Granose* wheat flakes. With Post and Kellogg producing and promoting their tasty, grain-filled products, by the 1950s, breakfast cereals became a traditional part of the American diet.

In 1939, ready-to-eat cereal consumption averaged 4.4 lbs. per person annually. By 1994, this statistic had jumped to 14.8 lbs. per person. [27]

Today, ready-to-eat breakfast cereals are served in 9 out of 10 American households.

The grains used in these cereals have much more omega-6 than omega-3 essential fatty acids. So, although they are viewed as a healthy choice, increased consumption can contribute to our overall essential fatty acid imbalance.

Corn Beef (What's the Beef with Cattle Eating Corn?)

At the same time cereal was becoming common place in households across the United States, technological developments were leading to cattle subsisting on grains, as well.

In the 1940s, more efficient grain harvesting machines, called *combines,* gave U.S. farmers the ability to produce more grain than the nation's population could eat.

With surplus grain reserves, and a new commitment to factory farming, corn became the primary source of live-stock feed, and the supply of grain-fed cattle soared.

To help illustrate the effect grain-based feed has on cattle, I would like to invite you to a snapshot of my childhood summer memories in the Northeastern United States: an outdoor cookout with the whole family gathered together. Immediately, I can smell the steak grilling. I can see the meat turning brown and fat turning opaque as it sizzled on the barbecue. But wait—if you grew up in Texas, your memories might be *colored* a bit differently.

In Texas, when steaks are grilled the fat becomes almost clear, rather than opaque.

This simple observation, and understanding, about the difference in a grilled steak's fat color is a major key to achieving our healthy weight. [28]

How can the color of steak fat contribute to a human's ability to burn fat?

To start, Texas is too hot to grow corn, so Texan cattle are fed grass. Not so big of a deal, right? Wrong! Studies show that grass-fed beef, such as Texas Longhorn beef, contains elevated levels of healthy omega-3 essential fatty acids.[29] The U.S. government recognizes this distinction and issues the label "USDA Approved 100% Natural Grass-Fed Beef."

Just like humans "are what we eat," so too are the livestock we raise for food. By feeding grains to livestock, which are heavy in omega-6 and light in omega-3 EFAs, farmers began to produce cattle that are also heavy in omega-6 and light in omega-3 essential fatty acids.

In our quest to produce more cattle and use excess corn supplies, the unintended consequence is a population that struggles to convert glucose (blood sugar) into energy, in addition to many other health challenges. [30-42]

Did You Know?

An Omega-3 Essential Fatty Acid Insufficiency May Effect Autism

While attending a medical conference, I heard a doctor tell about a family physician listening to the radio on the way to work. Dr. Mary Megson was being interviewed about cod liver oil (omega-3 essential fatty acids) helping unlock verbal abilities in autistic children. [43-44]

When he got into his office, he was told that there was an hysterical woman on the phone for him. The woman was his patient. A medical expert had just told the woman that her 6-year-old autistic daughter, who had never spoken before, would never utter a word in her life!

The doctor told the woman about the interview he had just heard and suggested that the woman give the girl one teaspoon of cod liver oil daily. He figured there was nothing to lose? According to Dr. Joseph Hibbeln, a psychiatrist at the National Institutes of Health, omega-3 essential fatty acids are like neuronal [brain] fertilizer. [4]

A few weeks later, the same woman called back, and appeared to be hysterical again. The doctor wondered if he had given the wrong advice. Upon speaking with her, however, he quickly realized that her hysteria and sobbing were due to elation, rather than worry. Moments earlier, the woman awoke her daughter, and her daughter said, "Mommy, I'm sorry I've never spoken before."

How Does a Fat Imbalance Relate to Healthy Weight Management?

What do incorrect ratios of omega-3 to omega-6 essential fatty acids have to do with weight management? Everything! The body gets energy by burning a fuel called glucose (blood sugar) within your cells.

Glucose must cross the cell membrane (plasma membrane) to reach the power generating organelles called mitochondria. The omega-3 fats make the cell membrane more flexible, allowing more fuel to cross the cell membrane for the mitochondria to convert to energy.

On the other hand, omega-6 fatty acids make the cell membrane more resistant to allowing glucose into the cell.

The medical terms associated with the resistance to the glucose getting into the cells include insulin resistance, hyperinsulinemia, metabolic syndrome X, insulin resistance syndrome and if severe enough, diabetes.

When the fuel has difficulty getting to the power generators inside the cells, often that excess fuel is stored as fat, which leads to the paradox of being overweight and over tired. I say a paradox because fat is a fuel. Think of the full diesel tanker that has run out of fuel. Just as the truck can't access the diesel fuel it is hauling, most obese or overweight people struggle with low energy because their bodies can't easily burn their fuel (glucose) and instead store it as fat. So because their cell membranes are too resistant, their bodies continue to accumulate more fat while their power-generating mitochondria are starving for fuel.

Another important consideration regarding omega-3 essential fatty acids is how it affects our brain's function as it relates to our eating behaviors. The brain is an astonishing 60% fat and requires ample omega-3 essential fatty acids for optimal function.

A balanced ratio of omega-3 and omega-6 essential fatty acids is necessary for a healthy brain, which is structurally composed of a 1 to 1 ratio (equal amounts) of omega-3 and omega-6 essential fatty acids. The growing brain, in womb or in childhood, thus must have adequate omega-3s. Studies show that lowered omega-3 EFAs, specifically DHA, inhibit the neurotransmitters dopamine and serotonin.[46] These brain chemicals, when lowered, trigger food addictions and cravings, in particular, the desire for sweets, chocolate, fatty, and salty foods. [47]

So, in the end, if omega-3 and omega-6 EFAs are not properly balanced, you'll not only struggle to burn glucose in your cells for energy, you'll be more likely to crave the unhealthy foods that lead to further fat accumulation. But, with only a few small changes, the cycle can be broken and you can be freed from feeling overweight and overtired.

Using Essential Fatty Acids to Fit Into Your Genes and Cut the Guilt

The bottom line is: you must consume more omega-3 essential fatty acids in order to fit into your genes and cut the guilt.

Currently, there are two primary ways to rebalance your omega-3 and omega-6 essential fatty acids consumption:

1) through a change in diet, or

2) by taking supplements.

Change in Diet

Much of the processed food and meat found in United States supermarkets has unnaturally high levels of omega-6 essential fatty acids. Consequently, increasing your omega-3 consumption through diet requires focus and commitment. To begin rebalancing your fat consumption, I recommend:

- Reducing the amount of grains you consume.

- Eating cold-water fish more often such as anchovies, salmon, sardines, and herring.

- Increasing the amount of nuts you eat, especially walnuts.

- When buying fish, be sure to choose low-mercury selections, such as:

  o Flounder and its relative sole, tend to be low in mercury levels.

  o Herring tends to be low in mercury.

  o *Mackerel is also a good source of omega-3 fatty acids.*

    ◊ King mackerel is relatively low in omega-3 fatty acids but high in mercury levels. The varieties such as Spanish, Atlantic and Pacific mackerel are high in omega-3 while being low in mercury.

  o Salmon: Alaskan wild salmon tend to have the lowest mercury level. Sardines are rich in omega-3 fatty acids and tend to be low in mercury. [48]

Taking Supplements

For people who are not inclined to change their diets to include more naturally occurring omega-3 EFAs, taking a supplement is the easiest way to ensure you are properly balancing your essential fatty acids.

There is quite a bit of confusion regarding whether a plant-derived source, such as flaxseed oil, or a marine-derived source, such as fish oil, is preferred. Although flax seeds and flaxseed oil have many benefits, they are not recommended as a therapeutic source of omega-3 fatty acids. Research shows that only fish-based omega-3 fatty acids have preformed EPA and DHA—and thus are more usable by the body. Flaxseed oil, on the other hand, contains alpha-linolenic acid (ALA), which the body must first convert into EPA and DHA. Thus, when you take flaxseed oil to increase your omega-3 consumption, your body has to complete a slow conversion process—with only a maximum of 15 to 20% of the flaxseed oil converting—before receiving the same benefits cold-water fish oil provides immediately.

Just as diet changes require diligence and attention to detail, individuals who decide to take supplementarily fish oil, should be equally discriminating about the supplements they purchase. Many capsules may contain environmental toxins that accumulate in the fish during their life span, so choosing *pharmaceutical grade* fish oils is crucial to ensure you avoid contaminants that could derail your health goals. Contrary to popular belief, fresh, non-rancid, cold-water fish oil does not have a bad "fishy" taste or smell, and pharmaceutical grade fish oil should not have a "fishy" smell or taste. There are several sources of high quality pharmaceutical grade fish oils without a fishy taste or smell such as Nordic Naturals, Inc. (800-662-2544, or visit their website: www. nordicnaturals.com).

So, how much fish oil should you take?

I recommend that people over 15 years of age include a daily supplement that contains a minimum of 500 milligrams of fish oil containing DHA and EPA. If you want to maximize your results while still being conservative, consider adding a total dose of 800 to 2000 milligrams of of omega-3 fatty acids per day.

Questions for Your Doctor

Because increasing omega-3 consumption aligns our bodies with a more natural essential fatty acid balance, most people should feel comfortable making this change without experiencing any negative side effects. However, because omega-3 essential fatty acids can reduce blood viscosity, discussing an increase in omega-3s with your doctor is crucial if you are using medications that are "blood thinners," taking aspirin, or anticipating surgery.

When a patient increases consumption of omega-3s, many progressive physicians will actually reduce the dosage of prescription blood thinners and still achieve the desired "blood thinning" goals by utilizing pharmaceutical grade fish oil in conjunction with the blood-thinning medications.

Definitions and Glossary

Cell membranes (plasma membranes) are the outer covering of our cells. The plasma membrane controls the exchange of materials between the cell and its environment, letting some substances pass in and go out while acting as a barrier against others.

Dietary fats can come from animal and vegetable sources. Animal fats such as butter and lard tend to be solid at room temperature. Vegetable fats like olive oil and sesame oil tend to be liquid at room temperatures.

Dietary oils are pressed from plants, such as corn, peanuts and olives. Oils are liquid at room temperature.

Fatty acids are dietary fats and oils otherwise known as lipids, which are vital nutrients our bodies need for health and daily functioning. Fats serve as building blocks of cell membranes and play key regulatory roles in many functions.

Essential fatty acids (EFAs) are fatty acids that our bodies can't produce, so we have to obtain them from food. The essential fatty acids can be divided into two main types: omega-3 and omega-6.

Omega-3 essential fatty acids aid the body in maintaining the cell membrane's fluidity and stability to produce energy, as well as the healthy development and functioning of the brain and nervous system. Omega-3 essential fatty acids can be found in some vegetable oils, such as flax and rapeseed (canola) oil, as well as fish oils. The omega-3 essential fatty acids are also in green leafy vegetables, nuts and seeds. When animals eat insects, vegetation, nuts or seeds, then the fat in those animals contains higher amounts of the omega-3 essential fatty acids.

Omega-6 essential fatty acids make the cell membrane more rigid. Insulin resistance, and related conditions such as metabolic syndrome X, and even type II diabetes can be caused when an over-abundance of omega-6 EFAs makes the cell membranes resistant to allowing your fuel, blood sugar (glucose), to enter the cells to be turned into energy. Omega-6 EFAs are found primarily in meats; sunflower and corn oils, and products made with these oils; and most grains. If animals (livestock) are fed grains, then much higher amounts of omega-6 EFAs are contained in the fat of those animals.[1]

DHA (docosahexaenoic acid) is an omega-3 essential fatty acid, found mostly in cold-water fatty fish such as Bluefin tuna, herring, mackerel, sardines, shellfish, and fish oil supplements. Actually fish do not naturally produce DHA, but obtain it from the algae they eat. DHA is the most abundant omega-3 fatty acid in the brain and retina of the eye. DHA promotes the healthy functioning of the brain and nervous system. Vegetarian diets commonly contain inadequate amounts of DHA, and vegan diets typically contain no DHA. Vegetarian sources of DHA can be from seaweed or algae.

EPA (eicosapentaenoic acid) is an omega-3 essential fatty acid (EFA) found in cold-water fatty fish such as Bluefin tuna, cod, herring, mackerel, sardines, shellfish, and fish oil supplements. Like DHA, fish don't naturally produce EPA, but obtain it from the alga they eat. Vegetarian and vegan diets commonly contain inadequate amounts of EPA. Vegetarian sources of EPA can be from or seaweed or algae. EPA helps the cell membrane to more easily allow glucose (blood sugar) into the cell to burn as fuel and has a natural anti-inflammatory effect on the body.

Chapter 7

Our Body's Survival Mechanism Needs Tweaking

Mitochondria—Maximizing Cell Function

To best understand mitochondria, imagine, if you will, twins whose parents are celebrated artists.

The children, whom we'll call Jack and Jill, have innate artistic abilities and have always loved to draw and paint. While they have equal natural talents, Jill is slightly more committed to her artistic abilities than Jack.

At first, their skill levels are similar: both excel in their school art classes, so their parents buy them paints, canvasses, and easels. When engaging in projects, however, Jill fills the canvasses with fervor while Jack creates more slowly.

One summer, their parents enroll the twins in an art camp, where instructors notice Jill's focus and dedication—and give her a bit more encouragement than other students. The positive reinforcement inspires Jill to work even harder at her craft.

Jack, on the other hand, receives no special attention; he is simply treated like all the other campers. Recognizing the praise his sister receives for her skill, Jack begins questioning his own abilities. When camp ends, Jack leaves feeling lightly discouraged. Though he continues to create artwork, he starts losing motivation. Jill, on the other hand, is excited, engaged, and fills countless canvasses throughout the year.

For the next several summers, Jack and Jill return to the same camp, and each year the differences in their skill and motivation levels grow. Jill relishes the praise and guidance she receives, while Jack is distracted and struggles to find his muse. Eventually, Jack convinces himself that he must not be a very good artist, so he stops painting altogether. Jill becomes a professional painter.

What divides these twins who began with the same talent, opportunities, and love for art? It was the classic case of domino reactions:

The better Jill became, the more praise she received and the more she painted. The more she painted, the better Jill became, the more praise she received and so on.

The more Jack questioned his talent, the less he painted and the less praise he received. The less praise he received, the more Jack questioned his talent, the less he painted and so on.

Mitochondria, our body's energy generators, work in exactly the same way.

When we perform aerobic activity, our bodies replicate more mitochondria. The more mitochondria within our cells, the more fuel we burn and the more energy we have to expend. The more energy we have, the more motivated we are to exercise and the more weight we lose.

Conversely, when we don't get sufficient aerobic exercise, we lose the fuel-burning mitochondria within our cells. Less fuel burning means less energy. The less energy we have, the less we are prepared to exercise and the more weight we gain.

But, overcoming this trend is not as difficult as it might feel! With just two hours a week of aerobic exercise, you can stop the downward cycle and begin reaping the rewards of our body's natural energy generators: mitochondria.

Definitions and Glossary

Mitochondria are organelles (little organs) within all of our cells with the exception of mature red blood cells. Mitochondria serve as our body's power-generating factories The human body is made up of over a hundred trillion cells, and every cell needs energy to perform its specific functions. That energy comes from the mitochondria located within the cells. The more mitochondria you have, the more fuel (glucose and fat) you can burn and the more energy you generate.

Symptoms of Low Mitochondria Counts

Fatigue   Excessive weight—overweight or obese

Depression   Insomnia

Aerobic exercise allows your body to replenish exercised muscles with the oxygen they need. Aerobic simply means 'with air' and when you perform such exercises, your body uses oxygen to create energy. Examples of aerobic exercise include walking, swimming, or biking.

Mitochondria and Energy

These organelles have their own replication machinery (DNA and RNA), which means they are actually able to reproduce and increase in number within your cells.

Most scientists believe that about two billion years ago, mitochondria started out as independent cells that excelled at digesting food and turning it into energy. At some evolutionary point, mitochondria began living inside inside larger cells and lost theability to live on their own. Meanwhile, they did not lose their ability to replicate or digest glucose (blood sugar) for energy.

Because of their unique life structure, mitochondria can increase in number and activity by as much as 50% just weeks after we begin a regular exercise routine.[1] Imagine the energy and fat-burning you would enjoy if the powerhouses of your cells grew by 50%!

Fortunately, their astonishing energy is within your grasp. You have the power to improve your metabolism, and it starts with only two to four hours of exercise per week.

Did You Know?

You Can Raise Your Metabolism.

Many people erroneously believe they are doomed to have a slow metabolism and will always gain weight more quickly than their peers. The truth is, despite your current metabolic state, regular aerobic exercise will increase your metabolism, even when you aren't working out!

Because we create more mitochondria each time we exercise, we immediately experience a direct correlation to our body's ability to burn energy. The mitochondrial effects of regular aerobic exercise are like changing your car's engine from four cylinders to eight: you'll burn more fuel and have more energy when you're moving, and you'll also increase your fuel use even when you're idle. Plainly put—the more mitochondria you have, the more energy you burn.

If you follow an exercise routine like the 16-week exercise guidance detailed in this chapter, your cells will replicate more mitochondria. Each of these mitochondria needs fuel, which means you'll burn more glucose for energy, instead of storing it as fat—even when you are resting.

The Power Generators Within

Each winter, black bears settle in for a season of rest and a break from their normal, active lifestyles. Their metabolic rates are cut in half and their bodies retain fat in preparation for months of near hibernation. The bears' adaptation protects them not from cold—but food scarcity.

Like the bears, our bodies have a built-in mechanism that allows us to survive periods of low food availability. Our energy conservation adaptation involves shutting down the fuel-burning mitochondria within our cells, so we burn fewer calories.

Historically, when cold winters, droughts, and other acts of nature made foraging and hunting food difficult for our ancestors, they minimized activities to get through the rough times. Their bodies helped conserve remaining fat stores by reducing the number of mitochondria within the cells. With fewer energy-producing mitochondria, they consumed less fuel and the stored fuel (fat) sustained them for longer periods. As our ancestors hunkered down awaiting the return of plentiful food sources, their metabolic adaptation put their cells into a *hibernation-like* mode and kept them from starving to death.

When spring or other changes increased the food supply, our ancestors again began the active search for nutrition. To survive under these circumstances, they needed enough energy for sustained activity or they would quickly become exhausted while hunting and foraging and again risk starving to death. Their bodies responded to the increased aerobic activity by creating more mitochondria. With more mitochondria came more energy and a greater ability to burn fuel and fat—since their bodies were no longer in conservation mode.

When our ancestors had little food available, their bodies responded by burning fewer calories. With nutritional abundance, their bodies burned more fuel and fat and created the energy needed to hunt and forage.

A pretty amazing adaptation, right?

But, how is it serving us in today's world?

Mitochondria and Weight Gain

Is Our Body's Survival Mechanism Killing Us?

One of the consequences of a modern, busy Western lifestyle is that too many of us let our cells, our bodies, get stuck in the *hibernation,* fat-conservation mode. Finding yourself stuck in *cellular hibernation* leads to the paradox of being both overweight and over tired.

The trigger for abundance or conservation is not the food we are consuming, but our activity levels. For our bodies:

> *Low Activity = Prepare for Starvation*
>
> *High Activity = Create Energy*

Triggered by our inactive lifestyles, our bodies believe our food sources must be scarce—even if we regularly overeat—so they start conserving energy and burning less fuel and storing any excess glucose as fat. So, the less we move, the fewer power-generating mitochondria our bodies create, the less energy we have, and the more stored energy (fat) we retain.

Using Mitochondria to Fit Into Your Genes

Fortunately, the cycle of more fat and less energy can be reversed relatively quickly. Because our bodies are designed to adjust from winter scarcity to summer abundance, you can increase your mitochondria (up to double) with just two to four hours a week of aerobic exercise for 12 to 16 weeks. In one study, even sedentary men and women with an average age of

67 who engaged in 30 to 40 minutes of aerobic exercise four to six times a week, increased their number of mitochondria by 53% and the amount of energy produced by 62% within only 2 weeks! [2]

Increasing the number and size of mitochondria within your cells happens when you exercise at around 65% to 85% of your maximum heart rate for at least 15 continuous minutes, three times per week, on alternate days. Use the information below to calculate your maximum heart rate and then your target heart rate zone.

Maximum Heart Rate (HRmax) is calculated by subtracting your age from 220.

Our maximum heart rate is biologically determined and declines as you age. Most people should exercise to bring their heart beats per minute to within an aerobic training zone, which is ideally between 65% to 85% of their maximum heart rate. To be safe, you should probably begin training at 65% of your maximum heart rate and as your aerobic fitness improves, gradually increase the intensity, working toward 85% of your maximum heart rate. [3]

Find exercises you enjoy.

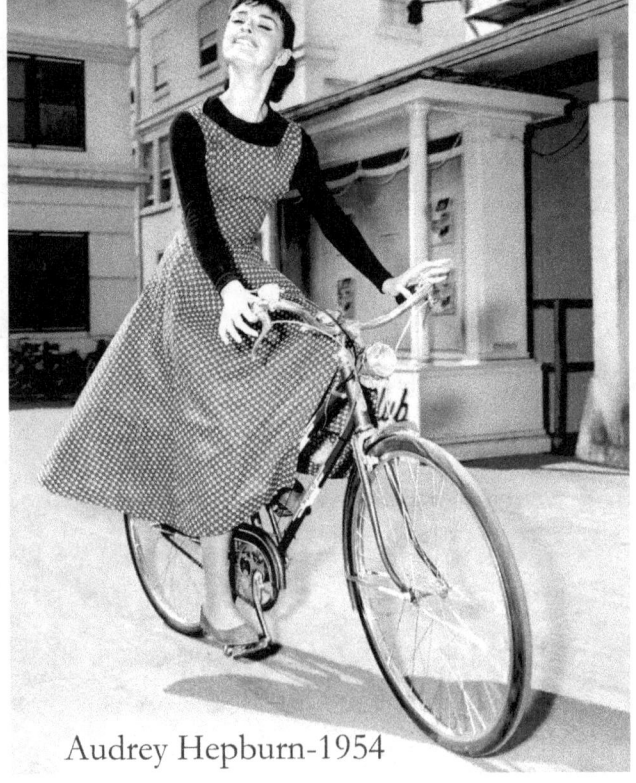

Audrey Hepburn-1954

Please refer to the example shown for a forty-year-old person on the *Calcuate Your Target Heart Rate* Zone chart that follows:

CALCULATE YOUR TARGET HEART RATE ZONE

To perform aerobics effectively, you need to calculate your target heart rate zone. To do so, subtract your age from 220 to find out your maximum heart rate.

For example, the maximum heart rate for a person 40 years old is:

220 minus 40 = 180 beats per minute

Then multiply your maximum heart rate by 65%:

180 X 65% = 117 beats per minute—117 beats per minute will be the lower range of the zone.

Now, work out your higher range by multiplying your maximum heart rate by 85%:

180 X 85% = 153 beats per minute—153 beatsper minute will be the upper range of the zone.

In the above example, the 40-year-old person has a target heart rate zone of 117—153 beats per minute.

Realize that your heart rate will vary somewhat while exercising, despite your best efforts to exercise at a steady pace. I recommend you predetermine a range of 5 to 10 beats per minute within your target range as your goal for that workout session. Please remember to make sure the 5 to 10 beats per minute range you decide on is still within your safe target range. Once your exercising brings your heart rate to your desired target rate range, start the clock. A good time frame to use is between 20 to 40 minutes.

To manually check your heart rate during a workout, begin by slowing your pace so you can concentrate more.

1. Gently place your index and middle finger on the inner part of your wrist,

2. Find your pulse,

3. Count the number of beats in 10 seconds then multiply the number by 6.

That final calculation is your heart rate.

I recommend, however, using an automatic heart rate monitor, so you can concentrate on exercising effectively to burn more fat, rather than heart rate calculations. Many exercise machines include heart rate monitors, and you can also purchase your own monitor at sporting goods and health related stores.

Types of Aerobic Exercises

When jumpstarting mitochondrial growth with aerobic exercising, make sure to choose exercises that allow you to increase your heart rate to your specific target zone and maintain it within that zone for at least 20 minutes. Walking, bicycling, swimming, or using an elliptical exercise machine, treadmill, or stationary bicycle are all healthy choices.

If a regular exercise routine is new to you, be honest with yourself and explore what will work, considering your lifestyle and your personality. Make it fun and not a chore! Many people vary the types of exercise they do from session to session to avoid overworking a particular set of muscles and to escape the boredom of always doing the same exercises. If time is an issue, consider a treadmill or a stationary bicycle located in front of the television, so you can view the evening news or your favorite shows while you exercise. If you love to get outdoors, consider what is practical within your particular circumstances.

Are you a social creature? Would you like the opportunity to get out of the house and meet folks with similar interests? There are gyms, health clubs, and group training programs that can fit most budgets and personalities.

Whether you speed walk to the store, take an aerobics class at the gym, or ride a stationary bike while watching television—you will reap the benefits of the increased number of mitochondri as long as you get to your target heart rate and maintain it for at least 15 to 20 minutes, four times per week.

Exercise With Friends

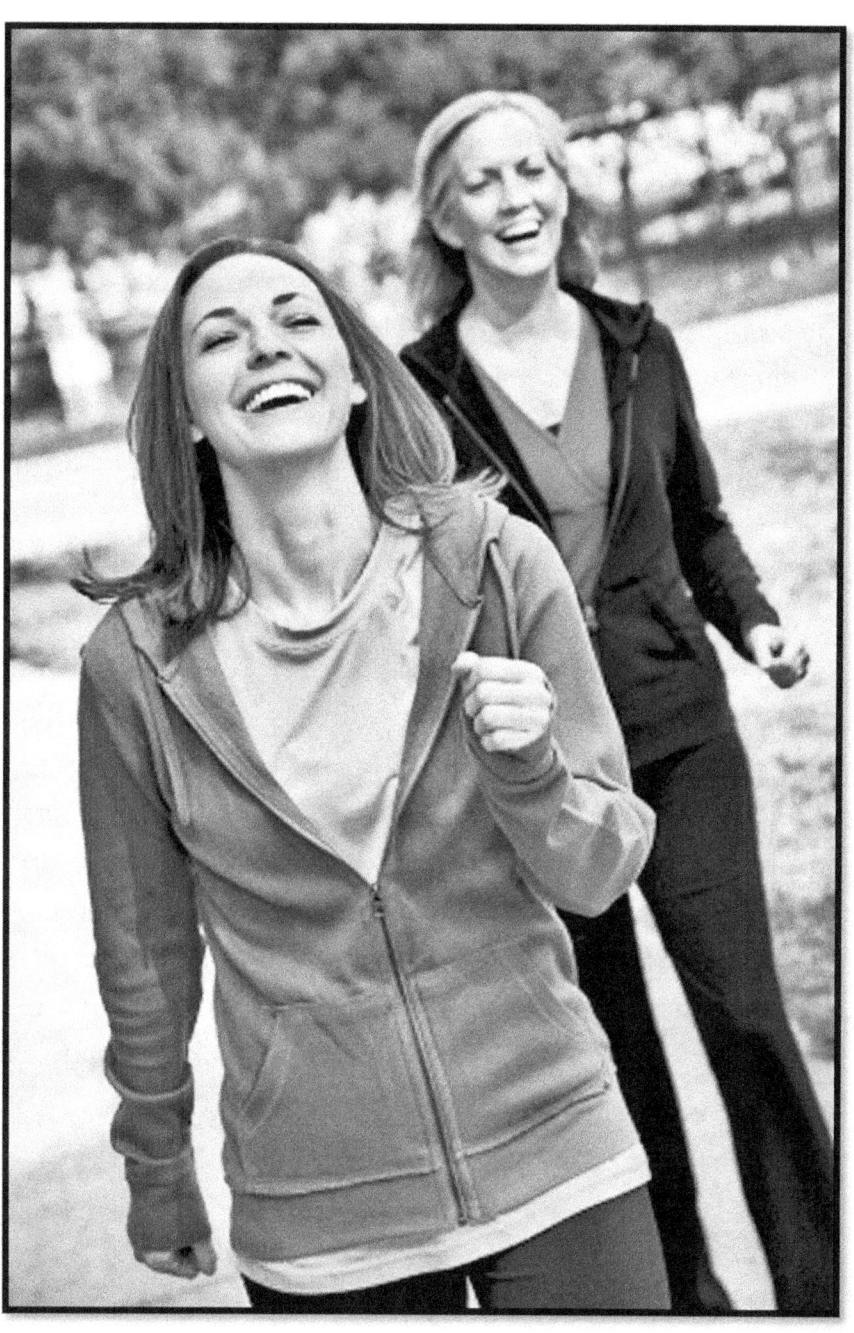

Questions for Your Doctor

You should always check with your physician before beginning a new aerobic exercise program.

In addition to general medical clearance, you may want to address any common musculoskeletal aches and pains that can derail exercise programs. If sprains, strains, joint discomfort, or other musculoskeletal issues make exercising difficult or painful, you should talk with your doctor about the full range of available treatments.

I don't consider living on anti-inflammatory medications or analgesic (pain dampening) medications a solution—a temporary fix, perhaps—but there are likely therapeutic options you haven't considered.

During my many years as a physician and an expert on musculo-skeletal conditions, as well as a professor of human anatomy and physiology, I have observed an interesting obstacle to fitness: Many people cannot resolve their health problems because they don't know their therapeutic options.

If your list of therapeutic options is too limited, your musculo-skeletal conditions may prevent you from unleashing the power of mitochondrial energy through exercise; however, do not be discouraged. You have not tried every viable therapy, unless you have considered all the options presented below. You will probably find that there are few physcians knowledgeable about the vast array of available therapeutics methods. And if your clinician follows more traditional approaches to weight management, they may not be able to give you a referral or even be supportive in your pursuit of other therapeutic approaches. At times, you may have to research on your own to locate and evaluate practitioners of the following therapies in your area, but with persistence and commitment, you can find the answers you need to build a successful exercise routine.

Reasonable Therapies to Consider Incorporating into your Exercise Healthcare Lifestyle:

Acupuncture, which is part of a broader healing approach known as Traditional Chinese Medicine (TCM), offers an array of therapeutic modalities, which can improve musculoskeletal problems by balancing underlying weaknesses. Additionally, acupuncturists may use needles, electricity, cold laser, heat or any combination to provide almost instant relief of pain and inflammation. TCM treatments can also include the use of herbs, diet, lifestyle modifications, addressing mental/emotional well-being, and manipulation of misaligned joints of the body.

The fascinating history of Acupuncture (Traditional Chinese Medicine).

The cultural background that gave birth to Traditional Chinese Medicine is rich as well as intriguing.

There are at least three theories to explain how acupuncture was developed. You choose which one to accept.

1. Wounded warriors who survived their wounds, found certain health conditions improved from the puncturing of their bodies by sharp weapons at specific points. These points were charted and this was the beginning of acupuncture.

2. Weavers and tailors pricked themselves with sharp objects and found certain health conditions improved from the puncturing of their bodies at specific points.

3. Acupuncture had a enthralling origin as described by Chee Soo in his book, *The Tao Of Long Life, The Chinese Art of Ch'ang Ming.*[4]

"*Ch'ang Ming* was developed by the Taoists between 10,000-5,000 B.C., on the basis of the guidelines and foundations handed down to them by the 'Sons of Reflected Light,' a sect of people reputed to have been over seven feet in height, and who wore a type of clothing never before been seen in China.

Where they came from is still a mystery, and perhaps we may never know the answer to this riddle. Upon arriving in China they began to choose artisans and craftsmen from every known profession, selecting those of the highest intelligence. Having collected this band of people together they began to instruct them in many different arts and crafts far in advance of anything else that existed in those far-off days.

Among the skills passed on were silk-weaving, pottery, glass and gunpowder making, and metal working; but most important of all was the enormous range of health arts. The health arts that the 'Sons of Reflected Light' brought to China eventually came to be known as the 'Eight Strands of Brocade' (*Pa Chin Hsien*), and even to this day, after thousands of years have passed, they are still known by that name. One of the most specialized sections, and one of the most well known is Acupuncture (*Hsia Chen Pien*)...".

Modern science confirms that acupuncture points are 'energy portals' with low electrical resistance. This establishes "a bridge between Western and Chinese medicine." [5]

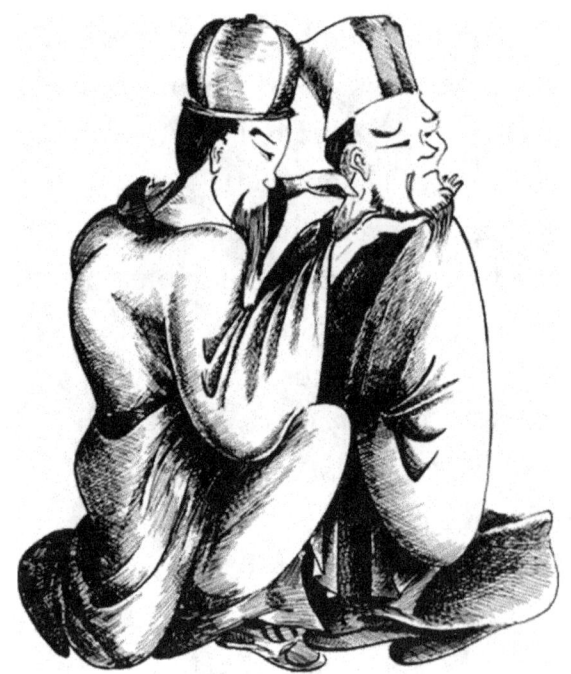

This print was taken from the original and discovered at the Tai Chung Medical School in Taipei, China, and is estimated at more than 3,000 years old. It was inscribed on the breastplate of a tortoise shell. It illustrates a form of ancient spinal adjustments.

Applied kinesiology is a system that evaluates structural, chemical, and mental aspects of health using manual muscle testing with other standard methods of diagnosis. Treatment may involve specific joint manipulation or mobilization, various myofascial therapies, cranial techniques, meridian and acupuncture skills, clinical nutrition, dietary management, counseling skills, evaluating environmental irritants and various reflex procedures.

Chiropractic or **osteopathic manipulation** corrects structural misalignments of body joints that can compromise musculoskeletal function and cause pain and degenerative changes. Physicians practicing this therapeutic modality may have a D.C. (Doctor of Chiropractic) or D.O. (Doctor of Osteopathy) degree and M.D.s who are physiatrists.

Glucosamine sulfate is a nutritional therapy that may help repair injured tendons, ligaments, and cartilage. [6] A rule of thumb is to take 10 milligrams per pound of body-weight for at least six weeks. Although this is an over-the-counter supplement, you should talk to your doctor before beginning any new medications.

Muscle activation technique (MAT) can improve musculo-skeletal function and reduce pain and dysfunction by resetting the muscle proprioceptors, which are sensory nerve ending in muscles, tendons, and joints that provides a sense of the body's position by responding to stimuli from within the body.

Orthopedics focuses on preventing and correcting deformities, disorders, or injuries of the musculoskeletal system, including bones, joints, tendons, and ligaments.

Physiatry uses physical agents, including light, heat, cold, water, electricity, therapeutic exercise and mechanical apparatuses to help treat and rehabilitate disease, injuries and disabilities. Practiced by medical doctors (MDs) and osteopathic doctors (DOs), this medical specialty is also known as physiatrics, physical medicine, and rehabilitation.

Physical therapy or **physiotherapy** is the treatment of disorders of the muscles, bones, and/or joints by means of physical agents such as heat, light, water, electricity, manual and electronic massage, and exercise.

Podiatry is a medical specialty that diagnoses and treats diseases, injuries, and defects of the foot and ankle. Podiatric medicine may use surgery, mechanical, physical and adjunctive treatments. Physicians practicing this specialty have a DPM degree, meaning Doctor of Podiatric Medicine. Be sure to be checked to see if you need foot orthotics for ankle pronation problems.

Prolotherapy utilizes specialized injections of to help rebuild over-stretched or damaged tendons, ligaments, and cartilages. Also called non-surgical Regenerative Therapy, this treatment has been used successfully since 1958 and is considered very conservative because it relies on medications rather than surgery. Former Surgeon General, Dr. C. Evertt Koop highly recommended this therapy.

"I had been diagnosed by two separate neurological clinics as having intractable pain. I obtained complete relief from prolotherapy." [7]

Neurology is a field of medicine that diagnoses and treats the nervous system and disorders affecting it. Therapeutic modalities may include pharmacology, surgery, or referrals to a physical therapist or physiatrist.

Therapeutic massage improves circulation, relaxes muscles, and aids healing through rubbing and kneading of the body. There are over 200 massage technique variations, and each helps different body systems, including the lymphatic, circulatory, and meridian (acupuncture pathways). Some of the most commonly practiced massage variations are deep-tissue, myofascial, neuromuscular, massage acupressure, Rolfing, shiatsu, sports, Swedish, and trigger point.

Chapter 8

Optimize Your Body's Metabolism

Thyroid Function

If your home stays warm in the winter and cool in the summer, there is a good chance the comfortable climate is regulated by an HVAC system: heating, ventilation and air conditioning. These deceptively complex functions work together to create the temperature you desire and can malfunction in a variety of ways, including:

1. Lack of fuel,

2. System blockage and,

3. Faulty thermostat.

1. **Lack of fuel:** Our thyroid glands are similar to a home's HVAC system. The thyroid controls the body's heating unit, also known as the metabolism. Your HVAC system may run on a variety of fuels, but your thyroid requires one in particular: iodine, which is the basis for thyroid hormones. Whether addressing our thyroid or HVAC unit, without adequate consistent fuel, the heat will not function properly.

2. **System blockage:** What happens if you have the proper fuel, but the system is not supplying the heater? Something is blocking the free flow of fuel. In our homes, many blockages can occur, creating the same results: The house will not remain at a comfortable temperature. In our bodies, that blockage occurs when the thyroid hormone, T4 is not converting to the more active, usable form, T3. Without this conversion, our metabolism will not function properly.

3. **Damaged thermostat:** In our homes, we set the preferred temperature by adjusting the thermostat. But, if the thermostat is not functioning properly and the readings are askew, we will be uncomfortable, because the actual temperature will be different than what the thermostat indicates. Like an inaccurate thermostat, many of the commonly used lab

tests and medications many physicians use when looking for and treating thyroid problems can also give incomplete or inaccurate readings. Ensuring you have the most up-to-date thyroid testing is crucial to keeping you healthy and optimally running.

Just as maintaining a comfortable temperature in your home is dependent on the technical functions of an HVAC system; so too is your properly functioning thyroid.

In this chapter, I will explain the complex, interconnected thyroid, and how mastering its myriad of complications can improve your quality of life, and help you fit into your genes and cut the guilt.

Symptoms of an Underactive Thyroid

- Weight gain
- Fatigue
- Intolerance to cold temperatures
- Crying for no apparent reason
- Female hair thinning
- Morning headaches
- Dizziness
- Inflammation
- Blurred vision
- Slow healing
- Infertility
- Hoarseness

- Depression
- Insomnia
- Dry skin
- Overall weakness
- Menstrual irregularities
- Muscle cramps
- Poor memory or "brain fog"
- Arthritis-like pain
- Slow speech
- Coarse skin
- Constipation
- Carpal tunnel syndrome (wrist pain)

- Learning disabilities and poor concentration [2-3]

- Elevated cholesterol and triglycerides

- Decreased pain threshold and increased intensity of pain [1]

- One additional, probably unexpected symptom of low thyroid function is, *an addiction to exercising.*

But wait, you may be thinking, didn't the last chapter tell me that I need to exercise in order to increase my mitochondria?

Yes—that's exactly right.

To achieve your ideal weight, exercising is good for you and a fundamental component of healthy weight control. Excessively exercising, however, dances the delicate balance of health and can also be an important diagnostic clue to your health's true state.

If one of the only ways you can feel good is by exercising, you may have a sluggish metabolism—hypothyroidism. People with low-thyroid function may try to compensate and end up addicted to exercise, since exercise can temporarily "jump start" our metabolism. If you can't get yourself going—especially in the morning—until you exercise, pay careful attention to the information within this chapter.

How an Underactive Thyroid Contributes to Weigh Gain

An underactive thyroid gland that is either ignored, missed, or mismanaged may not be responsible for all the stumbling blocks on your road to achieving a healthy weight; however, you can be certain of the following fact: If your thyroid gland is not functioning optimally, it may sabotage all your other best efforts at weight-loss management. Because your resting metabolic rate (RMR) is controlled by your thyroid gland, a poorly functioning thyroid causes a reduced resting metabolic rate, resulting in about 500 to 600 fewer calories burned *each day* compared to someone of equal body mass with a normal metabolic rate!

Basically, burning so many fewer calories is the same as eating an extra dinner every day—of course losing weight will be challenging!

Additionally, excess refined sugar consumption may suppress thyroid function, and a low thyroid often triggers carbohydrate cravings. Sub-normal thyroid hormone levels decrease the "feel good" neurotransmitter serotonin, while eating carbs boosts our serotonin levels. So, you eat more refined carbohydrates to boost serotonin levels, which in turn lower your thyroid hormone levels, triggering your body to crave more carbs—creating a vicious cycle. [4] In the long run, a sluggish thyroid can hinder your ability to achieve a healthy weight in the following two ways, by:

1. Lowering your metabolism, which leads to more stored fat; and
2. Stimulating the sweet tooth or "carb carnivore" within.

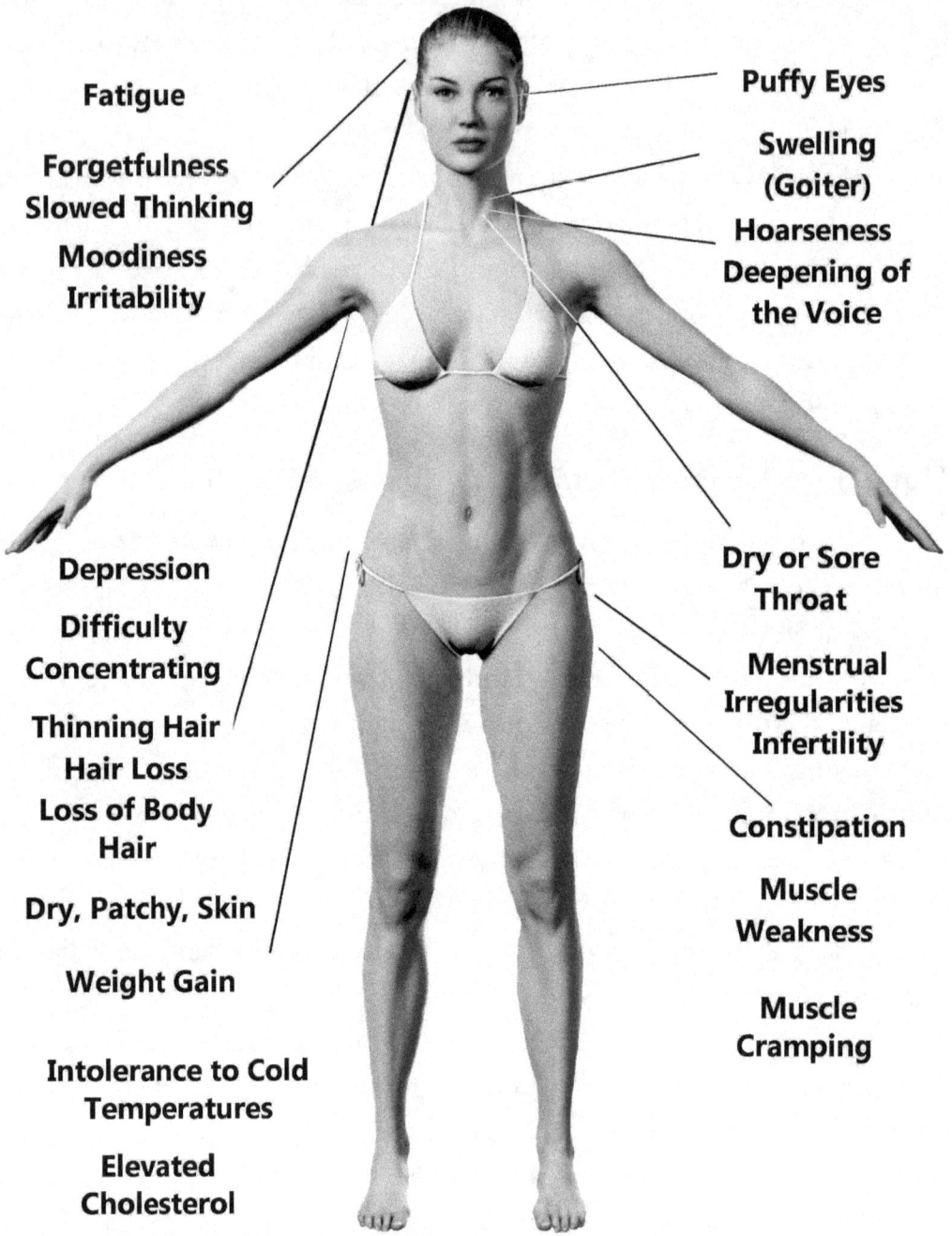

Fatigue

Forgetfulness
Slowed Thinking

Moodiness
Irritability

Puffy Eyes

Swelling
(Goiter)

Hoarseness
Deepening of
the Voice

Depression

Difficulty
Concentrating

Thinning Hair
Hair Loss
Loss of Body
Hair

Dry, Patchy, Skin

Weight Gain

Intolerance to Cold
Temperatures

Elevated
Cholesterol

Dry or Sore
Throat

Menstrual
Irregularities
Infertility

Constipation

Muscle
Weakness

Muscle
Cramping

Signs and Symptoms of Low Thyroid Function (Hypothyroidism)

Why a Simple Conversion Can Sabotage Your Health

Despite a diminutive size, the thyroid gland holds great responsibility for your health and metabolism—and experts believe our American society is suffering from a hypothyroidism epidemic. In 2008, the fourth most most popular prescription medication in the U.S. was a thyroid drug, with over 81 million prescriptions dispensed to treat underactive thyroids. [5]

And millions more people likely have undiagnosed thyroid gland dysfunction:

- David Brownstein, M.D., author of the book "Overcoming Thyroid Disorders," believes that *50% of the population may have undiagnosed, underactive thyroids.* [6]

- The FDA and American Health Partners, conservative sources, estimate that *over 13 million Americans are undiagnosed for low thyroid* and that one out of every eight women will develop some type of thyroid dysfunction.

You might notice that the estimated number of thyroid sufferers differs within the medical world.

Why?

Unfortunately, capturing a single, concrete answer is difficult because the parameters and tests for thyroid dysfunction vary. To help combat the confusion, however, later in this chapter are provided a discussion of the numerous thyroid tests you can request and the reasons for underdiagnosis. No matter how you look at it, the various estimates speak to the same concern: Many of us are unknowingly suffering from underactive thyroids.

- A sluggish thyroid (hypothyroid) can be overlooked if you mistakenly think your lethargy is just due to getting older and slowing down.

- People often are incorrect to believe they are overweight because they just eat too much, when their weight management goals are actually stymied by a low metabolism.

- Your metabolism may be in slow motion because your body is having trouble making or getting the right type of thyroid hormone.

An Overview of Thyroid Gland Function

Your thyroid produces two hormones, T4 and T3, which are the body's major metabolic hormones and effect every cell in the body. Unfortunately, T4 is not easily used by our body's cells, so in order for us to function well, we must convert the T4 to the active and useable T3.

Regrettably, many people miss out on their optimal health potential because their bodies have difficulty making this conversion. Without adequate T3, you will experience a sluggish metabolism, meaning you cannot efficiently burn your fuel for energy and will store it as fat, instead.

A wide variety of factors can cause difficulty converting T4 into T3, including:

Less-than-Optimal Nutrient Levels of Any of These

Iodine, iron, selenium, chromium, zinc, vitamins A, B-2, B-6, and vitamin B12 (see Chapter 10 for much more on B12), and vitamin D (the sunshine vitamin)

Medications

Beta blockers,	Birth control pills [7]
Estrogen [7]	Iodinated contrast agents
Lithium Phenytoin	Theophylline

Hormone Imbalances

Estrogen imbalances

Low adrenal gland function (non-Addison's hypoadrenia)

Growth hormone deficiency

Environmental Toxins

Fluoride, chlorine, bromine

Lead, mercury, pesticides

Antibacterial soaps containing triclosan, triclocarban (TCC) [8-9]

Other Factors

Stress [10]

Obesity

Diabetes – high blood sugar or elevated insulin levels

Surgery   Cigarette smoking

Alcohol   Radiation exposure

Unfermented soy   Fasting

Cruciferous vegetables, (broccoli, cauliflower and cabbage)[11]

As the above lists reveal, many common factors can slow down your metabolism and thus inhibit your body's ability to convert fuel to energy. In theory, eliminating as many of these low-thyroid-function contributors should be our clinical goal.

If you are experiencing symptoms of low thyroid function, we encourage you to address the underlying causes of your low thyroid, as the steps you take will enhance many other aspects of your health as well. But, do not put off achieving your health goals, either. Your metabolism may need the proper prescription thyroid medication and dosage to accelerate into the next gear.

Get your metabolism up to par with medications now, while you continue to change your lifestyle to support a healthier thyroid function. An open-minded clinician will reduce your thyroid medication levels if your other efforts kick in. Treating a hypothyroid condition with the new medical protocols is the easiest hormonal imbalance to address and gives patients spectacular results!

Did You Know?

The Path to Healthy Weight Could be Just a "Handshake" Away

In addition to the battery of tests that can confirm hypothyroidism, new information tells us that a postural cue can also signal an underactive thyroid or an improperly managed thyroid condition.

Think about the natural rotation of your hand when you reach out for a handshake with your right hand: your palm faces to the left and the thumb points upward. This natural state is called the "handshake position" or "vertical position."

If you were to lower your hand to your side from the handshake position, your palm would face in towards your body and rest flat against your hip or thigh. Put *both* hands at your side in this manner, and you are standing with normal posture, a position which should feel comfortable and natural.

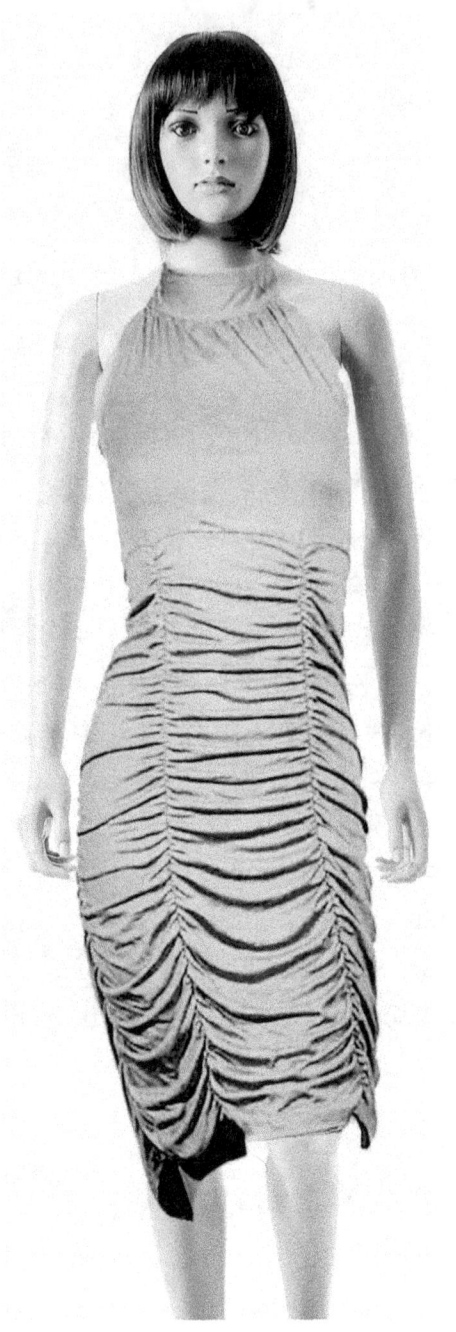

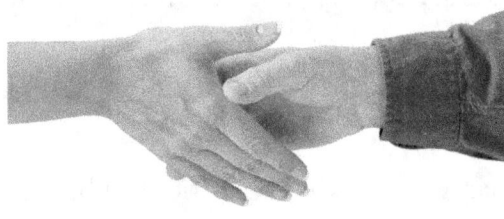

Unfortunately, not everyone is living within their normal, healthy state. For many people, when they stand with their hands at their sides, their palms do not face in towards the thighs, but instead, face backward (posteriorly).

An *Absent Handshake Sign* is when you stand or walk with your arms relaxed by your side and the palm faces posteriorly, the thumb points to the thigh and the fifth finger (the pinky) is always opposite from the thigh—an abnormal postural position of the arm.

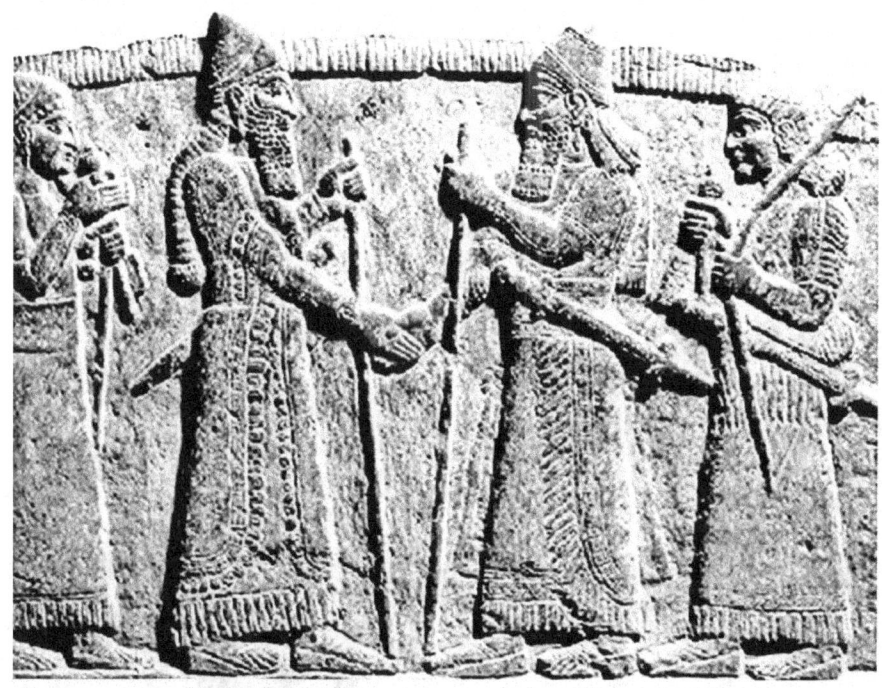

Marduk-Zakir-Schumi v. Babylon: 885-819

THE HANDSHAKE POSITION
AS OLD AS TIME
AS MODERN AS TODAY

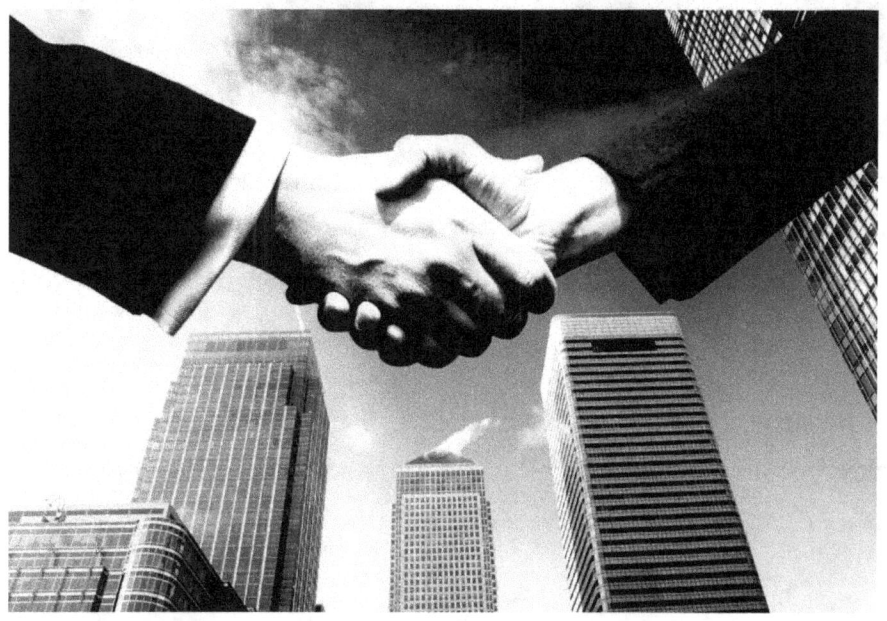

Absent Handshake Sign shown below
is an **Abnormal Postural Position.**

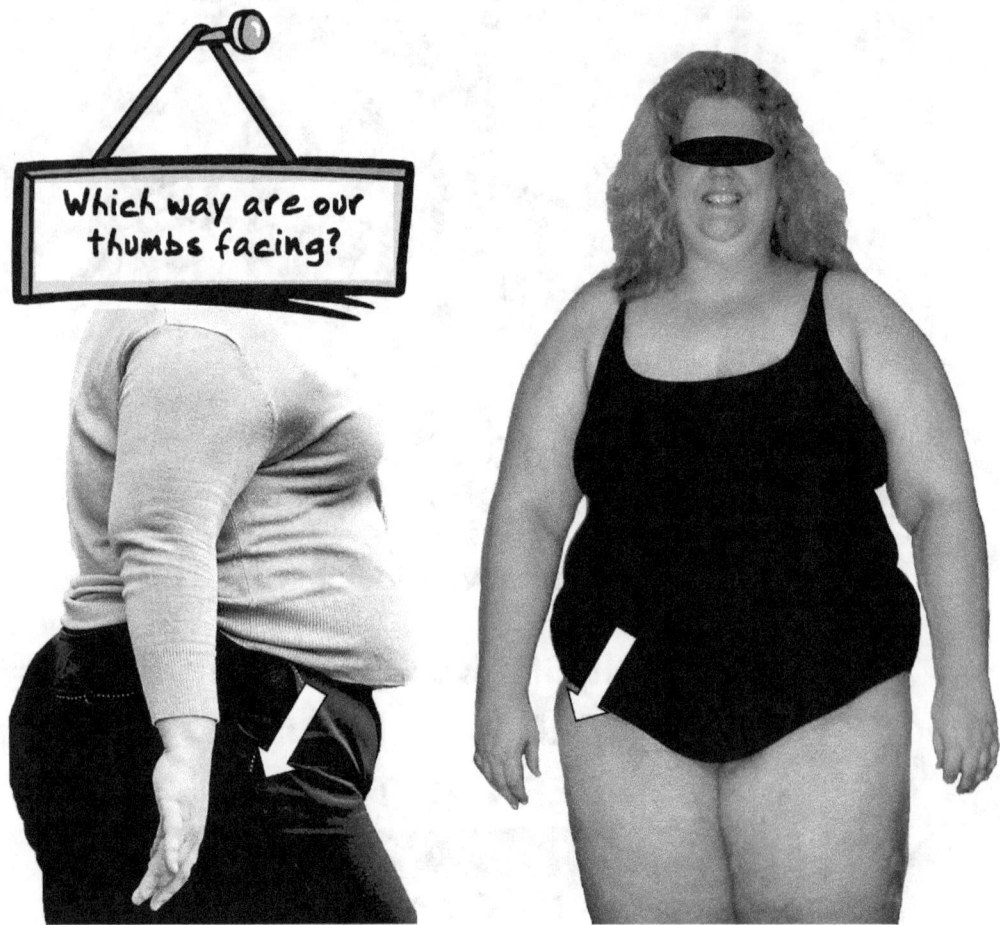

So what does this palm-direction detail have to do with your thyroid? The absence of this normal postural position may signify a sluggish thyroid. **If the Handshake Sign is absent bilaterally**, suspect an *underactive thyroid* and resultant sluggish metabolism.

A connection between posture and thyroid imbalances probably seems odd, but when you take a holistic view of health, the link becomes quite clear. When a healthy person stands, their arms should be in the functional, or normal position. According to noted author and physician,

I.A. Kapandji, this position "corresponds to a state of *natural equilibrium* between the antagonistic muscle groups so that expenditure of muscular energy is at a minimum." [12] In other words, your body is designed to stand in the *Handshake Sign* position, so maintaining this should take the least muscle energy expenditure, as you are in the body's natural state. *If the normal Handshake Sign position is absent, however, that is an indication that the teres minor—a muscle in the shoulder blade area—may have weakened, causing your hand to rotate to the abnormal "palm facing backward" position.*

From lower neck injuries to damaging your shoulder muscles, your teres minor muscles can be weakened in many ways. But, if you or someone you care about is experiencing an *Absent Handshake Sign* on both the right and left hands, the very likely cause of the teres minor muscle weaknesses is an imbalance of the acupuncture circuit (meridian) which is named the *triple warmer* or *triple heater*. Since this specific acupuncture circuit is associated with both this muscle and also the thyroid, a functional weakness of the thyroid gland will also trigger a "grade 4" muscle weakness of the teres minor muscles and an *Absent Handshake Sign*. [13]

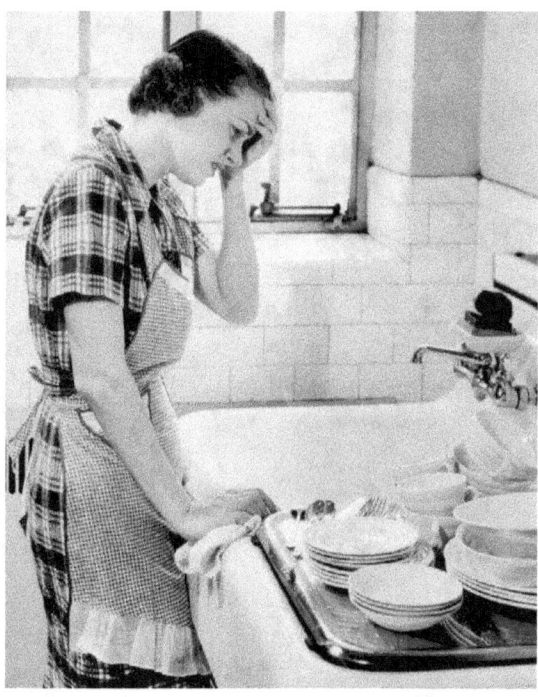

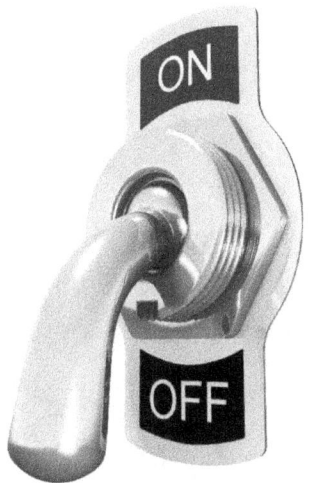

The *Absent Handshake Sign* is easy to
remember with this memory *gizmo:*

The '5 Ts' Rule

Thumbs facing inward

Towards the

Thigh makes us suspect

Thyroid

Trouble

With experts asserting that two thirds of people who have a low thyroid may not know they have the disease, the absence of the normal *Handshake Sign* may be just the easy tool we need to help people achieve greater health. Once a person knows they have a thyroid problem, with treatment, a healthly and productive life can be enjoyed. Here are just a few examples of world leaders with thyroid conditions on the following pages.

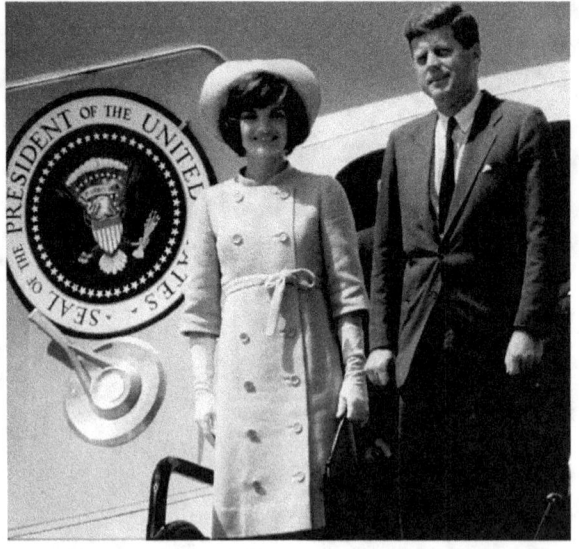

John F. Kennedy "was diagnosed with a subnormally functioning thyroid gland in May 1955. He took iodine throughout his Presidency and (liothyronine [T3] 2 5 mcg twice daily)." [14]

Jackie Kennedy also took thyroid medication. [15]

Look at the *absent handshake sign*. Remember the "5 Ts Rule"—
Thumbs **T**owards the **T**hight suspect **T**hyroid **T**rouble.

President of Brazil   President of Argentina
Dilma Vana Rousseff   Cristina Elisabet Ferandesde Kirchner

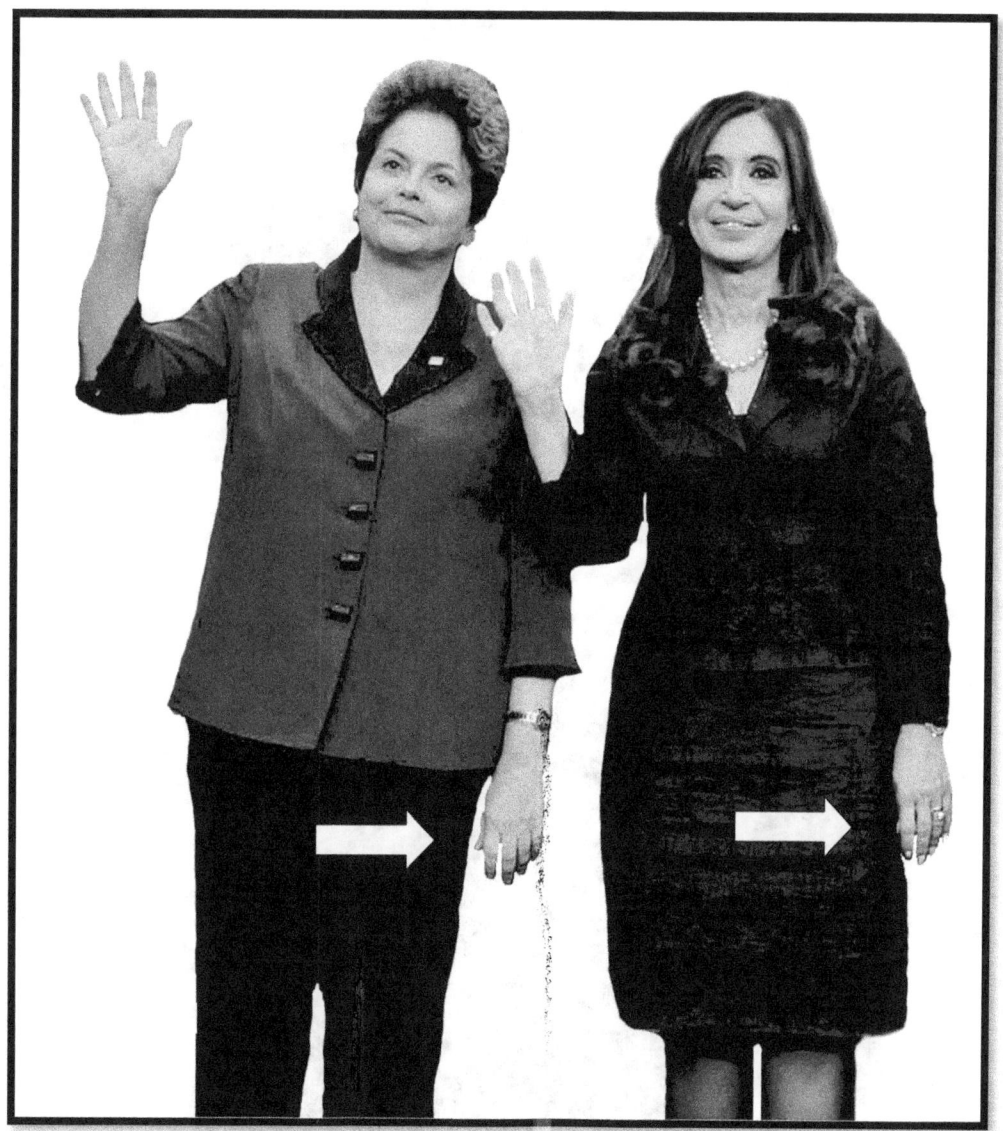

Both female presidents have a medical history of thyroid problems.

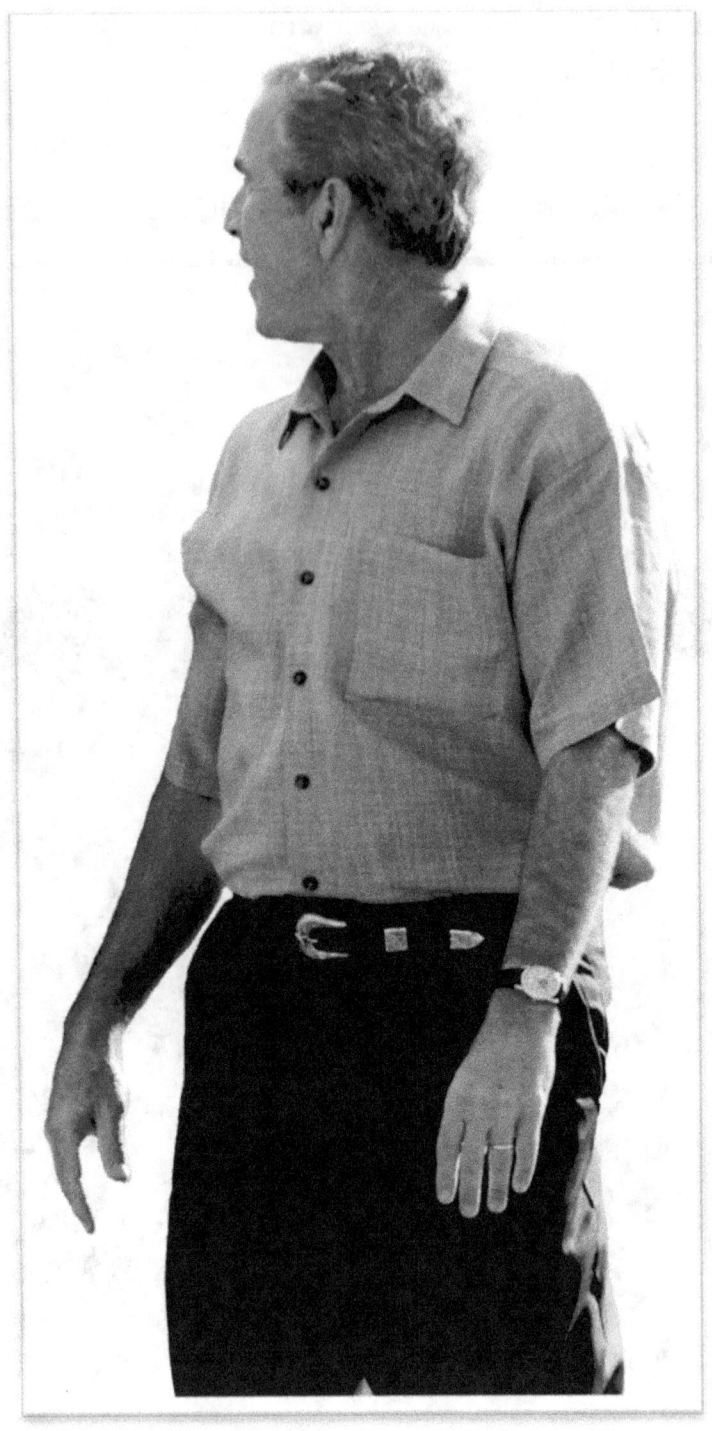

It's not official, but what's your guess about President George W. Bush?
Both his parents have thyroid problems.

Questions to Ask Your Doctor

Over the past several years, the "normal ranges" of the thyroid function blood tests have changed. If your physician has not performed a thyroid blood profile on you in over five years, ask for a new test. When evaluating a patient's thyroid function, physicians often use a simple thyroid blood profile, which contains a minimum number of tests. Because many people's thyroids function "normally" but not "optimally," ask your physician to order a comprehensive thyroid blood profile, which should include—at the minimum—the following tests:

- Thyroid stimulating hormone (TSH) Test
- Total T4/Total thyroxine
- Free T4/Free thyroxine
- Total T3 /Total triiodothyronine
- Free T3/Free triiodothyronine
- Reverse T3

With the above battery of tests, you and your doctor can comprehensively identify potential ways to improve your thyroid's function—and your metabolism. If you are already on thyroid medication such as thyroxine, which is commonly prescribed under the brand name thyroxine (Synthroid®), ask your doctor to conduct the fuller panel of blood tests above to more accurately determine the proper dosage to prescribe.

Guidance

Dr. Broda Barnes, a medical physician and researcher, published a book in 1976 entitled, *Hypothyroidism: The Unsuspected Illness,* in which he revealed that many patients with symptoms of a low thyroid had normal thyroid blood tests. When he checked their metabolism by objectively measuring their basal temperatures, however, the readings were subnormal. In response, Dr. Barnes put them on thyroid medications and their symptoms improved and the subnormal basal temperatures normalized. [16] The *Barnes Temperature Test* is a reasonable way to screen oneself at home for a low metabolism/low-thyroid function.

Conducting the Barnes Temperature Test

Before conducting this at home test, be sure you have a sensitive and accurate thermometer. [17]

The preferred Barnes temperature test method is to take your axillary (armpit) temperature with an accurate thermometer. Do not use an oral temperature test since any infections or inflammation of the nose, sinuses or mouth mucosa can skew the results. Using an *accurate* electronic digital thermometer is imperative, so ensure you use an up-to-date, properly functioning tool. One readily available tested model is Walgreens model VT-820W5T. [18]

An alternative to an electronic digital thermometer is the Galinstan basal thermometer. Galinstan basal thermometers are widely available and sold under the brand name Geratherm®. Like mercury thermometers, Geratherm® thermometer consists of silvery liquid in a glass tube, but they do not pose the health risks of mercury.

- If using a Geratherm® thermometer, shake it down before going to bed.
- Go to sleep without an extraneous heat source such as a bed partner (spouse or pet) right next to you.
- Do not use an electric blanket, heating pad or a heated waterbed since they will affect your body's temperature. You can wear nightclothes and use blankets, since these items will not alter the test.
- Wake up 10 minutes earlier than you usually do and put the thermometer in the middle of your armpit before rising out of bed.
- Try to use as little body movement as possible since all muscle movement raises your temperature.
- If using a digital thermometer, leave it in place until it beeps.
- Wait eight minutes if you are using an old-fashioned, mercury type thermometer or the basal Geratherm thermometer.
- Check whether your basal axillary temperature before getting out of bed in the morning reads between **97.8 - 98.2 degrees F**.

- Chart your temperature for at least three days before making a conclusion and seeking medical advice.

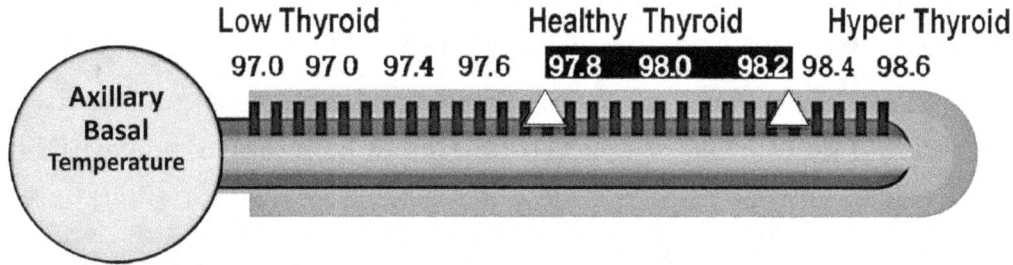

- If the thermometer reads your axillary temperature as below 97.8 F degrees on at least three mornings, suspect low thyroid function, an inadequate dose of thyroid medication or perhaps the incorrect medication.
- If the axillary temperature reads above 98.2 degrees on at least three mornings, suspect an overactive thyroid or excessive thyroid medication.
- Menstruating women should take their temperatures on the first four days of their cycle (menstrual flow) and average the numbers.[19]   In mid-cycle, there is a typical rise in temperature with ovulation.
- Post-menopausal women may complete this home test at any time, as their body temperatures are no longer affected by ovulation.

Another easy screening for a sluggish thyroid is to check for an *Absent Handshake Sign*. Revisit the "Did You Know?" section of this chapter to learn a quick way to see if you or someone you care about may be suffering from undiagnosed thyroid problems.

If your symptoms, the Barnes temperature test and/or an *Absent Handshake Sign* lead you to believe you may be suffering from hypo-thyroidism, see the "Questions to Ask Your Doctor" section for tests that will help determine your thyroid health. Additionally, if you are already taking thyroid medication but still have signs of hypothyroidism, your dosage is likely too low or you may not be using the ideal medication for your body. Insist your doctor performs the comprehensive set of tests, because the *commonly used abridged set of tests can be misleading*.

Keep requesting tests and adjustments to your medication until your Barnes temperature test reads in the normal range and your symptoms subside.

Further Scientific Information

The Complex World of Thyroid Function

Ultimately, when it comes to addressing thyroid function, the rising prevalence of thyroid-based weight problems and diminished quality of life can be traced to three distinct issues: lifestyle, under-diagnosis, and under medicated.

Lifestyle

As I discussed earlier in the chapter, many different lifestyle and environmental factors from birth control pills to stress can impact thyroid function and conversion of T4 to T3 (the more active form). Two relatively recent influences, however, may be having a disproportionate effect on thyroid health: environmental toxins and iodine deficiencies.

Multiple sources of environmental contaminants act as thyroid disrupting chemicals (TDCs) and are theoretically involved in our modern pandemic of hormonal dysfunction. According to a 2009 Associated Press article, our drinking water has been tainted by at least 271 million pounds of pharmaceutical ingredients, which U.S. manufacturers have *legally* dumped in water ways.[20] And at least six of the chemicals now found in the public drinking waters at municipalities throughout the United States inhibit normal thyroid function.[21] Bottomline—do not drink tap water unless you first treat it. You can purchase a reverse osmosis filter or a water distiller for your kitchen at a modest price—a small cost to protect your general health and thyroid function.

-Iodine Deficiencies

Although experts disagree on the reason why Americans have prevalent thyroid problems, one leading argument is based on suboptimal levels of the mineral iodine in our diet. Iodine is one of the most common mineral deficiencies in America today. A study released by the Centers for Disease Control and Prevention in September 2006, found that more than one-third of women in the U.S. have low iodine levels. They based their findings on the U.S. recommended daily allowance (RDA) for iodine—only 0.15 to 0.20 milligrams per day—a relatively minute amount that can help prevent goiter and cretinism, but probably not enough to support healthy thyroid function. Because the optimal requirement of iodine has never been studied—and the RDA's goal for iodine was to prevent goiter and cretinism—we cannot rely on that recommended daily allowance for our optimal health and a fined tuned metabolism.[22] For optimal health I recommend a daily dose of at least **6.25 milligrams of elemental iodine, with 40% iodine and 60% iodide as potassium salt.**

The thyroid gland contains about 80% of the body's iodine, which it uses to make thyroid hormones. After the thyroid, the ovaries have the second largest concentration of iodine in the body.[23] The reason women have a higher incidence of low thyroid function than men, may be due to the ovaries' iodine requirements, since their bodies have two uses for the available iodine in their diets.

Iodine's important connection to healthy thyroid function was widely recognized in America during the first half of the 20th century. Most physicians used iodine supplementation for hypothyroidism. The medical references and protocol of that time, had a *minimum* prescribed dose of 6.25 mg of elemental iodine and the *recommended* daily intake for iodine supplementation was between 12.5 to 37.5 milligrams of elemental iodine. Compare that medical standard to today's recommended daily allowance (RDA) for iodine of only 0.15 to 0.20 mg per day. Do the math and you will see physicians were commonly prescribing elemental iodine doses that were 80 to 187 times higher than today's recommended amounts.

During the second half of the 20th century, some misinformation resulted in decreased use of supplemental iodine.[24-26] A report published in 1948 and later referred to in medical journals, claimed the commonly prescribed doses of iodine would cause the thyroid to become underactive.

The animal studies on rats referred to were never duplicated in humans! Many times since, the validity of that conclusion has been shown false, yet far too many clinicians still believe the recommendations of that

that 1948 report.[27-29] Instead, iodized salt became the standard for iodine supplementation. Unfortunately, iodized salt provides iodide at levels 200 to 500 times *less* than the amount of iodine previously recommended by physicians.

As iodine supplementation decreased, our diets also affected our iodine intake. In the 1960s, one typical slice of bread in the United States contained the full RDA of 0.15 mg iodine. Over the last 20 years, however, iodine was replaced by bromine, which actually blocks thyroid function and may interfere with iodine. Add fluoridated drinking water—which suppresses thyroid function by blocking iodine absorption by the body's iodine receptor sites—and high cholesterol diets that increase the body's excretion of iodine,[30] and it's no wonder the National Health Nutrition Survey from the Centers for Disease Control and Prevention found iodine levels declined 50% in the U.S. from 1971 to 2000. [31]

Under Diagnosis

Nothing seems more straightforward than treatment of hypo-thyroidism. We have robust assays to diagnose the condition and an effective replacement in the form of T4 and T3 hormones. However, the field appears to be in some turmoil and clinical endocrinologists are under increasing pressure from disaffected patients who believe their symptoms indicate hypothyroidism despite normal thyroid function tests. Consider the following: A group of patients recently lodged a petition with a Member of Parliament and the United Kingdom's General Medical Council, as "a formal complain against the clinical practice of the majority of the medical profession with regard to the diagnosus and management of hypothyroidism on four counts:

[Count 1]

Overreliance on thyroid blood tests and a total lack of reliance on signs, symptoms, history of the patient and a clinical appraisal.

[Count 2]

The emotional abuse and blatant disregard by the majority of general practitioners and endocrinologists over the suffering experienced by untreated and/or incorrectly treated thyroid patients and their lack of compassion over the fate of these patients.

[Count 3]

Stubbornness of general practitioners and endocrinologists to treat patients suffering from hypothyroidism with a level of medication that returns the patient to optimum health. In addition, the unwillingness to prescribe alternative thyroid treatment for patients on individual grounds, such as Armour® Thyroid.

[Count 4]

The ongoing reluctance to encourage debate or further research on hypothyroidism." [32]

The active substances produced by the thyroid were first extracted in 1893 and physicians have used them ever since to treat obesity. Today, however, many physicians shy away from claiming thyroid prescriptions can be used to combat excess weight. Part of their reluctance may be due to the large number of patients suffering from underactive thyroid function and weight issues whose thyroid problems have gone undiagnosed. Why are so many of these "borderline" low-thyroid function patients overlooked? Often it's because the blood test standards used to measure the "normal range" for thyroid levels have changed since 2003. Many physicians are not updating the medical records by retesting. Without a test proving low function, doctors may believe weight gains are caused by other factors.

Before 2003, the "normal range" in clinical laboratory standards for the thyroid stimulating hormone (TSH) test (the primary blood test used by conventional doctors to diagnose thyroid disorders) ranged from 0.5 to 5.0 IU/mL, with hypothyroidism being above 5.0. and hyperthyroidism below 0.5. When a policy change occurred in 2003, however, the new guidelines for measuring acceptable TSH levels became far narrower, from 0.3 to 3.0 IU/mL.

This significant change in optimal thyroid levels means if your TSH blood test revealed a number above 3.0 but below 5.1, before 2003, your thyroid was considered "normal." Now, a lab result of 3.1 and above indicates an *underactive* thyroid, and doctors will pursue treatment to lower your TSH. Since the lower end of the normal range was also extended, you can be given a higher dosage of thyroid medication to bring the TSH down close to the 0.3 range, rather than the previous 0.5 limit. Many thyroid experts now recommend a TSH level of 0.1 if the patient continues to present symptoms of low thyroid function.

Another reason many people do not realize they suffer from a sluggish thyroid is because few doctors use the fuller battery of available tests to diagnose the disorder. As previously discussed, a set of tests—not just the TSH blood test—is required to gain a full and balanced understanding of an individual's thyroid function.

Essentially, the generally used test most clinicians order measures the level of thyroid stimulating hormone (TSH) and not the T4 and T3 hormones your body needs for optimum functioning. Although a TSH imbalance can signify thyroid problems, other health complications, like pituitary gland issues or elevated antibodies, can distort your TSH readings. If your doctor relies only on the TSH blood test, you may not receive an accurate assessment of your thyroid health, which is yet another reason why so many people are not diagnosed for hypothyroidism when they should be.

Under Treatment

One of the challenges when treating patients with sluggish thyroids is running complete, appropriate, cutting edge, diagnostic tests in order to find the subtle examples of a less-than-optimally functioning thyroid. Sadly, many of the patients diagnosed with low thyroid function are not monitored properly. Studies show that only 60% of patients taking thyroid medication have their TSH hormones within the normal range. Thus, 40% of patients taking thyroid medication for their subnormal metabolism— millions of Americans—are still hypothyroid. And when you consider this statistic is only based on TSH levels, with more rigorous testing, the number of people treated correctly would likely fall way below 60%. [33]

When treating underactive thyroid glands, determining the correct dose and combination of T4 and T3 hormones is vital. Unfortunately, many clinicians undertreat low thyroid conditions because patients are not properly monitored or receiving a full range of testing—barely bringing all the thyroid hormones into the borderline low end of the normal range. State-of-the-art thyroid-hormone-replacement therapies shoot toward the mid-to-upper-end of the normal range as their goal, because patients' weight-control and overall health response to this type of thyroid treatment is much more impressive and presents fewer health risks.

Under treating patients with sluggish thyroids will not kill them immediately, but the individuals are robbed of their vitality and wellness, may struggle to maintain a healthy weight, and increase their chances of cardiovascular disease. And the risk of serious health issues is a reality. The *Annals of Internal Medicine* published the Rotterdam study, detailing that older women with even subclinical hypothyroidism were nearly twice as likely to have blockages in the aorta and heart attacks. [34]

While under treating hypothyroidism can be deadly, overtreating a low thyroid simply quickens the patient's heart rate and can be corrected in hours with no lasting harm. Clinicians may instruct their patients to check their resting pulse at home and call the doctor if it becomes too fast, at which point they will lower the dosage of the medication. Studies now document that patients with "borderline" or "subclinical" low thyroid function have significant negative changes in their bodies. The conventional criteria for the diagnosis of "subclinical" hypothyroidism are an above range TSH level and an "in range" free T4 level.

"Listen, the goal of therapy is not to have a normal TSH or normal T4. The goal is to have a normal patient."

Thyroid Power by Richard and Karilee Shames [35]

Treatment protocols

The protocols for the management of low thyroid function is slowly changing.

As the definition and diagnosis of normal thyroid function is changing, so too are the treatments for an underactive thyroid.

Traditionally, physicians prescribed a T4 medication and monitored the patient's response by repeating the TSH blood tests (a pituitary gland hormone). Relying on the change in TSH levels to adjust the dosage, however, can create inaccurate results. This is because of the interaction between the pituitary and thyroid glands:

- The pituitary gland makes TSH, which controls the thyroid.

- The body's cells do not readily utilize T4, so our body converts T4 to the more active T3.

- But *the pituitary gland is very sensitive to T4.*

So, while the pituitary's sensitive reaction to the medication may result in normal TSH readings, the thyroid still may not be producing the optimal amount of T4 and T3 for our body to truly be healthy.

Memory Gizmo-When thinking of thyroid hormone prescriptions, remember:

If the Doc says just T4,
There's a good chance I'll need more.
If the Doc says T4 and T3,
That's a combo great for me!

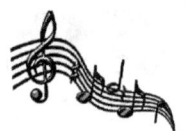

Medication Options

Treating thyroid problems with both T4 and T3 is not new; the approach simply went out of fashion when synthetic drugs came to market in the 1970s. In fact, since the late 1800s, medications with approximately 80%—T4 (thyroxine) and 20%— T3 (triiodothyronine) made out of cleaned, dried, and powdered thyroid glands from pigs have been used with great clinical response. These combined T4/T3 natural medications are still sold under several brand names, including (Armour®Thyroid), (Nature-Throid™)

by Forest Labs, (Westhroid™) by Western Research Labs/Time Caps, and and (Qualitest™) by Time Caps Labs.

In the 1970s, natural thyroid extracts were largely replaced in clinical medicine by a synthetic medication, most often prescribed as thyroxine (Synthroid®). These days, most physicians are reluctant to prescribe natural glandular extracts because they are led to believe the medicines are impure and inconsistent from dose to dose. [36] Also, there was the argument that a synthetic version was healthier because it was produced in a laboratory.

An article in the *New England Journal of Medicine* disputed these claims, reporting that patients with a low thyroid function showed greater improvements in mood and brain function if they received treatment with Armour® thyroid rather than Synthroid®. [37] The authors concluded, "Treatment with thyroxine [T4] plus triiodothyronine [T3] improved the quality of life for most patients." In other words, if you are diagnosed with hypothyroidism (low thyroid function and your doctor prescribes only a T4 drug, such as thyroxine (Synthroid®), you are likely not receiving the most complete treatment available. You may have to work to get the exact medication you need, because many physicians:

- Are hesitant to prescribe natural thyroid, like Armour® thyroid.

- May be using limited clinical laboratory testing methods.

The new protocol for managing underactive thyroid is to prescribe a combination of T4 and either a sustained-release (SR) T3 or T3 taken twice day; a comprehensive approach reflecting the complex nature of thyroid problems. A compounding pharmacy can prepare the (SR) medication. If your physician isn't using these combination hormone treatments for your sluggish thyroid, please ask him or her about it and ensure you receive the answers you need. Considering low T3 not only slows your metabolism— the imbalance can contribute to everything from depression to hair loss— finding the thyroid balance you need may unlock many aspects of the healthy life you deserve. [38]

(Physicians can easily convert your present thyroid medication to a T4 and T3 equivalent using the table in the reference section.) [39]

Definitions and Glossary

Metabolism is the term used to describe the process by which food is converted into energy.

Basal body temperature or **core body temperature** is the body's lowest temperature, typically found during sleep.

Thyroid gland is a small, butterfly-shaped pad that wraps around the front of the esophagus and windpipe at the base of the neck. This proportionately diminutive gland is the master controller of your body's metabolism.

Thyroid hormones are the body's major metabolic hormones, and they consist of two closely related iodine-containing compounds: T4 (*thyroxine*) and T3 (*triiodothyronine*). Although the thyroid only makes about one teaspoon of thyroid hormone per year, these hormones affect every cell in the body.

T3 (*triiodothyronine*) is the most active thyroid hormone.

T4 (*thyroxine*) is a hormone produced by the thyroid that your cells do not easily use. In order for your body to function properly, T4 must be converted to the more active and useable form, T3.

Thyroid stimulating hormone (TSH) is a hormone made by the pituitary gland and it controls the amount of thyroid hormone the thyroid produces. TSH has an inverse relationship with thyroid function. Low thyroid function triggers a higher release of TSH, while an overactive thyroid causes a reduction in amount of TSH released by the pituitary gland.

Hypothyroidism results from the thyroid gland producing too little thyroid hormone.

Hyperthyroidism results from an overactive thyroid gland producing too much thyroid hormone. Please note, in this book we will only focus on *hypothyroidism* and its influence on weight gain, because an overactive thyroid is most often accompanied by unexplained weight loss.

Graves' disease is an inflammatory disorder of the thyroid gland that causes an overactive thyroid, commonly associated with protrusion of the eyes (exophthalmos).

Hashimoto's disease is an autoimmune disease caused by antibodies attacking the thyroid gland, causing damage that results in hypothyroid (low thyroid) function.

Goiter is an enlargement of the thyroid gland causing massive swelling to the front of the neck. An iodine deficiency is one of goiter's primary causes.

Iodine and **Iodide**: There is often confusion when the terms iodine and iodide are used. Their chemical properties differ, in that *iodine* is the elemental atom with the symbol (I), whereas *iodide* is a negative ion of iodine (I⁻), which means it has a charge.

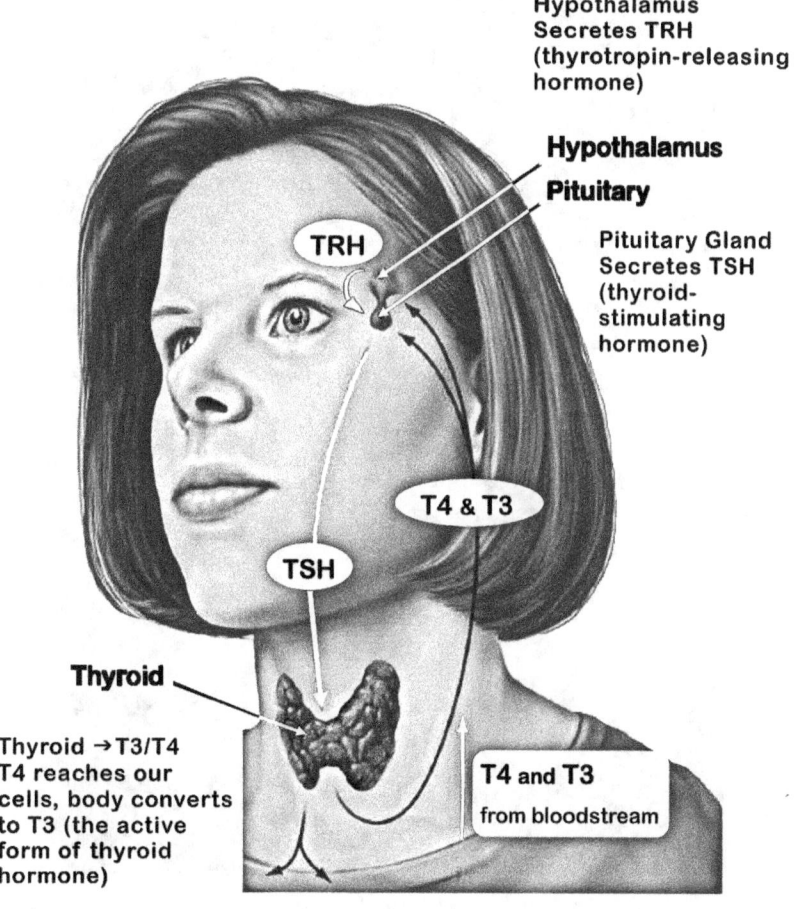

Hypothalamus
Secretes TRH
(thyrotropin-releasing
hormone)

Hypothalamus

Pituitary

Pituitary Gland
Secretes TSH
(thyroid-
stimulating
hormone)

TRH

T4 & T3

TSH

Thyroid

Thyroid → T3/T4
T4 reaches our
cells, body converts
to T3 (the active
form of thyroid
hormone)

T4 and T3
from bloodstream

HYPOTHYROIDISM

It's Only a Word, Not a Sentence.

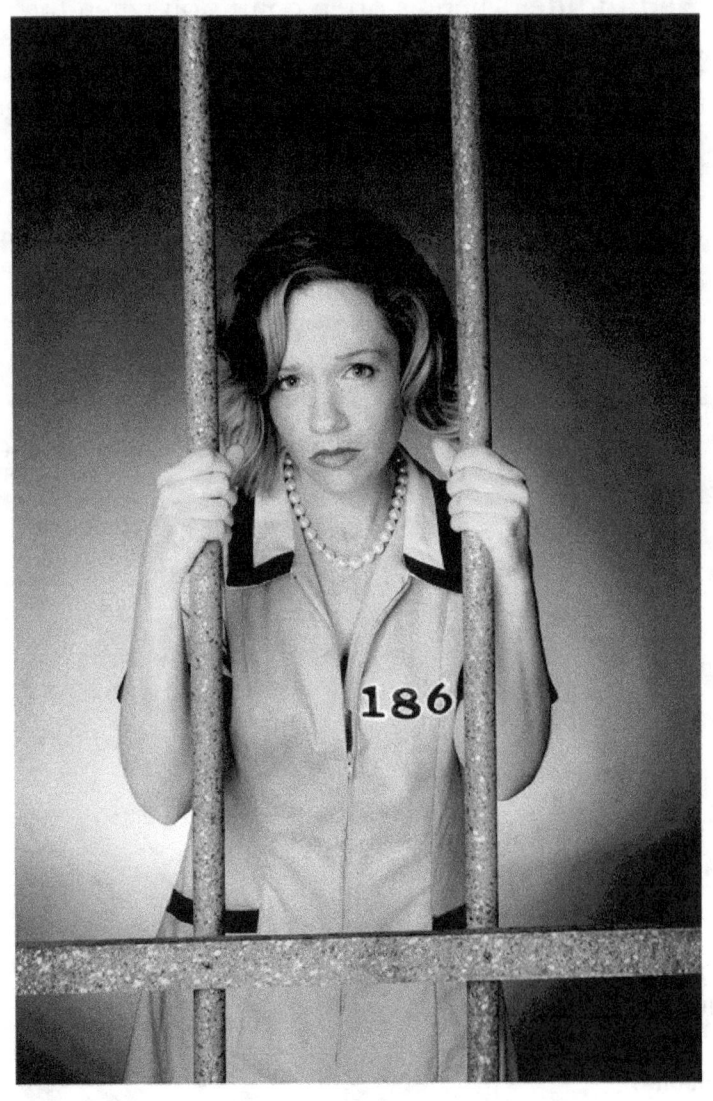

Chapter 9

Over Stressed and Overweight

Adrenal Glands and Chronic Stress

Once, I witnessed a lecturer hold up a glass of water and ask, "How heavy is this glass of water?" Answers from the audience ranged from 5 ounces to 1.5 pounds. Considering a liter of water has an absolute weight of approximately 2.2 pounds, the guesses were reasonably accurate. The speaker, however, was not interested in identifying the *absolute* weight of water, but the relative weight. The *absolute* weight will not change; it's an intrinsic aspect of H_2O. On the other hand, when it comes to lifting a glass of water, the *relative* weight depends on how long you try to hold it:

- A minute would not be a problem.

- An hour would probably make your arm ache.

- A day would cause severe discomfort and lasting physical injury.

In each case, the *absolute* weight of the glass of water remains the same, but the heavier it seems to become and the more there is potential for pain and damage the longer it is held aloft. Without rest, the burden increases and sooner or later you simply won't be able to carry on. But, imagine instead of a day straight you had to hold the glass aloft for a day *total*, and you were given a year to complete the task. By breaking up the challenge into manageable increments, the task becomes less daunting, right? [1]

Stress management functions in the same way.

As humans, stress is an inherent part of our lives, whether we are running from a predator or driving in rush hour traffic. How we carry our burdens, however, affects our long-term health.

Similar to lifting the glass of water, you must have a break between stressful experiences in order for your body to recover, move forward, and prepare for the next challenge.

Finding Balance in a Stressed-Out Society

What do you think of when you hear the word "stress?" If you're like many people, negative images and feelings immediately flood your mind as you picture a variety of overwhelming or tense circumstances.

Contrary to this common idea, however, stress is not intrinsically good or bad. Instead, stress is simply our body's reaction to a variety of physical and emotional stimuli—and we are genetically designed to experience it.

In fact, your bones and muscles depend on physical stress in the form of regular, weight-bearing exercise in order to keep from growing weak and atrophying. You also need occasional emotional and mental stressors—like getting a new job, watching your favorite sporting event, or even falling in love—because these events excite the brain's pleasure centers, bathing them in the "feel-good" neurotransmitter dopamine.

A healthy, satisfying, engaging life demands—and creates—stress.

Like the example of the glass of water continuously held aloft, problems only arise when your body doesn't have time to take a break from regular stress.

Acute Versus Chronic Stress

In 1936, Dr. Hans Selye received a Nobel Prize for discovering that when our bodies experience stress, our physiological responses are the same, regardless of the origin or type of stress.

When we face a stressful event, whether real or imagined, our body's first response is normally to shut down the appetite and pause the digestive process. These changes allow energy to be diverted toward handling the crisis: Blood flow and neurological energy are redirected from our gastrointestinal tract to the skeletal muscles, heart's arteries, lungs, liver, and brain. We are ready to transform into the fight-or-flight response (*sympathetic mode*) essential for survival. The body is genetically programmed to react to stress by triggering this survival response to gear up as if we are in the middle of an endangering emergency.

So, you may be asking, if we are designed to handle stress, why is it an issue today? The problem is, as Dr. Selye's research shows, the same response is set in motion even by the common everyday stresses of a "burning the candle at both ends" type of lifestyle. Modern stressors are often more frequent and sustained than in hunter-gatherer days, but our bodies are still similarly reacting.

Historically, humans did not often survive long enough to experience chronic stress. Instead, our ancestors would either have perished from the events causing the stresses—such as severe injuries or illnesses, starvation, animal attacks, or warring humans—or would have lived through the traumatic event and quickly recovered from the acute stress.

Imagine the stresses our ancestors would have faced:

There's no water available, so I must travel to find some before I die of thirst.

The weather is too hot/cold/windy/stormy, etc., so I have to find shelter.

That wild animal is about to attack my family, so we need to run away as quickly as possible.

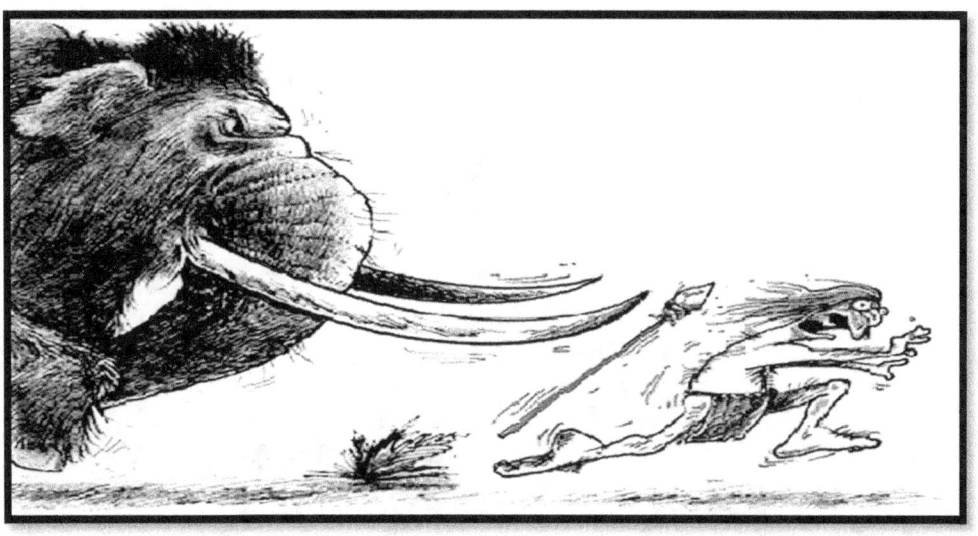

Now compare those life or death problems with typical stressors today:

My alarm didn't go off and now I'm going to be late to work!

The baby sitter cancelled last minute and I don't have anyone to provide the childcare I need.

The economy is down, and my retirement accounts have been decimated.

My marriage has been feeling strained lately—in fact, for years.

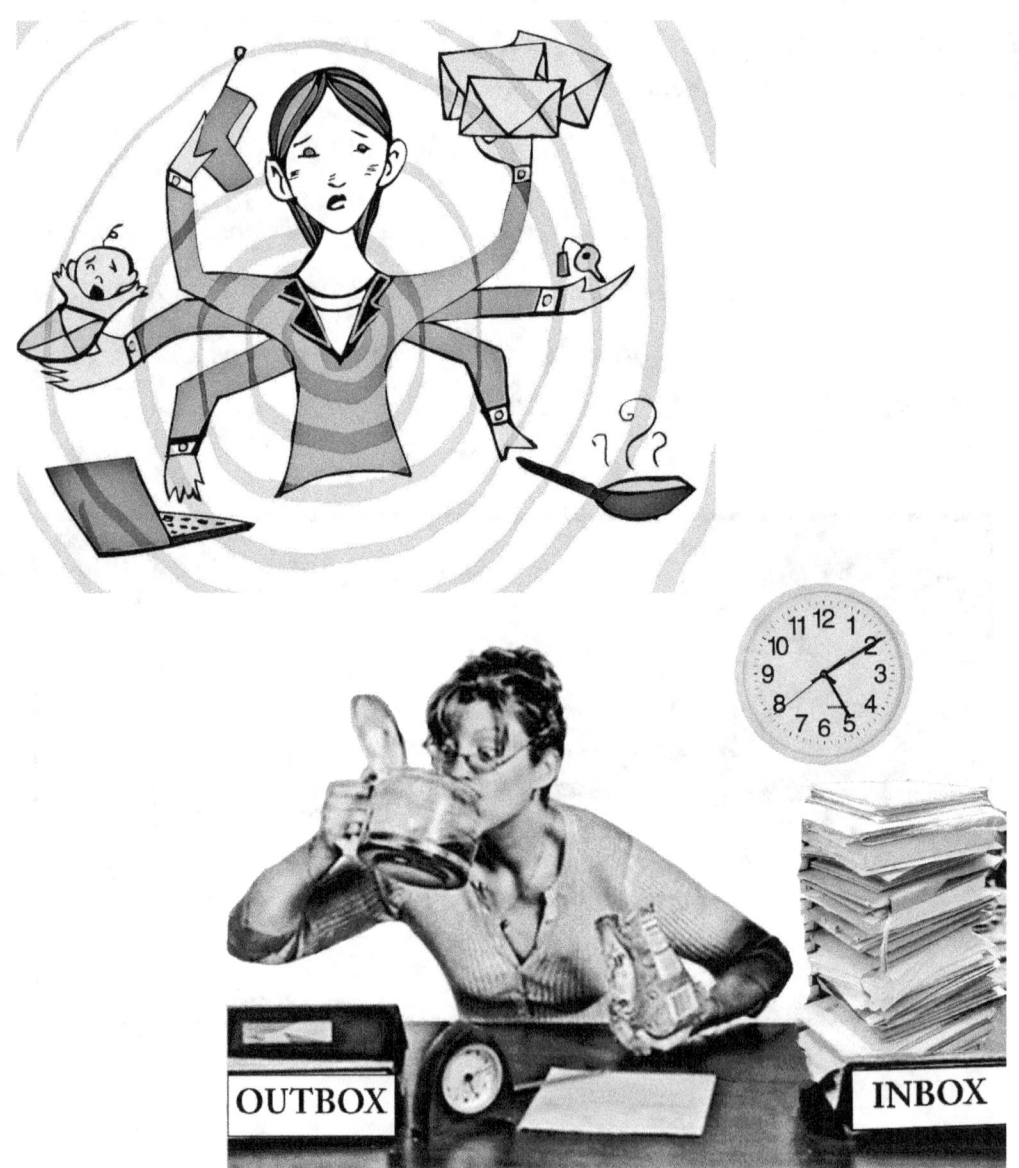

In addition to showing that our bodies have the same reactions to all stress, Dr. Selye also made us aware that stresses from different categories are cumulative: each adds to the other. So when you're worried about something at work or home (mental stress) and you don't have time to grab anything but junk food for lunch (chemical stress), you **have** dealt a double whammy to the body. With all that stress at work or home, you're not sleeping well (physical stress), and you just finished shopping in an air-conditioned department store. You parked close to the store and within seconds you are in your car, which was sitting in the sun and its interior temperature is 110 degrees F (thermal stress).

Our adrenal glands cannot function effectively with such frequent, overlapping stressors creating the near constant need for stress hormones and system regulation. After years of overreaction, the glands become exhausted—while our bodies struggle to find a balance between the "fight-or-flight" (sympathetic) and the "rest-and-digest" (parasympathetic) responses. All these forces combine to form one stressed-out person and endocrine system—and prevent you from truly fitting into your genes.

Symptoms of Adrenal Fatigue Syndrome

1. Abdominal fat deposits and weight gain resulting in what is called "central obesity," an "apple-shaped figure," and upper body android fat distribution.

2. Alcohol intolerance

3. Alternating diarrhea and constipation

4. Fear, anxiety

5. Cravings for sweets

6. Cravings for salt or salty foods—lack of the adrenal hormone aldosterone, leads to salt wasting from the kidneys into the urine, hence the craving for more salt

7. Difficulty building muscle

8.   Dizziness that occurs upon standing, postural dizziness and low blood pressure (low aldosterone related)

9.   Dry and thin skin

10. Excessive hunger

11. Fatigue worsens with exercise and is relieved by rest

12. Feelings of frustration

13. Food and/or inhalant allergies

14. Generalized weakness

15. Headaches

16. Heart palpitations

17. Hypoglycemia (low blood sugar)

18. Impaired thyroid gland function results in lowered metabolism (stress can block the conversion of T4 to the active form of thyroid hormone which is T3 (see symptoms of an underactive thyroid in Chapter 8)

19. Inability to concentrate

20. Indigestion

21. Insomnia

22. Irritability

23. Lack of energy

24. Lightheadedness—especially when getting up suddenly

25. Light sensitivity, squinting in bright light, must wear sunglasses or eyes hurt

26. Low blood pressure

27. Low body temperature

28. Mental depression, moments of confusion

29. Muscle loss

30. Nervousness

31. Premenstrual syndrome (PMS)

32. Poor memory

33. Poor resistance to infections

34. Scanty perspiration

35. Sexual dysfunction in women, since the female body produces most of its androgens in the adrenal glands

36. Tendency towards inflammation

37. Unexplained hair loss

38. Uterine fibroids

Guidance

How do you know if adrenal fatigue syndrome is preventing you from fitting into your genes? To begin, review this chapter's list of symptoms and ask yourself how many of them you are experiencing. If you are affected by more than 33% of the symptoms, seek out an adrenal fatigue syndrome evaluation conducted by a properly trained clinician. See the "Questions to Ask Your Doctor" section for guidance on how to find a physician who truly understands the disorder, rather than someone only familiar with the more severe adrenal malfunction, Addison's disease.

Before searching for treatment from a qualified clinician, you can verify if your symptoms are related to adrenal malfunction by conducting the following three self-screening tests:

Ragland's Sign (Blood Pressure Test)

Equipment needed: An accurate blood pressure kit.

Procedure: Take your blood pressure while laying face up on your back (supine). Then, stand up and immediately take your blood pressure again. Your systolic (first) number should have risen 8 to 10 mm. If the number did not rise or dropped, you may have adrenal fatigue.

Rogoff Sign Test (Pupil Dilation Test)

Equipment needed: A flashlight or penlight, and either a mirror or someone to help you perform the test.

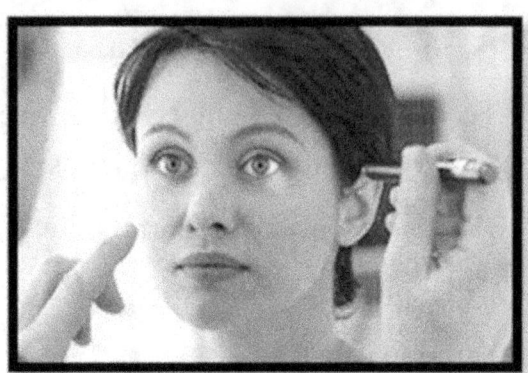

Procedure: If you are doing the test alone, look into the mirror and shine the flashlight into one of your eye's pupil, which is the dark hole located in the center of the iris (the colored portion of your eye). Shine the light into your eye and not into the reflection of your eye as seen in the mirror. The mirror is there so you can observe your eye's pupil response to the light. If you have someone to assist you, have them shine the light into one of your eyes. Your pupil should contract in response to the light. Continue shining the light into the same eye, and after 30 seconds, if your pupil is not continuing to contract or it contracts at first but within 30 seconds dilates (widens) again, you most likely have adrenal fatigue.

Why does this happen?

During adrenal insufficiency, there is a suboptimal level of sodium and an abundance of potassium in the body. This mineral imbalance causes an inhibition of the sphincter muscles of the eye. These muscles normally initiate pupil constriction in the presence of bright light. However, in adrenal fatigue syndrome, the pupils actually dilate when exposed to light.

Self-Ordered Adrenal Lab Testing

You can order for yourself the "Diurnal Cortisol DHEA-S saliva test kit" by contacting ZRT Laboratory at 866-600-1636. For NY and CA residents please read the information about self-ordering this lab test given in the reference section of this chapter. [6]

Dim Light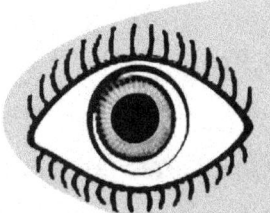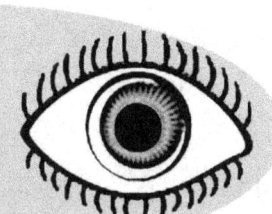

Normal Response to Light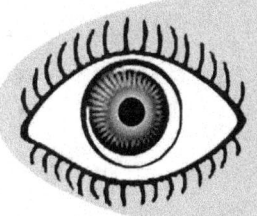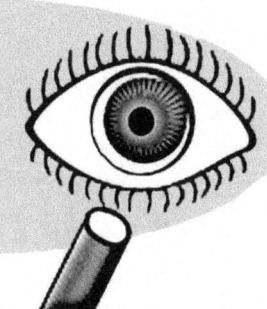

Pupils Dilate After 30 Seconds (+) Rogoff Sign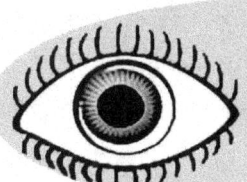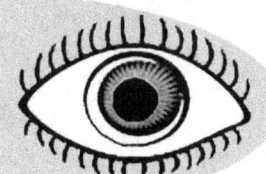

Questions to Ask Your Doctor

If you believe adrenal fatigue syndrome may be causing you to respond to chronic stress by overeating, you must find a physician who is skilled in diagnosing and treating this disorder. As was stated, most doctors are more familiar with Addison's disease—a severe adrenal gland deficiency—than adrenal fatigue syndrome or hypoadrenia.

One of the best ways to find a clinician with this type of expertise is to contact either Genova Diagnostics,[7] Diagnos-Techs,[8] or ZRT Laboratory;[9] three medical laboratories that specialize in testing functional imbalances such as adrenal fatigue syndrome. You can go to either of their web sites and use the Practitioner Directory to find physicians across the United States familiar with *adrenal fatigue syndrome.*

Once you find the right doctor to address your concerns, if not already done, you should insist that they run adrenal fatigue syndrome lab tests. These should include checking your cortisol and DHEA levels. Often, salivary hormone testing is used to show the circadian cortisol pattern. Another method uses urine analysis, but it sacrifices information of cortisol's circadian fluctuations. Normal cortisol levels, when measured by saliva testing, should start off high in the morning then begin to drop at noon, continue to go down at dinnertime and be the lowest at bedtime.

If your lab test results are abnormal, the trained clinician can prescribe a therapeutic regime. DHEA levels should be stable throughout the day, so a single sampling is used. Here, the levels vary between men and women, and your age. The labs will help your physician determine what levels should be considered normal.

Did You Know?

"I'm just so tired" is the most common complaint that brings a person to see his or her primary care physician.

Malaise is the medical term for this type of exhaustion and in plain language means, "I'm sick and tired of being sick and tired." There are a least 383 medical conditions that manifest malaise symptoms. Yet, all too often, long-term stress is the true culprit. Chronic stress eventually lowers our adrenal hormone levels; when that happens, our "get up and go" gets up and leaves!

So, after your physician has ruled out life-threatening diseases as possible causes of your malaise, think seriously about your adrenal glands.

But when addressing stress, remember there is stress and there is distress. As I mentioned earlier in the chapter, "good stressors" or challenges in life can motivate us by exciting the pleasure centers in the brain that are then bathed in the "feel good" brain chemical dopamine. The problem, however is that in our modern lifestyles we often have a hard time recognizing—and managing—chronic stress.

How Chronic Stress Contributes to Weight Gain

Our bodies are naturally designed to respond to acute, short-term stress by decreasing hunger and digestive activity. But, chronic stress disrupts (deregulates) this normal body response and actually triggers cravings for fat, sugar, and carbohydrate-laden foods. Consequently, chronic, long-term stress is a very common culprit sabotaging our healthy weight goals.

As researchers Torres, Nowson, Adam and Epel state:

"Chronic life stress seems to be associated with a greater preference for energy and nutrient dense foods, namely those that are high in sugar and fat" [10]… "it appears the obesity epidemic may be exacerbated by the preponderance of chronic stress, unsuccessful attempts at food restriction, and their independent and possibly synergistic effects on increasing the reward value of highly palatable food." [11]

In plain English, when we couple high levels of long-term stress with junk foods, obesity results!

Furthermore, not only does chronic stress cause unhealthy cravings, it's the trigger mechanism for fat accumulation in the abdominal region. Known as visceral obesity and also commonly called "belly fat", this type of weight gain gives a person the "apple figure" body appearance.

The authors of a Dutch study found that "chronically high ambient levels of stress and the availability of high caloric foods" heighten the risk of abdominal fat.[12] And unfortunately, visceral fat is particularly dangerous, because it increases your chances of suffering from diabetes (type II diabetes), heart disease, hypertension, and stroke-separate from obesity. [13]

Abdominal fat is caused when the stress hormone cortisol and insulin which are released by eating sweets, both increase. Thus, chronic stress causes weight gain in three dangerous, interconnected ways:

1. Deregulating the body's hunger mechanisms

2. Triggering cravings for sweets

3. Releasing the adrenal hormone cortisol, which combines with insulin to cause abdominal fat

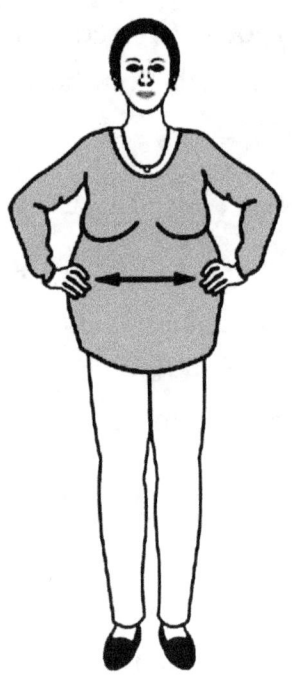

"Apple Shape" of Fat Distribution

The combination of high cortisol + low DHEA contributes to excess fat accumulation around the upper body and waist

The Hormonal Stress Responses

The Autonomic Nervous System:
Parasympathetic and Sympathetic

The human body has an *autonomic nervous system* that controls our: glands, smooth muscle, and cardiac muscle. The autonomic nervous system controls processes that maintain our body's balance, which is known as *homeostasis*. The autonomic nervous system is also known as the general visceral motor system and the involuntary nervous system.

The autonomic nervous system has two divisions: the sympathetic and parasympathetic. The sympathetic part mobilizes the body during extreme situations, whereas the parasympathetic performs maintenance activities and conserves body energy. These two divisions counterbalance each other's activity—and most of our glands and organs are innervated by (or connected to) both the parasympathetic and sympathetic.

Parasympathetic: Rest and Digest

Our autonomic nervous system's parasympathetic part is concerned with keeping the body's energy use low and involves digestion, defecation, and diuresis (urination). Parasympathetic activity is illustrated, for example, in a person who relaxes after a meal. In that state of parasympathetic relaxation, blood pressure, heart rate, and respiratory rates are low, but the gastrointestinal tract is active. The parasympathetic activity also induces stomach acid production and *satiates our appetite.*

Over 90% of all parasympathetic nerve fibers are derived from the vagus nerve, which puts us into the "rest and digest" function mode when stimulated. And, part of our appetite's shutting down process after we have eaten—or the "shutting off your appetite" command—actually comes from signals carried to the brain from the digestive tract by the vagus nerve. This command is triggered by the digestive tract in response to mechanical pressure from the food we eat and food-released brain-gut chemicals. *If we are stuck too long in the sympathetic stress mode, our parasympathetic-carried signals telling us we are full may not get to the brain.*

Sympathetic: Fight or Flight

Our autonomic nervous system's sympathetic division, on the other hand, is involved with exercise, excitement, emergencies, and embarrassment. Its activities are illustrated by a person who is threatened: The heart rate increases, breathing is rapid and deep, blood sugar (glucose) increases and gastrointestinal function decreases. To best use our limited human resources, the body shunts blood from the gastrointestinal tract to the muscles, heart, lungs, and brain to maximize the effectiveness of our emergency survival mode. Up to 50% of all sympathetic effects acting on the body are caused by the sympathetic nervous system triggering the adrenal glands to release the hormones *norepinephrine* and *epinephrine* (adrenaline). In other words, this is certainly an example where the nervous system and the hormonal system dance arm-in-arm to accomplish life-sustaining effects.

Chronic Stress and Appetite

Our autonomic nervous system (the sympathetic and parasympathetic), influence our appetite and digestion. The "rest and digest" parasympathetic branch signals us to eat and digest our food. The "fight or flight" sympathetic, on the other hand, gladly sacrifices our appetite and digestive chores in order to shunt the body's efforts to run or fight to save our lives in times of peril.

The inner part of the adrenal glands, called the medulla, works as part of the sympathetic nervous system and focuses on secreting and regulating the two previously mentioned hormones: epinephrine, and norepinephrine.

Under chronic, long-term stress, the body's sympathetic nervous system releases a chemical called "Neuropeptide Y" (NPY), a key element in stimulating our appetites. NPY is the most potent food-intake-stimulating chemical known. Therefore, *chronic stress triggers our appetites, especially for sweets, and causes fat to accumulate.*

On the other hand, high cortisol levels released due to *acute stress, actually shut off our appetite.*

On a normal day, we should have a healthy rhythm of cortisol rising and falling: The body produces more cortisol in the morning, giving us the energy we need to begin our busy day. In the evening, our cortisol level should drop by about 90%, so we can relax and wind down.

Cortisol, know also as hydrocortisone (17-alpha-hydrocortisterne).

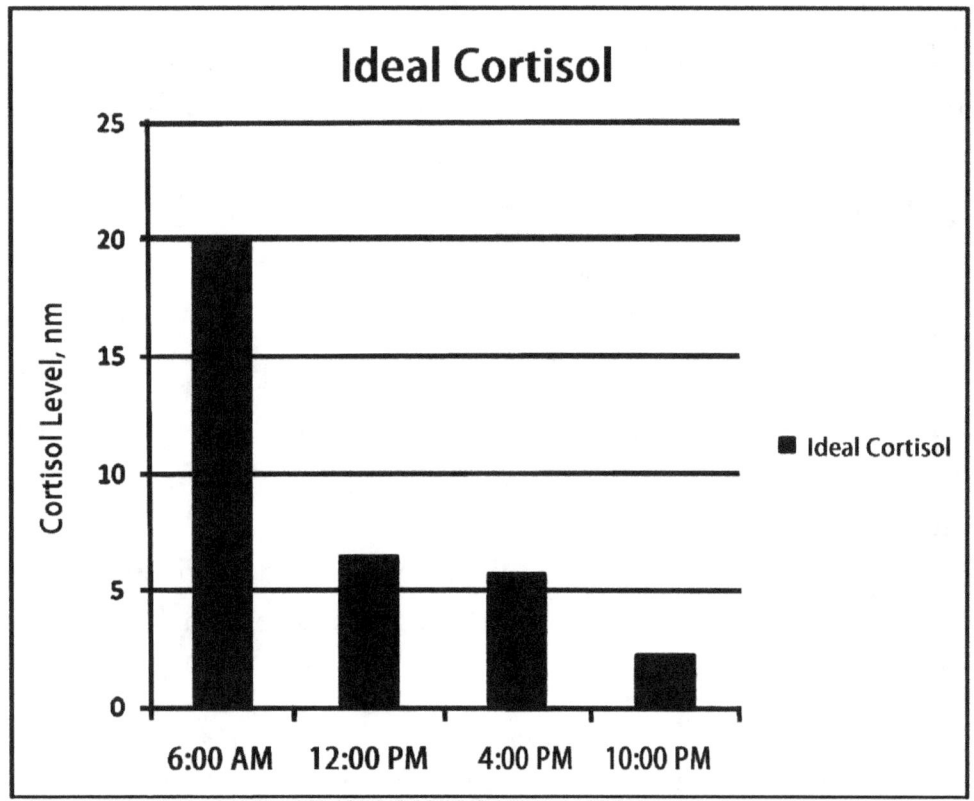

Unfortunately, in our modern society, this hormonal balance is not the norm. Scientific research reveals that elevated cortisol levels are much too commonplace. The instinctual, classic fight-or-flight stress does not cause most weight problems, because in those situations the stressful event is quickly resolved. Unlike acute stress, modern-day chronic stress is ongoing and may not be resolved without long-term effort. As a result, chronic stress disrupts our cortisol balance by consistently overrunning our bodies with this hormone.

Elevated cortisol has the following effects on our bodies:

- **Triggers craving sweets**: Stress increases cortisol levels, which initially dampen hunger. Once the stress has eased, our hunger hormones kick in and scream, "Refuel!" At this point, our stress-related, elevated cortisol leads to sugar cravings because cortisol impairs our tissues' insulin dependent uptake. In response, our body craves the sugar (fuel) we need, ultimately driving people to reach for the unhealthy sweets (candy bars, ice cream, etc.) in order to get more glucose (blood sugar).

- **Stimulates fat deposits and can result in weight gain**: The higher our cortisol levels, the more abdominal fat we gain. Because our abdomen's fat tissue has more cortisol receptors, it is more responsive to stress and ultimately gives us the 'apple-shaped' figure linked to many diseases.

- **Triggers fat storage**: Together, insulin and cortisol activate an enzyme called lipoprotein lipase, which readies our body to store fat.

- **Impairs thyroid function**: Cortisol impairs the conversion of the T4 thyroid hormone, to the more active T3 form. As a result, our body is unable to maintain healthy levels of T3.

- **Decreases progesterone production** and competes with progesterone receptors, leading to estrogen dominance, fat accumulation, potentiating premenstrual syndrome (PMS), uterine fibroids, and breast cancer.

- **Increases blood pressure**: Blood pressure naturally increases in response to stress. When challenged by threatening events, we need blood pumping to our muscles and brain so they can respond as powerfully as possible.

- **Increases protein breakdown that can lead to muscle loss**: Cortisol converts proteins to glucose as an extra energy source. The body's process of converting proteins into a useable carbohydrate (glucose) in the liver is called gluconeogenesis, which makes more energy available to handle a stressful situation or threat.

- **May cause poor memory**: High levels of cortisol may make thinking about or retrieving long-term memories difficult, which also explains why people often become confused in a severe crisis. [14]

Adrenaline (epinephrine): In order to deal with stress, the body also raises the level of another adrenal gland hormone called *adrenaline* or *epinephrine*.

Adrenaline has these effects on our body:

- Stops or greatly **slows** down movements of the **gastrointestinal tract** and digestive secretions.

- **Inhibits insulin secretion:** Insulin allows sugar to enter the cells to be burned for fuel. Lower insulin levels reduce blood sugar supplies to most of our tissues, except the brain, retina, and liver; these tissues use non-insulin dependent transporters to bring the blood sugar (glucose) into the cells. Because of their isolated glucose relationships, our brain remains able to focus while the rest of the body is starving for sugar.

- **Increases blood sugar levels:** Our blood sugar levels increase when adrenaline (epinephrine) breaks down the liver's stored sugar (glycogen) into circulating blood sugar (glucose).

Adrenal Glands—Stress Central

At the heart of our stress response are the adrenal glands: two walnut-size glands that sit above each kidney and are the body's major responders to stress. Despite their small size, the adrenals are involved in regulating virtually every aspect of body function; they are the command post. Two adrenal hormones, cortisol, and DHEA (dehydroepiandros-terone), have genetic influences on the body and are involved in carbohydrate, protein, and fat metabolism. DHEA and cortisol must always remain in a proper ratio for the body to function optimally. When cortisol levels are elevated and DHEA is low, we are in what is known as the *chronic stress response.*

The combination of high cortisol and low DHEA is often a major contributor to excess fat accumulation around the thighs, waist, and hips. In fact, these people may be slender except for those "problem" areas. If you or someone you know has excess fat only in their midsection, you are witnessing a revealing sign of adrenal dysfunction and hormone imbalance, specifically an elevated ratio of cortisol to DHEA from chronic stress.

Crash and Burn

Imagine a horse racing in the Kentucky Derby. The jockey whips his mount from the start of the race and shoots ahead at break-neck speed. Under near constant whipping, the horse at first pulls away from the others for stride after stride and seems unstoppable. Eventually, though, the horse cannot maintain his unnatural fast speed. No matter how much the jockey encourages his mount, the horse is exhausted and must stop.

Like the over-exerted racehorse, when you push your adrenal glands too hard by experiencing chronic, unabated stress, they will eventually grow exhausted.

Though I have written extensively about high cortisol levels and hyperadrenal function, the greatest problems occur when you experience the inevitable crash and burn from pushing your adrenal glands in this manner.

In my clinical practice I actually saw more patients with low cortisol than with high cortisol levels. Often, the person with high cortisol levels is stressed but, at least in their mind, dealing with it. The person with exhausted adrenals and low cortisol has crashed, and they want their life back. Remember the Folgers' coffee slogan from the 1980's, "The best part of waking up is Folgers in your cup!?" Does the slogan, "America Runs on Dunkin," sound familiar?

After a long-hard day in the "can do" mode, we feel ready to kick back and relax. *Hooray, it's that time again, Happy Hour!* A cocktail, glass of wine or beer will do the trick and help relax us from a stressful day. Studies show that consuming a small amount of alcoholic beverages is healthy—perhaps one of the reasons is because alcohol eases us into the rest-and-digest mode and aides our ability to digest a meal without overeating or craving sweets.

Hey, don't criticize my coffee and cocktails. I can live like that! And many do. Yet after years of using caffeine, nicotine, and alcohol while whipsawing between the rest-and-digest-parasympathetic and fight-or-flight-sympathetic modes, our body eventually becomes worn out and sluggish. We call this *adrenal fatigue syndrome or hypoadrenia*, not to be confused with Addison's disease, which is a rare and life-threatening deficiency of the adrenal glands.

Since cortisol can provide euphoria, some people with adrenal fatigue syndrome will indulge in certain patterns of behavior to shock the adrenals into action. Squeezing more and more from the adrenal reserve undoubtedly ends in more severe adrenal fatigue.

Commonly, the person with adrenal fatigue may be addicted to caffeine, sugar, and salty foods. Drugs such as cocaine or amphetamine and nicotine also stimulate the adrenals. Behavioral patterns that whip up the adrenal glands include anger and work related drama. So, the "drama queen" may actually be acting this way to get a "cortisol" rush just to feel normal. Strenuous exercise also stimulates cortisol release, and the exercise "addict" may be compensating for adrenal fatigue syndrome. Also, people with low thyroid function can be addicted to exercise.

As I stated in the chapter on low metabolism, exercising is a great, fundamental way of achieving your healthy weight; it can also be an important diagnostic clue. If one of the only ways you can feel good is by exercising, you may have adrenal fatigue syndrome and/or a sluggish metabolism (hypothyroidism.) So the key for optimal adrenal functions is to have cortisol in the healthy range. Adequate cortisol levels are critical for the body to adapt to stress. Normally, if cortisol is too high, we must tone down the stresses in our lives. Also, be aware that it is only a matter of time before "burning the candle at both ends" takes a toll and the adrenal glands exhaust themselves and low cortisol ensues. With low cortisol, our vim and vigor vanishes!

Definitions and Glossary

Stress is defined as any change or challenge in life, and is not intrinsically good or bad.

Acute stress is an intense, short-term reaction by the body's survival mechanism that triggers our systems to focus energy on reacting to a perceived threat. Commonly this is known as the "fight or flight" response and is the type of stress we most often encounter in day-to-day life, such as dealing with road rage.

Chronic or **long-term stress** seems never ending: a bad marriage or an extremely taxing job. This type of stress is a hormonal event affecting every cell in the body. Unlike acute stress, which is a short-lived response to an immediate threat, chronic stress involves long-range responses to a variety of ongoing, negative types of stress, including:

- **Physical stress**: pain, not enough sleep, too little or too much exercise

- **Emotional stress**: anger, jealousy, hatred, fear, or loneliness

- **Mental stress**: vanity, worry, insecurity

- **Chemical stress**: poor nutrition, toxic chemicals

- **Thermal stress**: too hot, too cold, and sudden changes in ambient temperature

- **Electromagnetic stress**: cell phones, computers, electric blankets, computers, microwaves, etc. Electromagnetic fields (EMFs) fields are invisible fields of electric and magnetic force result from the flow of current through wires or electrical devices and increase in strength as the current increases.

Magnetic fields are measured in units of gauss or tesla. Most electrical equipment has to be turned on, i.e., current must be flowing, for a magnetic field to be produced. Electric fields, on the other hand, are present even when the equipment is switched off, as long as it remains connected to the source of electric power.

Both electric and magnetic fields decrease *exponentially* as the distance from the source increases.

A simple way, therefore to reduce the stress of electromagnetic waves is to use a gauss meter. This is an inexpensive tool you can use to survey nearby electromagnetic fields radiation levels (EMFs) from fans, electrical appliances, wiring and power lines from cell towers, microwave beams, high power tension lines, televisions, florescent lights, Wi-Fi and other common sources. Gauss meters are available at some local hardware stores or are found through the internet.

Since Electromagnetic field energy decrease as the distance from the source increases, simply relocate the EMF emitters; even a few inches of repositioning can dramatically help reduce your exposure. [2]

Adrenal glands or **suprarenal glands** sit on top of the kidneys. In response to stress, they produce several hormones that influence our eating habits and fat build up.

Adrenal fatigue syndrome (adrenal burnout) is often caused by chronic stress and occurs when the adrenal glands have reduced hormonal production. Unlike Addison's disease, which is a rare and potentially fatal condition, the adrenals are not as severely underactive with adrenal fatigue syndrome. Instead, the adrenal glands function on a suboptimal level, creating up to 40 symptoms, most commonly fatigue, light sensitivity and getting dizzy or light headed when standing up quickly from a seated or laying position. Adrenal fatigue syndrome is also known as non-Addison's hypoadrenia, hypoadrenalism, and neurasthenia. [5]

Addison's disease is a severe, life-threatening deficiency of the adrenal glands and should not be confused with tired adrenal glands, which we can call adrenal fatigue syndrome or hypoadrenia.

Adrenaline (epinephrine) is an adrenal gland hormone released when our bodies are stressed and switch to the "fight-or-flight" sympathetic nervous system response. This hormone ensures we are physiologically ready to respond to danger, whether we have to run or fight for our lives, by causing:

- Blood glucose (blood sugar) levels to rise

- Blood vessels to constrict

- Blood to be diverted to the brain, heart, and skeletal muscles

Autonomic nervous system controls glands, smooth muscle, and cardiac muscle, which are the processes that maintain balance in the body, known as homeostasis. The autonomic nervous system is also known as the general visceral motor system and the involuntary nervous system. There are two divisions of the autonomic nervous system: the sympathetic and parasympathetic.

Cortisol is one of the adrenal gland hormones and has been called the "stress hormone," because it is released when we experience stress.

DHEA (dehydroepiandrosterone) is a hormone released by the adrenal glands. DHEA decreases body fat, shuts off our appetite; increases muscle mass; improves energy, vitality, sleep, premenstrual symptoms, and mental sharpness; and helps the thyroid hormones function more effectively. In the U.S., DHEA is available without a physician's prescription. If excessive amounts are taken, DHEA may raise testosterone levels and oily skin and acne can result. A simple decrease in the amount taken reverses this.

Sympathetic nervous system is part of an automatic, behind-the-scenes system that triggers our body's "fight or flight" responses, so we are able to handle and face dangerous, crisis-ridden, or stressful situations as they arise. When this system is engaged, blood is pumped to the muscles and brain and shunted away from our digestive system and skin. Our heart pounds and our pupils open wide to better see whatever may be coming at us.

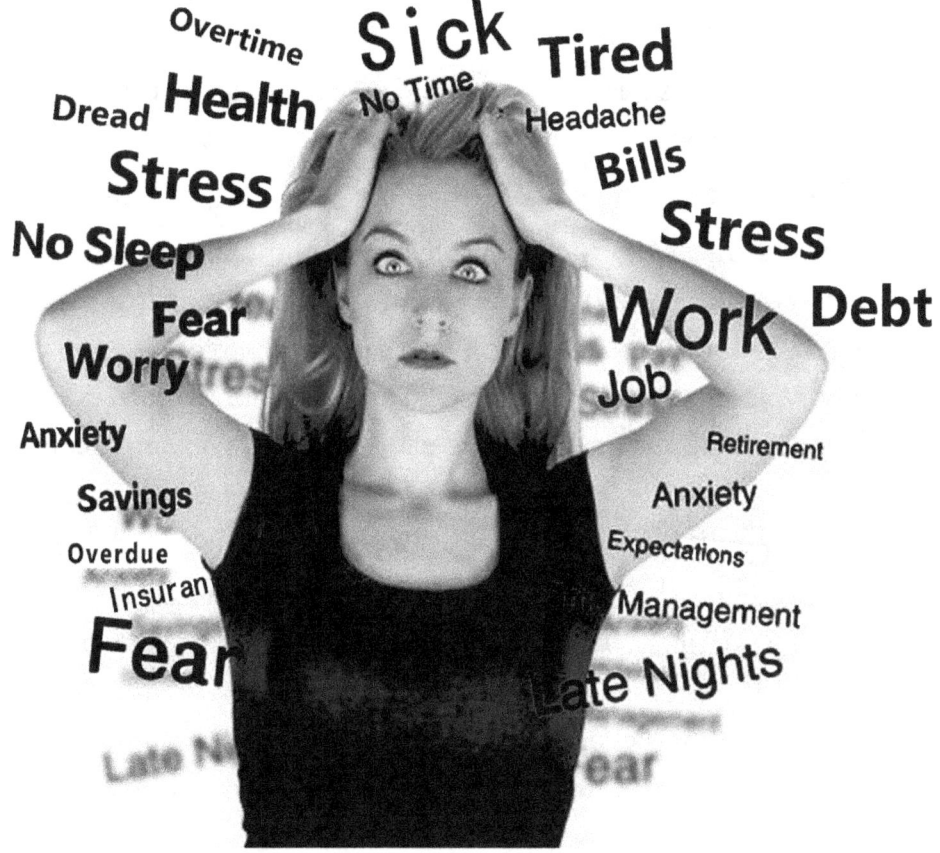

Parasympathetic nervous system keeps the body's energy use low and involves the '3 Ds': digestion, defecation, and diuresis (urination). This system's functions can be summarized as "rest and digest" and is illustrated, for example, in a person who relaxes after a meal. In a state of parasympathetic relaxation, blood pressure, heart rate, and respiratory rates are low, but the gastrointestinal tract is active. The parasympathetic activity also induces stomach acid production and satiates the appetite.[3]

Eating when calm and relaxed, in a parasympathetic mode, leads to better digestion of food, eating less food and also can curb our sweet tooth! Perhaps one day we will do a brief breathing exercise before each meal to switch us from the sympathetic to the 'rest and digest' para-sympathetic mode.

Pharmacological dose or **supraphysiologic dose** involves taking large quantities of an active ingredient, in doses that exceed the levels normally found in the body.

Physiological dose is the amount of a substance the body needs (such as a hormone, mineral, or vitamin), and replace what is lacking, to achieve levels normally found in the body.

Neurotransmitters are chemicals that control the flow of information from one part of the nervous system to another. These chemicals direct every thought, mood, and emotion. They shape our personality, as well as modulate our experience of pain and pleasure. Neurotransmitters control our food carvings, appetite, energy levels, sex drive, and our sleep.

Examples of neurotransmitters that influence our weight include:

- **Dopamine** produces feelings of pleasure when released by the brain's reward system. Low levels of dopamine can trigger cravings for sweets. Dopamine creates the "high" feeling associated with drug use, sex, eating certain foods, and even shopping. Elevations of dopamine are also connected with addictions, such as nicotine, cocaine, and other substances that produce a feeling of excited euphoria by increasing the brain's dopamine levels.

- **GABA** (gamma-aminobutyric acid) is the chief inhibitory neuro-transmitter in the central nervous system. GABA calms us down. Drugs that increase the available amount of GABA in our systems typically have relaxing, anti-anxiety, and anticonvulsive effects. Alcohol; barbiturates, and herbs, like valerian root and skullcap, are common GABA increasing substances.

- **Norepinephrine** (noradrenaline) effects the 'fight-or-flight' response; increasing heart rate, triggering the release of glucose from energy stores, and increasing blood circulation to the body's skeletal muscles. Low levels of norepinephrine increase our appetite for sweets.

- **Serotonin** imparts a feeling of wellbeing and satiates our appetite. Low levels of serotonin increase our appetite for sweets and eating carbo-hydrates, especially white sugar and white starch foods, because they raise serotonin levels. The over-the-counter substances 5-HTP (5-hydroxy-tryptophan) and tryptophan are chemical precursors to serotonin and quickly raise a person's serotonin levels. [4]

Caffeine raises levels of epinephrine (commonly known as adrenaline), and triggers our "flight-or-fight" sympathetic mode. Caffeine also increases dopamine levels. Furthermore, caffeine blocks adenosine, a neurotransmitter. Blocking adenosine, similarly raises the levels of dopamine. In the United States, 90% of adults consume caffeine daily and it is the most widely used drug in the world.

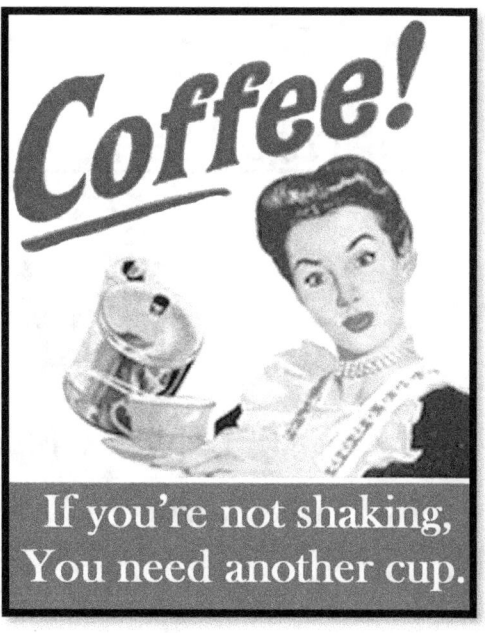

CHRONICALLY ELEVATED CORTISOL

STRESSED BUT COPING.

I'M A 'CAN DO' PERSON.

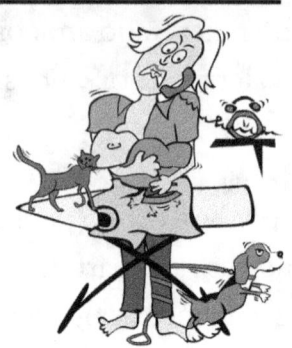

STEEP DROP IN CORTISOL

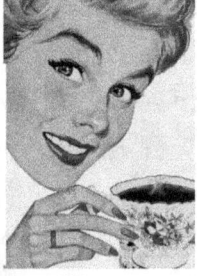

STRESSED AND BY AFTERNOON, I JUST COLLAPSE. BUT WITH SOME SMOKES & COFFEE I MAKE IT THROUGH THE DAY.

I HAVEN'T HAD MY COFFEE YET

DON'T MAKE ME KILL YOU

CORTISOL IS LOW ALL DAY

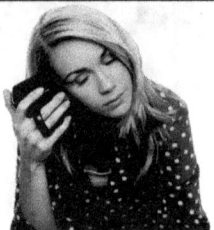

THE CAFFEINE & NICOTINE ARE JUST NOT ENOUGH ANYMORE. HELP !

Chapter 10

To B12 or Not to B12 —That is the Question

Using Sublingual Vitamin B12

Imagine a talented, yet temperamental, Broadway actress. You can't brashly ask her to show up at the theater—she needs a limousine, plush backstage area, and assistants who cater to her every whim. She is a larger-than-life international star whose abilities are unparalleled, and if her specific inflexible demands are not met, she simply refuses to go on stage.

Because otherwise talented cast members can't fill the space left by her absence, they too begin to falter in their roles. So, although her requests may seem rigid and frustrating, everyone's success depends on meeting this finicky, influential individual's needs. In the end, without her powerful presence, the production will fall flat.

Like this Broadway prima donna, vitamin B12 is uniquely skilled, elusive, and requires specific circumstances in order to perform.

Vitamin B12 is needed for the production of crucial neurtransmitters, including dopamine and serotonin, but you can't ask this famous star of blood and brain to simply show up and perform its duties. Long before reaching its performance debut (the stomach) vitamin B12 plays hard-to-get, appearing in significant quantities in just eight foods: liver, sardines, clams, mackerel, herring, croaker, snapper and flounder.

And, like the diva in her limousine, you must arrange special transportation for B12 if you want it to work. As the most-sizable-known vitamin molecule, B12 is 'larger than life' for our bodies, and relies on intrinsic factor, a chemical made in the stomach, to help transport it through the walls of our small intestine. Without adequate intrinsic factor, our bodies simply cannot absorb B12 on their own.

Though its needs and requirements may be greater than other vitamins, B12's critical role in supporting our body's functions makes acquiescing to these wishes in everyone's best interests.

After all, when it comes to a Broadway performance or a healthy life, the show must go on.

Definitions and Glossary—to describe commonly misunderstood terms.

Vitamin B12 is the largest and most-structurally complex vitamin molecule known, and has the chemical name *cyanocobalamin*. Neither plants nor animals are independently capable of making vitamin B12. Only bacteria have the enzymes required for making this vitamin, so animals must get vitamin B12 directly or indirectly from bacteria.

Intrinsic factor (IF) is a chemical that attaches to vitamin B12 and allows it to be absorbed into the body through the small intestine. Intrinsic factor, also known as gastric intrinsic factor (GIF), is produced in the stomach lining by the same cells (parietal cells) that make stomach acid. Without activated intrinsic factor, your body will not absorb adequate levels of B12, no matter how much is in your diet or vitamin pills.

Sublingual Vitamin B12 is a form of vitamin B12 that enters the bloodstream directly, bypassing the need for intrinsic factor. Taken by placing a tablet under the tongue or between the cheek and gums, the medication is absorbed through your mouth's many blood vessels and made available for immediate use by your body.

Pernicious anemia is a pathological manifestation of severe vitamin B12 deficiency most often caused by loss of the stomach's parietal cells, which subsequently causes an inability to absorb vitamin B12. Many clinicians *mistakenly* assume that if pernicious anemia is not present, then that person has an optimal level of B12. If you don't have a vitamin deficiency disease such as, scurvy (vitamin C), beriberi (vitamin B-1), or pellagra (vitamin B-3), is taking a multiple vitamin foolish? Of course not.

Symptoms of Vitamin B12 Deficiency

- Excessive food cravings

- Lack of energy

- Sluggish metabolism

- Tingling and numbness in the feet and hands due to peripheral neuropathy

- Memory loss

- Dementia

- Depression [1-2]

- Muscle aches

- Muscle weakness

Vitamin B12 Deficiency: A Hidden Epidemic

When it comes to a vitamin B12 deficiency, many people believe if you take a multivitamin or are not anemic, then you must be just fine. Unfortunately, that assumption could not be further from the truth.

Unlike many vitamin deficiencies, *low B12 is often caused by suboptimal stomach function, rather than failing to ingest sufficient doses of the vitamin itself.*

Are you …?

Over the age of 40

As we age, our stomachs produce less acid. With each decade the likelihood you will suffer from this deficiency goes up 10%. In other words, 50% of people in their 50s, 60% of people in their 60s, and 70% of people in their 70s have low stomach acid and therefore low vitamin B12. [3]

Taking stomach acid-blocking or acid-neutralizing medications, either over-the-counter or by prescription [4]

Although these medications may help sooth heartburn or gastro-esophageal reflux disease (GERD) by limiting your stomach acid, they are also limiting the function of your intrinsic factor so your body can't properly absorb vitamin B12.

Suffering from chronic stress

The medical journal *Digestive Diseases and Sciences* found that mental stress decreased the output of stomach acid by up to 60% in approximately half the healthy volunteers, therefore causing suboptimal levels of vitamin B12. [5]

Vegetarian or vegan

Vitamin B12 isn't readily available in plants, so deficiencies are very common in individuals who do not consume meat, eggs or fish.

If you answered yes to one or more of the questions, you may be among the 40% of Americans with low levels of vitamin B12.[6] Considering the symptoms range from food cravings to depression to dementia, this unnecessary epidemic must be addressed and remedied.

Do I have your attention now?

How Does a Low Vitamin B12 Level Relate to Healthy Weight Management?

Less than optimal levels of vitamin B12 can sabotage our healthy weight goals in two primary ways:

1. Impedes thyroid function

Without adequate vitamin B12, your body's ability to convert your thyroid hormone T4 into the more active T3 form that your cells can use, will be hampered. Without adequate T3, your metabolism will be lowered. Your body will burn less fuel (food) and store the excess as fat.

2. Triggers craving junk foods

A vitamin B12 deficiency limits your body's ability to produce serotonin and dopamine. Our bodies release these neurotransmitters when we ingest carbohydrates and sweets—which represented dense nutrition to our hunter-gatherer forebears—so the low levels that result from a suboptimal level of vitamin B12 can trigger cravings for sweets, comfort foods, and alcoholic beverages. By combining a sluggish metabolism with unhealthy cravings, a vitamin B12 deficiency delivers a one-two punch that can make weight gain inevitable.

Guidance: Using B12 to Fit Into Your Genes and Cut the Guilt

I believe everyone should consider trying sublingual vitamin B12. Even if you are one of the rare people whose levels of vitamin B12 are already ideal, because B12 is a water-soluble vitamin, any excess is harmlessly secreted in the urine. The downside to trying this absorbable form of vitamin B12 is at the most, $15.00 urinated away. The upside is a whole new lease on life.

Sublingual B12 supplements typically come in doses of 500 to 1000 micrograms per tablet. (1,000 micrograms equals 1 milligram.)

One tablet per day, under the tongue, is the normal trial dose. If you want to try the more potent form of this nutrient, which may increase the positive benefits you experience, the stronger version of sublingual B12 is the methylcobalamin formula. Remember, taking regular B12 vitamin tablets won't work if you have stomach issues; they must be labeled *sublingual* B12 tablets on the bottle.

If your physician is cooperative, other options are either B12 injections or intranasal B12 gel. *B12 injections are the preferred method to use* but require a doctor's prescription.[7]

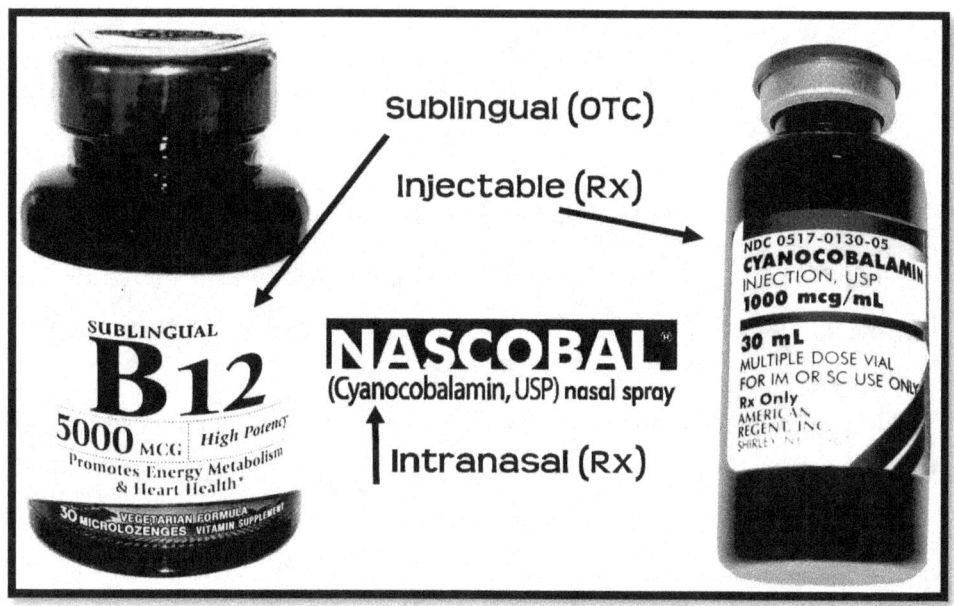

Questions for Your Doctor

The concept of suboptimal levels of vitamin B12 being a common health problem may be in some physicans' "blind spot." You may discuss this topic with your physician, including the use of B12 injections or intranasal B12 gel, and share with him or her the list of *152 medical journal references* on this topic that I have included.[8]

Did You Know

Vitamin B12 Supplements May Reverse Dementia

I was teaching a class on human physiology at a state college in Florida when the topic of vitamin B12 came up. As I have explained in this chapter, I emphasized the difficult nature of B12 absorption and suggested sublingual vitamin B12 supplements, especially for senior citizens.

About six weeks later one of my students asked to speak with me after class. She began crying as she shared this amazing—yet, not rare—story.

My student was in her 50s and her mother had been placed in a special type of assisted living facility due to her dementia. After hearing my lecture she went out and purchased sublingual B12 and instructed the staff at the facility to give her mother this vitamin. Within weeks, she received a phone call from the nursing home's physician, who said her mother was ready to leave the facility. The elderly woman had snapped out of her dementia, was cognitively normal, and wanted to go home.

More Facts about Vitamin B12 and Intrinsic Factor

If low levels of vitamin B12 affect at least 40% of adult Americans, why do so few people know their weight challenges may result from this easy-to-fix deficiency?

For decades, suboptimal vitamin B12 deficiencies got caught in the "peripheral vision" of medicine. Physicians empirically knew that many of their patients over the age of 40, for some reason, felt more vim and vigor after receiving vitamin B12 injections.[9-10] Injectable B12 bypasses the need for intrinsic factor to get the vitamin into the body. But health insurance companies questioned the use of B12 injections when the laboratory tests were normal for pathologically low B12. Severe B12 deficiency causes pernicious anemia that easily shows up on basic blood tests. But can there be negative health consequences of suboptimal levels of vitamin B12 without pernicious anemia being present?

Why, yes, of course!

Our bodies require this water-soluble vitamin for normal brain and nervous system function including the creation of dopamine, serotonin, and norepinephrine. Additionally, B12 is involved in the metabolism of all cells and effects DNA, blood, and energy production.

Without adequate B12 absorption, your entire body may be compromised.

In order to harness this powerful vitamin, the cells in our stomach make a chemical called intrinsic factor that attaches to B12 and allows it to be absorbed through the small intestine's lining so our bodies can utilize it. Intrinsic factor is a glycoprotein produced by the parietal cells of the stomach—the same cells that make stomach acid.

Despite advertisements that make us believe we all suffer from too much stomach acid, a high percent of middle aged people and older seniors actually have too little stomach acid.[11-21] Because the cells that make the stomach acid also make intrinsic factor, poor stomach function not only impedes digestion, it causes low vitamin B12. Without adequate intrinsic factor, you could consume an endless supply of vitamin B12 in your diet or vitamin pills and your body would still not absorb adequate levels.

In addition to aging, many lifestyle choices may contribute to poor stomach function and the resultant, suboptimal vitamin B12 levels, including:

- Diets with heavily cooked foods

- Difficult-to-digest foods, such as fried foods or processed meats

- Foods containing artificial preservatives and/or additives

- Soft drinks, which contain high amounts of phosphorus, high-fructose corn syrup, and/or white sugar

- Combining foods that have different digestive needs, such as fruits for dessert after eating a heavy meat meal

- Eating foods we **are** not genetically designed to eat—from a part of the globe our ancestors were not from. For example, people with a Scandinavian background may not digest oranges well since there are no orange trees in Scandinavia.

Oranges Trees in Scandinavia? No Way.

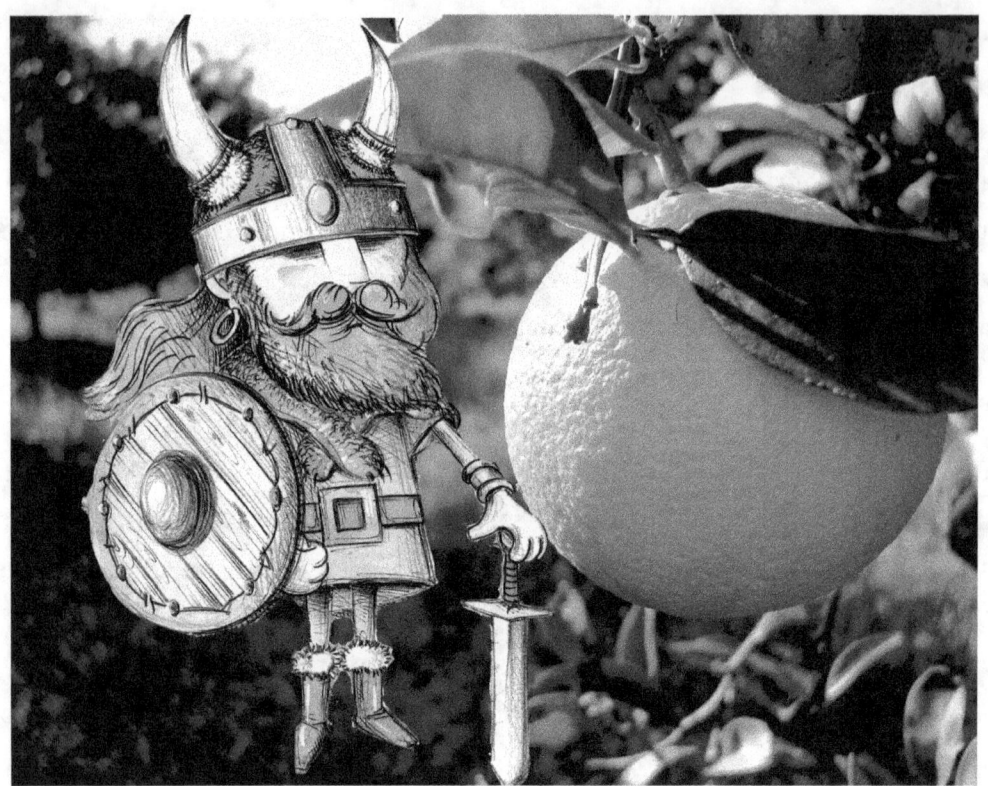

*Suboptimal vitamin B12 levels may be caused by eating foods we **are** not genetically designed to eat—from a part of the globe our ancestors were not from. For instance, people with a Scandinavian background may not digest oranges well since there are no orange trees in Scandinavia.*

Chapter 11

Ladies, Meet Progesterone, the Hormone Your Body Loves

Turning Fat into Energy by Reversing Estrogen Dominance

Estelle and Preston were lead singers in a world renowned band. When they shared the spotlight equally, their voices and instruments blended perfectly, producing genuinely moving music. But after years working together as a band, a misguided music director believed Estelle was more talented and charismatic than Preston. Hoping to increase profits, the music director convinced Estelle to drop her longtime partner and start a solo career.

Unfortunately, Estelle's individual efforts were nothing compared to the sonic brilliance created when both musicians worked together. Her voice sounded shrill without the accompaniment of Preston's voice. The once complex, enchanting guitar melodies were now frilly and frivolous without Preston's bass lines to ground them.

In other words, the unique qualities that made Estelle so compelling were unfulfilled without a balancing musical force. Though talented, she was not a strong solo star, but was truly powerful as half of a duo. Estrogen and progesterone work the same way in women's bodies. Together, they lower the chances of getting breast cancer, support pregnancy, can prevent or reverse osteoporosis, and help women maintain a healthy body weight. But, when estrogen dominates, its unique attributes can ruin a woman's wellness and potentially shorten her life.

Estrogen Dominance: A Growing Epidemic

Women's bodies have naturally evolved to keep estrogen and progesterone in balance, with levels fluctuating through various hormonal stages, including pregnancy and menopause.

During prime reproductive years, progesterone prepares the uterine lining for the implantation of a fertilized egg, among other responsibilities.

Estrogen, is a female hormone involved in ovulation, and also helps ensure a women's body is prepared for pregnancy by triggering fat accumulation. At menopause, as progesterone and estrogen levels diminish when fertility is no longer a concern, their delicate balance should nonetheless remain.

For most of human history, the way our hormones varied with our reproductive needs was a blessing, but now it can be a curse. In our modern society by age 35, *half* of all women in the United States are low in progesterone (also known as estrogen dominance), revealing a true epidemic. And over the past 40 years, female-related illnesses that are believed to share a common link to estrogen dominance have risen dramatically: [1]

◊   Endometriosis affects 10% of all perimenopausal women.

◊   Premenstrual syndrome affects approximately 30% of women.

◊   Uterine fibroids affect approximately 25% of women, age 35 to 50.

◊   Breast cancer in the U.S. affects about one in eight women.

Like so many of our modern health problems, prevalent estrogen dominance cannot be blamed on a single factor. Instead, this debilitating imbalance has a variety of causes, including:

-   Birth control pills, which stop the body's progesterone production by preventing ovulation
-   Hormone replacement therapy that only includes estrogen and not bioidentical progesterone
-   Obesity, in which fat cells cause the conversion of other hormones into estrogen
-   Environmental pesticides, including those found on commercially grown fruits and vegetables [2, 3]
-   Exposure to xenoestrogens (external estrogens) such as those found in herbicides, and petrochemicals common in cosmetics, glue, and plastics.

Toxins commonly found in cosmetics can especially effect young women just entering puberty [4-8]

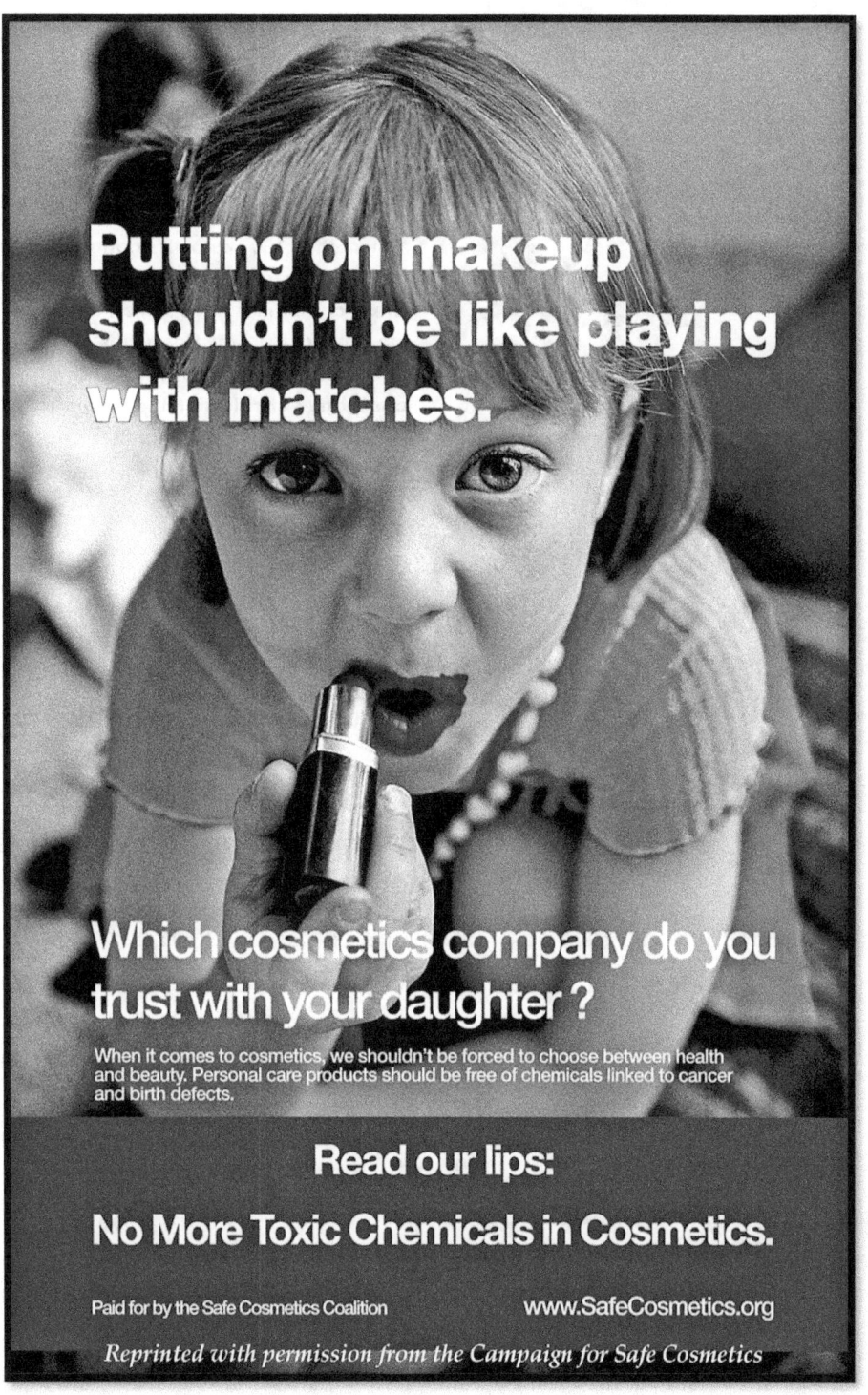

Reprinted with permission from the Campaign for Safe Cosmetics

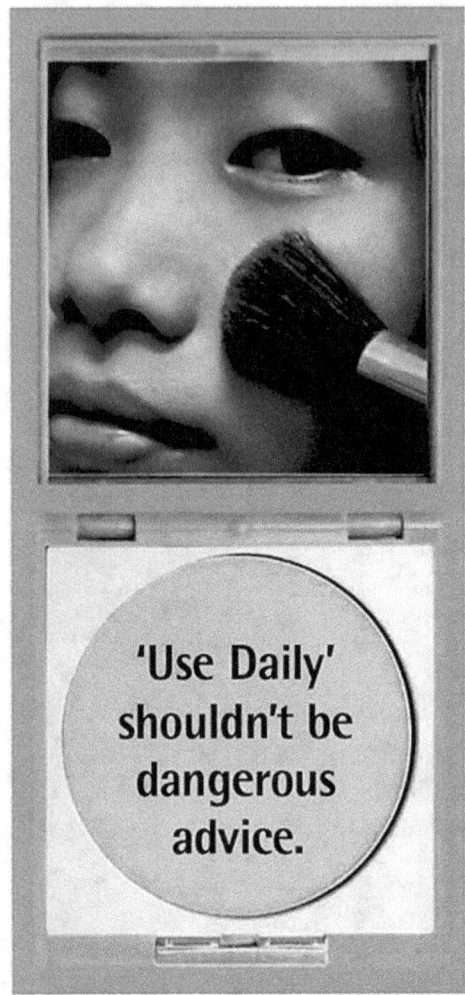

150 cosmetics companies agree: Beauty products don't need to be toxic.

Every day, we use as many as 25 personal care products on our bodies. Some of the chemicals in these products are linked to cancer, infertility and birth defects—and most have never been evaluated for their health effects.

More than 150 cosmetics companies are leading the way in cleaning up their industry. These companies have signed a pledge—the Compact for Safe Cosmetics—to remove hazardous ingredients. Now, all cosmetics companies should sign the Compact and prove that their concern for their customers is more than just skin deep.

Has your favorite brand pledged to make safe products?

The Campaign for Safe Cosmetics
www.SafeCosmetics.org

'Use Daily' shouldn't be dangerous advice.

Reprinted with permission from the Campaign for Safe Cosmetics

When you consider the fact that estrogen dominance not only contributes to weight gain, but also makes women 80% more likely to suffer from breast cancer, this is an epidemic that must be stopped. [9]

Definitions and Glossary—given early in the chapter to share key definitions.

Estrogens are a group of hormones formed in females by the ovaries, placenta, adrenal glands, and fat (adipose tissue). Higher levels of estrogens are associated with weight gain and fluid retention.

Progesterone is the actual specific chemical name for the hormone produced in females in the ovaries after ovulation, and to a much lesser extent, in the adrenal glands. It is sometimes referred to as natural or bioidentical progesterone. During pregnancy, large amounts of progesterone are also produced in the placenta. Although men do produce progesterone, their bodies do so at lower levels in the adrenal glands and the testes.

Progestins, **progestogens** or **gestagens** are a classification of chemical compounds that include drugs related (synthetic analogues) to the naturally occurring hormone, progesterone. Although chemically related, the synthetic versions have a number of unwanted side effects the natural hormone does not. Additionally, the chemically similar but not identical copies, lack many of the miraculous positive effects of bioidentical progesterone. Be aware that many physicians *erroneously* believe that synthetic progestins, such as those in birth control pills as well as the medication Provera®, are actually progesterone. Progestins are often called "progesterone", even in scientific papers! This confusion is so pervasive that progesterone is blamed, due to misunderstanding, but without evidence, for the sins of Provera® (medroxyprogesterone acetate). Their categorization is perhaps somewhat like fossil fuels: Natural gas, coal, gasoline, petroleum, and oil shale are all classified as fossil fuels, but certainly they are not all chemically the same.

Provera® (medroxyprogesterone acetate) is a very commonly prescribed synthetic progestin. Many doctors *mistakenly* think this medication has essentially the same effects on the body as that of the natural hormone progesterone.

Prometrium® is a prescription version of "bioidentical" progesterone in an oral pill.

Symptoms of Suboptimal Progesterone Levels

- Weight gain with fat deposition at the hips and thighs, giving a "pear shaped" fat distribution. Also known as "gynecoid", or "gluteo-femoral" fat distribution [10]

- Craving sweets   - Depression

- Breast swelling   - Premenstrual mood swings

- Water retention   - Uterine fibroids

- Fibrocystic breasts   - Heavy or irregular menstruation

- Loss of libido (sex drive)   - Low body temperature

How Low Progesterone Levels Contribute to Weight Gain

One of the many effects progesterone has on 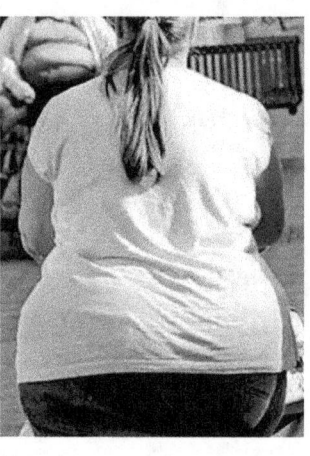 the female body is to promote turning fat into energy, whereas estrogen triggers the body to accumulate fat, resulting in a "pear shaped body."

Estrogen dominance causes weight gain in a variety of ways, including:

1. Triggers fat accumulation in the hips and thighs ("pear shaped" figure)
2. Leads to fluid retention and breast swelling
3. Interferes with thyroid function
4. Impairs blood sugar control and triggers the craving of sweets

Did You Know?

Progesterone Can Help Regenerate Thinning Bones

Progesterone is a powerful hormone. In addition to converting fat into energy, helping you lose weight, and drastically lowering your risk of breast cancer, bioidentical progesterone can also help reverse osteoporosis.

I first learned about progesterone's bone-strengthening benefits while hosting a weekly, call-in radio show from 1992 through 2002. The program discussed current health topics and issues, and experts in various health care fields frequently joined me as guests. Among my most popular visitors was John R. Lee, M.D., who was featured on the show 10 times starting in 1993. At that time, his message regarding hormone replacement therapy for women challenged the mainstream medical position: Doctors were recommending estrogen therapy to prevent menopausal symptoms, as well as osteoporosis (thinning of the bones). Ahead of the league, Dr. Lee pointed out the detriment of this approach, as estrogen only *slows down the loss of bone* (as opposed to preventing it) and only for the first five years of use. Estrogen slows bone loss by retarding the replacing of old, worn out bone. Bioidentical progesterone, on the other hand, stimulates the bone building cells—osteoblasts—and can actually create new, healthy, strong bone rather than simply slowing its loss.

The bulk of the material our bones are made from is not really alive; but rather, the cells within the bones, such as osteoblasts, are the actual living part. Continually rebuilding itself as old bone material wears out, osteoblasts create new material so our bones stay strong.

The medical establishment was slow to accept and adopt this realization. After several years of teaching human anatomy and physiology to future medical clinicians, I read through the latest edition of our textbook and found they announced that bioidentical progesterone stimulates osteoblasts to make new bone. Dr. Lee's assertions may have been doubted at first, but I was excited to see that future health clinicians would now be educated about the important role progesterone can play in treating osteoporosis.

Guidance

Ultimately, finding the proper balance between estrogen and progesteroneis best achieved under a well informed doctor's care. I recommend you seek a physician knowledgeable about the information in this chapter if you find you are:

- Having weight management challenges as well as some of the other listed symptoms of low progesterone or estrogen dominance
- Taking estrogen without bioidentical progesterone
- Taking a progestin and are unsure whether it is bioidentical progesterone

Should you struggle to find a physician who understands and acknowledges the differences between bioidentical progesterone and synthetic progestins, you can contact one of the medical laboratories specializing in estrogen and progesterone testing.

I recommend ZRT Laboratories. Not only do they accept saliva samples from patients without a physician's prescription,[11] they have a list of skilled doctors available on their website. You can visit www.zrtlab.com or call 866-600-1636 to learn more about where to find a clinician in your area who can help you uncover and treat estrogen dominance.

At every stage, I believe an informed patient is best prepared to pursue their greatest lifelong health. For further understanding of estrogen and progesterone, you can also gain a wealth of knowledge by reading any of the four books by Dr. John R. Lee (JohnLeeMD.com):

- *What Your Doctor May Not Tell You About Premenopausal*

- *What Your Doctor May Not Tell You About Menopause*

- *What Your Doctor May Not Tell You About Breast Cancer* by John R. Lee, M.D., David Zava, Ph.D., and Virginia Hopkins

- *Dr. John Lee's Hormone Balance Made Simple* by John R. Lee, M.D. and Virginia Hopkins.

And do not let the titles stop you if you are a young woman; the information is valid—and important—for you, too.

Questions to Ask Your Doctor

As stated, estrogen dominance can increase your chance of getting breast cancer by 80%. Thankfully, these days, most doctors have started realizing the damage caused by traditional hormone replacement therapy (HRT). Hormone replacement therapy usually means an estrogen medication is prescribed alone or an estrogen is given along with a progestin, such as in the case of the drug Prempro. But, if your your doctor happens to be prescribing estrogen to you and not also bioidentical progesterone, you must ask him or her to change your medications, as the two hormones depend on each other. If you are taking a progestin-class drug and are not 100% certain it's bioidentical progesterone, you should also talk to your physician about the hormones you have been prescribed.

When bringing up these topics with your physician, especially when discussing progesterone, you may discover he or she was given inaccurate information by the pharmaceutical companies that make or promote the chemically altered copies of this hormone. As mentioned, most clinicians mistakenly believe that Provera, for example, is the same as the body's own hormone progesterone, but simply a synthetic version.

If your doctor has an indistinct understanding of how the progestin-class chemicals differ from one another, feel free to refer him or her to the further scientific section of this chapter, where I discuss the specific chemical differences. And if you can't get the precise answers and solutions you need from your current physician, see this chapter's *Guidance* section to learn how to find a clinician who will help you prevent estrogen dominance.

Estrogen Dominance

Empowering You with Greater Understanding

Using estrogen and progesterone to fit into your genes and cut the guilt, depends on understanding two important factors: 1) the role each hormone plays, and 2) the difference between bioidentical progesterone and synthetic progestins.

Estrogen and Progesterone

As mentioned earlier in the chapter, estrogen is involved in ovulation and helps ensure fertile women are prepared for pregnancy by triggering the body to accumulate fat. There are three major naturally occurring estrogens in women:

Estrone (E1) – Estrone is produced during menopause.

Estradiol (E2) – Estradiol is the predominant estrogen in non-pregnant females.

Estriol   (E3) – Estriol is the primary estrogen of pregnancy—when levels increase a thousand fold. Estriol has the weakest estrogenic activity, and now studies indicate that in regard to cancer risk, it may be the safest estrogen to use for postmenopausal estrogen replacement therapy.[12-13] Estriol is also the preferred estrogen for topical vaginal use.

Progesterone, on the other hand, is produced in the ovaries after ovulation and turns fat into energy. The word progesterone comes from "pro-gestation" since one effect of this hormone is to help prepare the uterine lining for the implantation of a fertilized egg.

Comparing the Effects of Progesterone and Estrogen

When speaking of the effects of hot or cold water on our body, we describe them separately; however, when hot and cold waters mix, they attenuate and their temperatures neutralize. In much the same manner, progesterone and estrogen's natural attributes balance each other. Consequently, if either hormone is off-balance, the countering hormone will attempt to correct the relationship, thereby resulting in further imbalance. For example, when proper levels of natural progesterone are absent, the body attempts to reduce the effects of estrogen by desensitizing the estrogen receptor sites to lessen estrogen's effects on the body. In other words, low levels of progesterone directly effect estrogen's activity within the body.

Now let's apply their balancing act in regards to eating.

Serotonin is the neurotransmitter that influences our sweet cravings. When serotonin levels are high, our sweet tooth is curbed; conversely, when serotonin levels are low, our sweet tooth is triggered. And eating sweets raises serotonin levels in the body.

What is one of the hormones controlling the effects of serotonin? Estrogen. Estrogen can increase the effects of serotonin by increasing the number of serotonin receptors and also increasing the secretion of serotonin. But, remember, when the proper level of natural progesterone is absent, the body diminishes estrogen's serotonin enhancing effects.

On the flip side, the chemical dopamine reduces our appetite. And both estrogen and progesterone can directly effect dopamine. How? Estrogen will increase dopamine's effect in the body, while low progesterone will decrease estrogen's effect on dopamine. So when progesterone is low, our sweet tooth and overall desire for pleasurable foods rises. And eating sweets and chocolate increases both serotonin and dopamine.

Their delicate balancing act and side effects are directly related and can play a large role in our ability to control our appetite and food cravings.

Historically, estrogen has been prescribed to menopausal women to combat unpleasant experiences, such as hot flashes and/or vaginal dryness. At menopause however, the ovaries stop making significant amounts of both estrogen and progesterone, so why would we only replace estrogen, thus upsetting women's natural hormonal balance? Solely prescribing estrogen causes estrogen dominance.

PROGESTERONE Bio-Identical	ESTROGEN
Protects against fibrocystic breasts	Can cause fibrocystic breasts
80% reduction in breast cancer	Increases risk of breast cancer
Helps use fat for energy	Increases body fat
Natural diuretic	Triggers fluid retention
Natural anti-depressant	Can cause depression
Help thyroid hormone action	Interferes with thyroid hormone
Normalizes blood clotting	Increases blood clotting
Restores Libido	Decreases libido
Normalizes blood sugar levels	Impairs blood sugar control
Helps prevent endometrial cancer and endometriosis	Increases risk of endometrial cancer and endometriosis
Builds strong bones	Only slows rate of bone loss for the 1st 5 years of use
Helps premenstrual syndrome (PMS)	Can cause PMS
Anti-inflammatory agent	

Progesterone and Progestins

Many experts, such as John R. Lee, MD, do not object to the use of estrogens for postmenopausal problems if used concurrently with bioidentical progesterone.[14] For instance, women with low levels of body fat may need to use estrogen hormone replacement therapy to alleviate hot flashes and/or vaginal dryness.[15-16] Although the use of estrogens may in these instances be necessary, estrogens should only be given along with bioidentical progesterone. But, herein lies the dilemma: Many people—even physicians—believe bioidentical progesterone and other progestins, such as the popular drug Provera®, are the same. They are not!

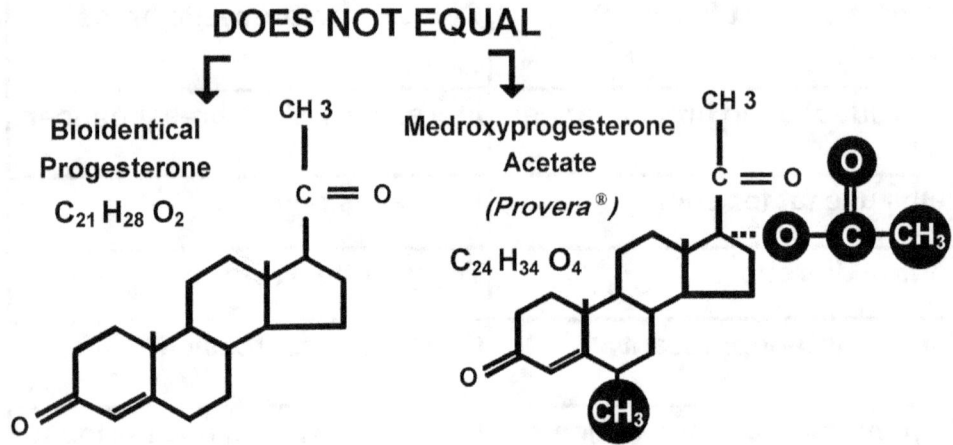

Just as oranges and apples are both fruits, but very different from each other, progesterone and Provera® are both in the progestin chemical class, but they are not chemically the same hormone. Although your doctor may believe a synthetic progestin and natural progesterone are the same, these medications have completely different chemical structures, and with their molecular alterations come a host of unwanted potential side effects not found with natural progesterone. Some of the negative effects of Provera®:

- Increased risk of breast cancer, *whereas bioidentical progesterone greatly reduces the risk of breast cancer* [17]
- Birth defects
- Thrombophlebitis, cerebral thrombosis (stroke)

- Depression
- Acne
- Hair loss
- Hirsutism (excessive growth of hair usually on a female's face and/or body)

Additionally, if you are taking a synthetic progestin along with estrogen, the combination can cause:

- High blood pressure (hypertension)
- Headaches
- Dizziness
- Nervousness
- Fatigue
- Premenstrual-like syndrome

Whereas, the real hormone progesterone does not cause any of these symptoms or side effects.

Consider this: Synthetic progestins are so powerful, they bind-up the body's progesterone receptor sites, thus blocking the healthy effects of the real or bioidentical progesterone. In other words, if you are taking a synthetic progestin, as in birth control pills for example and bioidentical progesterone at the same time, the synthetic drug will nullify the positive benefits of the bioidentical progesterone.

There are two forms of bioidentical progesterone available at present: Micronized progesterone—sold as the prescription medication Prometrium® in an oral capsule form only, and topical creams that are applied to the skin. Instead of hindering the body's systems, like their synthetic counterparts, bioidentical progesterone actually increases estrogen's effectiveness—whether it is a prescription or the body's own. Consequently, lower doses of estrogen are the typical rule when given along with bioidentical progesterone.

Thus, in most cases of women with excess body fat, when progesterone is added, the body's own (endogenous) estrogen is sufficient to alleviate the symptoms of low estrogen, such as hot flashes and vaginal dryness.

By balancing estrogen and progesterone with natural, bioidentical hormones, women are able to alleviate discomfort—and *fit into their genes* and *cut the guilt*.

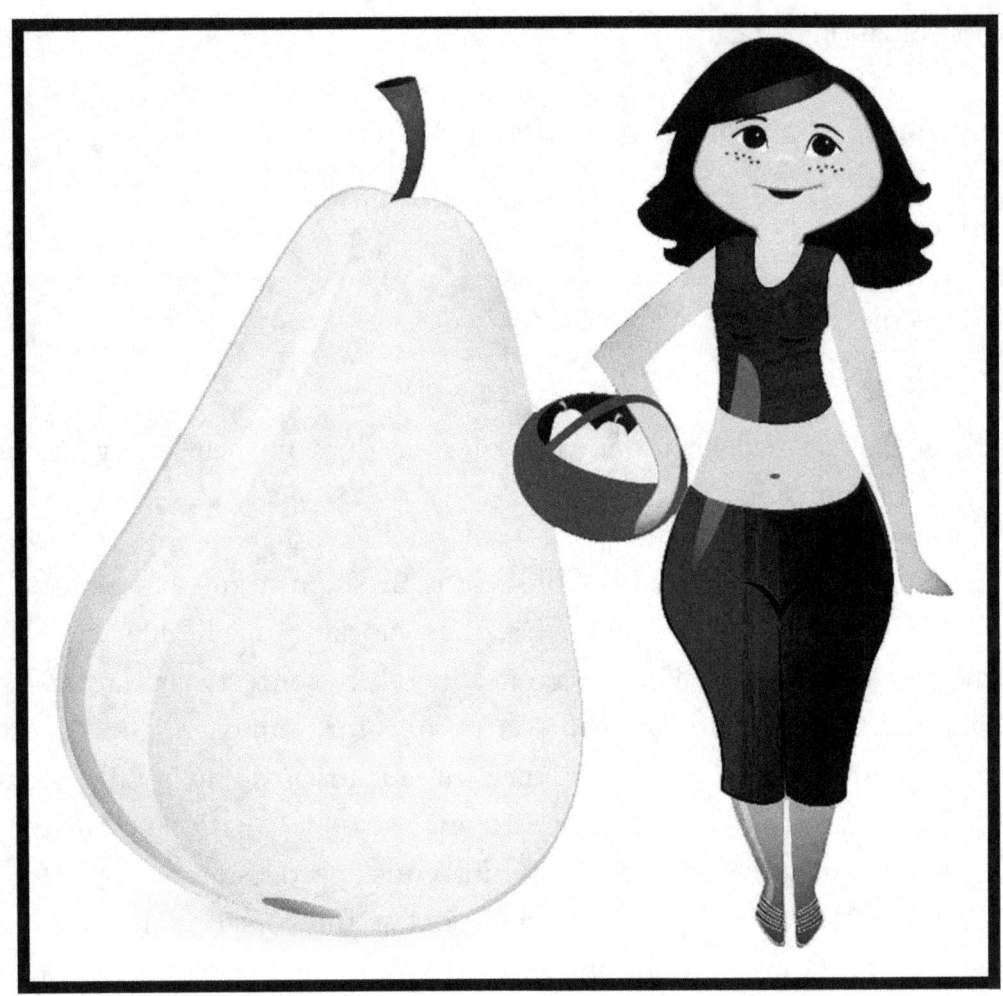

Pear Shaped Figure
(Fat Deposition in Hips & Thighs)
Caused by Low Progesterone
(Estrogen Dominance)

Chapter 12

A Sweet Tooth Can Be a Bitter Pill to Swallow

Have you ever gone camping in cold weather?

Without the comforts of home, you must rely on a fire to keep warm. When building and maintaining your fire, there are two types of fuel you can choose: leaves or logs. The leaves give a sudden burst of flames and heat—but even large quantities are burnt up too quickly, leaving you constantly scrambling to find more before your fire goes out. On the other hand, logs take longer to start and lack the instant-burning gratification the leaves provide. But, once ignited, they yield flames and heat that last much longer, so you are able to enjoy the experience, instead of running around trying to make sure you can find leaves to keep your fire going.

Your body's metabolism of sugars and carbohydrates is just like a campfire.

Refined foods, like those made with white flour and white sugar, are similar to leaves used for kindling: They offer a burst of energy and instant gratification, but when they burnout, we are quickly left searching for more.

Unrefined foods, like molasses and whole grains, are similar to logs: They offer your body dense nutrition, which is slow burning and provides lasting energy.

Refined foods stoke your sweet tooth and ignite cravings, whereas unrefined foods calm your appetite, minimize sweet cravings and keep you satiated for hours.

If you ever feel your sweet tooth is out of control—and you're having difficulty fulfilling the cravings—imagine you are desperately grabbing for leaves as your campfire dwindles. You now have a clearer and accurate picture of how your body reacts when its energy sources are depleted.

As you work to fit into your genes and cut the guilt, isn't it time you added some real fuel to the fire?

Our National Sweet Tooth is a Bitter Pill to Swallow

One hundred years ago, the average American adult ate about one pound of sugar, per year. Today, we consume about 150 pounds of sugar in the same amount of time! [1]

The average person eats about 20 teaspoons of sugar a day, with more than 99% of the consumption in the form of white table sugar and corn sweeteners. American adolescents consume an extra 15 to 20 teaspoons of sugar each day by drinking soda pop—which can increase their risk of obesity by up to 60%. [2]

A Broad Look at the Sugar Saga

Today, the food industry's sugar refinement or processing has changed the body's ability to deal with common sweets. In their natural form, sweet-tasting foods are always combined with other nutrients to help the body deal with the sugars they contain. Sugar cane, for example, is naturally sweet. But we process it and remove the molasses, where you'll find all the minerals, vitamins and enzymes. What remains is white sugar: a refined, super-concentrated sweetener stripped of the vitamins, minerals and other nutrients that help our body utilize this sweet food in a balanced and healthy way.

And sucrose ($C_{12}H_{22}O_{11}$), commonly called table sugar, is not the only sweetener contributing to the problem.

Corn sweeteners have actually replaced table sugar in many processed foods, such as soda pop and baked goods. One of the most common types is high fructose corn syrup (HFCS), which can disrupt the body's natural balance due to its large percentages of fructose—a type of sugar that may contribute to insulin resistance.

Choosing versus Craving

First, let's distinguish between fantasy and reality: Fantasizing about how a piece of pie would taste versus being ready to do almost anything to get your favorite sweet.

We are naturally inclined to enjoy sweet tastes. But when you are willing to make a midnight grocery store trip because you're out of ice cream, soda pop, cake, pie, or candy, then you have a sure sign your biochemistry is out of control.

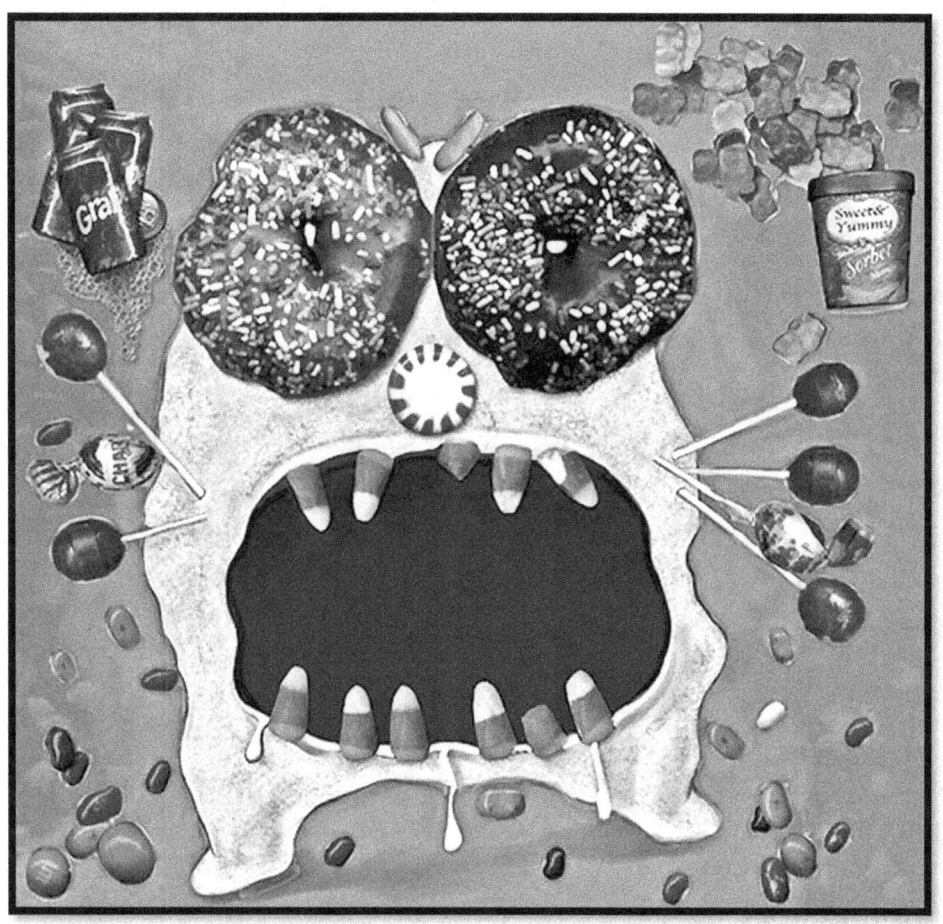

Our bodies are designed to maintain blood sugar (glucose) levels, because glucose is the brain's only required fuel other than oxygen. Low blood sugar can cause irreparable damage to the brain, so we are hard-wired to find sugar sources when our levels deplete. For healthy individuals, when their blood sugar levels drop, the body simply borrows stored sugars from the muscles and liver, and dumps them into the blood stream to provide fuel for the brain. Even if he or she has not eaten all day, a hormonally balanced individual will not actually crave refined carbohydrate foods as a source for glucose, because their bodies are able to successfully access the stored sugars.

For many people however, suboptimal nutrient levels have caused them to lose their delicate hormonal balance. As a result, when faced with low blood sugar, rather than using the body's reserves, cravings set in.

In order to protect the brain from damage caused by low blood glucose levels, we'll do whatever it takes to raise that level—and do it now. Most people with a sweet tooth satisfy their cravings with refined carbohydrates—white sugar and white flour—because they quickly raise blood sugar levels. But, like leaves in a campfire, these sugars burn out before providing the real energy the body needs. And once they're gone, we are again left scrambling to find more fuel.

Rely on refined sugars and carbohydrates too much, and you create a vicious cycle for your body: Low nutrient levels create intense, low-blood-sugar responses, which trigger nearly unmanageable sweet cravings. The quick-burning fuel provides a brief break from low blood sugar, but once exhausted, your body triggers sweet cravings to fuel the brain all over again, so you eat some more sweets ... and on and on.

But your health doesn't have to be this way.

By balancing your hormones and blood sugar, and choosing unrefined foods that add logs to your fire, not leaves, you can tame an out-of-control sweet tooth to fit into your genes and cut the guilt.

Definitions and Glossary (Shared early in the chapter to clarify key points.)

Refined sugars and **refined carbohydrates** have had vitamins, minerals, enzymes and other key nutrients removed in their processing. Common examples include white sugar and white flour, which are used in many snack foods and desserts, such as donuts, pastries, cakes, brownies, pretzels, soda pop and candies.

Although some processed foods using refined sugars and carbohydrates fortify their products with additional nutrients, they still lack many of the substances found in nature's own recipes.

When you obtain sugars and carbohydrates from whole foods, the rate of absorption dramatically slows down due to the other natural compounds bound to the sugars. When these same carbohydrates are obtained in a refined state, large amounts of insulin are released to manage the sugar surge, resulting in significant, negative health repercussions. [3]

Glucose or **blood sugar** is the principal, circulating sugar in our blood; major energy source of the body; and the only fuel our brain requires other than oxygen.

Hypoglycemia is low blood sugar.

Insulin is a hormone secreted by the pancreas and released into the blood when glucose levels go up, such as after eating. Without insulin, most cells are unable to use glucose for energy. Insulin satiates our appetite. In addition, insulin increases leptin release, which is also an appetite suppressant.

Pancreas is a gland near the stomach that secretes insulin and digestive juices (enzymes).

Liver is a glandular organ that secretes bile, stores and filters blood, and is involved in the conversion of sugars into stored sugar. The liver has over 500 known functions.

Adrenal glands or suprarenal glands each sit on top of a kidney. In response to stress, the two adrenal glands produce several hormones that influence our eating habits, blood sugar levels, and fat accumulation.

Carboholic is someone who consumes carbohydrates in excess, to the point of harming themselves.

Neurotransmitters are chemicals that control the flow of information from one part of the nervous system to another. These chemicals direct every thought, mood, and emotion. They shape our personality, as well as modulate our experience of pain and pleasure. Neurotransmitters control our food cravings, appetite, energy levels, sex drive, and our sleep. We know of about 100 neurotransmitters.

Serotonin is a neurotransmitter involved in many functions, including mood, appetite, and sensory perception. Low serotonin levels increase our appetite for sweets. Women make about seven times less serotonin in their brains then men do and this may explains why women crave sweets more than men.

Dopamine is a neurotransmitter that produces feelings of pleasure when released by the brain's reward system. Low dopamine levels can trigger cravings for sweets.

Prozac® and Sweets Raise Serotonin Levels

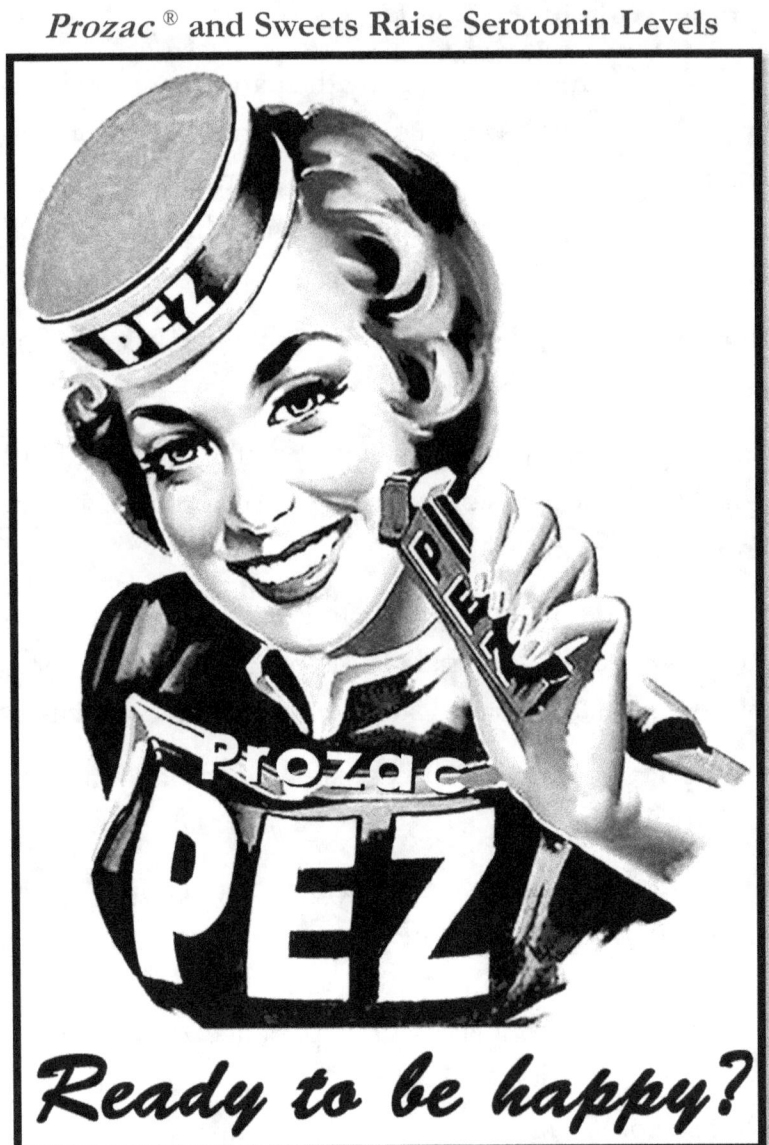

In the U.S. we eat more than 3 billion of the tiny "bricks" of candy annually.

(Source: Pez Company, Inc.)

Common Symptoms of Low Blood Sugar

Because our brains rely on glucose for functioning, the symptoms of hypoglycemia vary based on how low our blood sugar levels become. Although the most common experiences would be considered a "mild low-blood-sugar event," the effects can nonetheless devastate our ability to achieve true health.

Symptoms of a *mild low-blood-sugar* event occur most often with blood sugar falling below 70 milligrams/dL and may include:

- Extreme hunger, especially for sweets

- Feeling nervous

- Cold wet skin and/or excessive sweating

- A rapid pulse

- Numbness or tingling of the fingertips or lips

- Being shaky or trembling

- Nausea

Symptoms of *moderate low-blood-sugar* event occur most often with blood sugar falling below 55 milligrams/dL and may include:

- Changes in mood: anger, anxiety, irritability

- Inability to concentrate or think, confusion

- Fatigue, weakness

- Blurred vision

- Dizziness

- Headache

- Poor coordination

- Difficulty walking or talking, slurred speech

Symptoms of a *severe low-blood-sugar* event occur most often with blood sugar falling below 35-40 milligrams/dL and may include:

- Seizures or convulsions

- Loss of consciousness

- Coma

- Low body temperature

- Irreversible brain damage (if prolonged)

- Death

How an Unchecked Sweet Tooth Contributes to Weight Gain

Simply put, the seesaw experience of low blood sugar triggering sweet cravings causes many people to overeat AND choose high-caloric foods, low in overall nutritional value. Not only are you driven to eat too much, the very foods you turn to contribute to your ongoing struggle with blood sugar levels.

Eating to provide the body with adequate nutrition is necessary, but over-consuming foods, especially high-calorie, low nutrition foods, is disastrous to our health. On the other hand, expecting our bodies to ignore powerful survival instincts commanded by our brain is unrealistic. Instead, we must realign our cravings and nutritional needs by shutting down the misdirected, destructive urges.

For many people, overcoming the uncontrollable desire for refined carbohydrates—such as donuts, pastries, cakes, brownies, pretzels, soda pop, and candies—is a prerequisite to achieving their healthy weight.

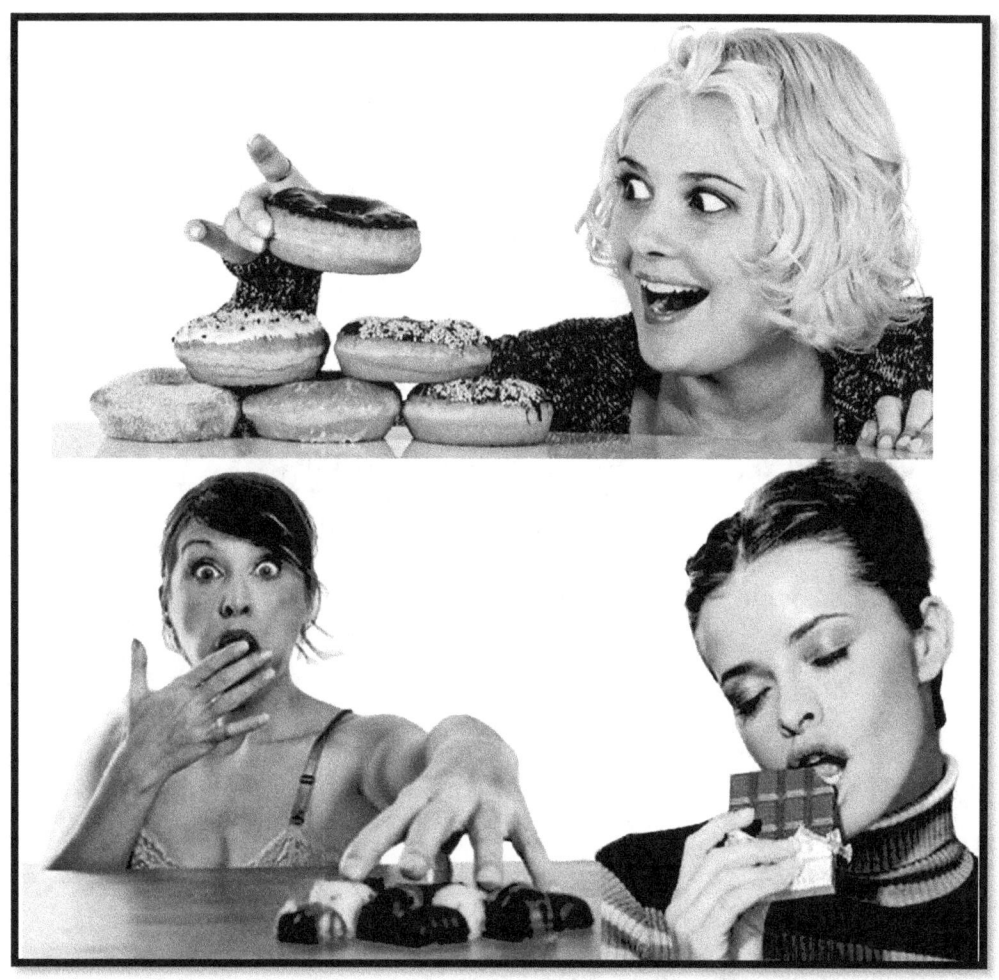

For many people, overcoming the uncontrollable desire for refined carbohydrates—such as donuts, pastries, cakes, brownies, pretzels, soda pop, and candies—is a prerequisite to achieving their healthy weight.

Did You Know?

Many Experts Believe Sugar is as Addictive as Tobacco? [4-6]

There is even a name for someone who is addicted to sweets: carboholic.

And as if weight gain isn't bad enough, refined sugars can cause a wide range of devastating health problems.

Author Nancy Appleton, Ph.D., compiled a list entitled "108 Ways Sugar Can Ruin Your Health," pulling data from a number of medical journals and other scientific publications. The following 10 examples of sugar's metabolic consequences represent less than 10% of the negative effects she compiled. According to Dr. Appleton's list, sugar can:

- Suppress the immune system

- Produce a significant rise in triglycerides

- Promote an elevation of harmful cholesterol (LDLs)

- Speed the aging process, causing wrinkles and gray hair

- Contribute to osteoporosis

- Cause food allergies

- Cause headaches, including migraines

- Alter the mind's ability to think clearly by increasing delta, alpha, and theta brain waves

- Cause depression

- Exacerbate premenstrual syndrome (PMS)

When we can no longer deal with refined carbohydrates in a healthy manner, the resultant condition of carboholic lifestyles has been euphemistically called "a sweet tooth." But as you can see from this list, there is nothing sweet about the damage refined sugars and carbohydrates can cause for our health.

Guidance

So, how do we cure the underlying imbalances that are actually responsible for our sweet tooth?

The first step is understanding that the cravings can be caused by two problems: low-blood sugar (hypoglycemia) or a serotonin-dopamine imbalance.

Determining whether "carboholic" sweet cravings are brought on by low blood sugar or suboptimal levels of dopamine and/or serotonin is easy. Purchase an inexpensive glucose meter ($25.00 is an average price) at your local pharmacy and use it to check your blood sugar level when in the midst of a "got to have a sweet" frenzy.

If your blood glucose level is below 80, then hypoglycemia is likely triggering your sweet tooth. The solution? You must strengthen the hormonal glands responsible for maintaining healthy blood sugar levels: the adrenal glands, liver, pancreas, and thyroid gland. (For information on the thyroid gland, please refer to chapter 8 on metabolism and for the adrenal glands, please refer to chapter 9 on stress).

If your blood glucose level is in the 80 to 90 range or higher, you probably have a dopamine and/or serotonin imbalance driving your hunger for sweets. This imbalance causes you to experience low blood sugar-like cravings, without actually suffering from hypoglycemia. Curbing your sweet tooth will depend on adequate dopamine and/or serotonin levels. Some ways you can increase these neurotransmitters to achieve your healthy weight are to use these nutritional supplements:

- **5-HTP** (5-hydroxytryptophan) and **tryptophan** raise serotonin levels. 5-HTP is made from the seeds of the West African plant, *Griffonia simplicifolia*. It is available over-the-counter in the United States. If a person is on prescription SSRI (serotonin selective reuptake inhibitor) or SNRI (serotonin norepinephrine reuptake inhibitor) medications, 5-HTP or tryptophan should only be used under the care of a clinician. Typical daily amounts taken are, 50-800 milligrams of 5-HTP or 1,000 milligrams of tryptophan, in divided doses. [7]

- **Hypericum perforatum**, an herb commonly known as St. John's Wort, has been shown to raise the levels of serotonin, norepinephrine and dopamine.[8-9] Since there can be interactions with some pharmaceuticals, such as SSRI (serotonin selective reuptake inhibitor) or SNRI (serotonin norepinephrine reuptake inhibitor) medications, inform your clinicians before taking St. John's Wort. The commonly used standard dose of St. John's Wort is 900 milligrams per day (given as 300 milligrams tablets or capsules, three times per day).

Mucuna pruriens, an herb also known as "velvet bean," "cowhage," "kapikachu," or "atmagupta" in India, can raise dopamine levels. This herb contains a precursor to the neurotransmitter dopamine, called L-Dopa.[10-11] When taking this herb, medical guidance is suggested. The correct dose varies and often clinicians start patients with a low dose of mucuna pruriens and then proceed to a higher dosage. The powdered mucuna pruriens dosage often used is 1 teaspoon daily.

Talking to Your Doctor

Be aware: Some clinicians are still unsure at what point they should start acknowledging a patient's low blood sugar symptoms as an actual health problem. Since low blood sugar episodes throughout the day are so common and most are self-treated by grabbing another sweet treat, dismissing low blood sugar as just "normal societal eating behavior" is understandable.

Though common the behavior may be, healthy, it definitely is not.

High blood sugar is a well acknowledged, serious health issue known as diabetes mellitus, commonly referred to as diabetes. Conversely, when addressing low blood sugar problems, unless you exhibit signs of severe low blood sugar, such as passing out, most physicians may be of little help in balancing your sweet cravings and getting your health in order.

Should you be experiencing an uncontrollable sweet tooth and symptoms of low blood sugar, have your clinician aid you by ordering thyroid tests, conducting adrenal function tests, and checking your vitamin B12 level.

Further Science Section:

Balancing Sugar to Balance Cravings

The brain lives on two basic biological foods: oxygen and blood sugar (glucose). These two 'nutrients' are so crucial for the brain's survival that the body has automatic mechanisms to ensure a constant and ready supply of both oxygen and blood sugar. Most tissues can shift to fats and proteins for energy in the absence of glucose, but glucose is the only nutrient that can be utilized by the brain and retina.12

Within the brain stem is the control center that automates our breathing. We breathe in and out without conscious thought. Imagine if we had to always remember to breathe—it just would not work. If we deny our brain oxygen for five minutes or longer, under most circumstances we will have permanent brain damage. By automating the respiratory system, our body ensures the brain will get the oxygen needed to fuel its processes.

Just as the brain stem automatically regulates our breathing, the hormonal system regulates our blood sugar levels. Between meals, our glucose levels should slowly drop. When the levels get below a certain point, we get hungry. If food is not eaten, the hormonal system kicks in and mobilizes stored sugars in the muscles and liver to be released into the blood stream.

The hormonal glands in charge of this process are the pancreas, the adrenal glands, and the liver. The thyroid gland also plays a role by regulating the rate of intestinal absorption of sugars. *If the adrenal glands, liver, pancreas, or thyroid are even marginally weak, the body won't regulate blood sugar efficiently.*

Processing Sugars

Ever wonder why you get a sugar rush? Most of our cells need help absorbing glucose, but the brain and the retinas are noted exceptions. Glucose can travel into their cells without a transporting agent, so when you eat concentrated or refined carbohydrates, the sugar truly does go right to your head (brain).

For the rest of the body's cells to receive adequate quantities of glucose, however, a helper called insulin is needed. Made in the pancreas, insulin is a hormone that allows glucose to be delivered into the cell across the cell membrane. When you eat sugars, the pancreas releases insulin into the blood to help cells access the sugar and convert it into energy. When the body senses a greater quantity of sugar being absorbed across the intestinal membrane and into the blood stream, it releases a correspondingly greater amount of insulin. Like so many of our body's processes, balance is the key to health.

But problems arise when we eat refined sugars.

We simply were not designed to handle these refined foods. Though our diets have changed, our bodies still assume the sugars we ingest come from fruits and other nutrient rich sources. So, when we eat refined carbohydrates our body overreacts. The mislead hormonal system believes we have ingested a huge quantity of foods containing complex carbohydrates, rather than a relatively small amount of food with highly concentrated, refined sugars and starches.

To handle the sugars, the pancreas releases a huge dose of insulin into the blood stream. Now, we have too much insulin circulating in the blood stream because our blood sugar (glucose) sensing mechanism was was tricked with refined cabohydrates. This hyperinsulinism (high insulin) causes a rapid transport of blood sugar into the cells. Then, the blood sugar level drops very quickly due to the overabundance of insulin in the bloodstream.

When the glucose is so quickly pulled by the high insulin levels from the bloodstream and absorbed into the cells, the body's hormonal system releases an emergency warning: The delicate brain must be protected from damage should the blood glucose level drop too far.

Now the pancreas kicks in again.

A hormonal message from the pancreas is sent to the liver informing that organ to release stored glucose into the bloodstream. The adrenal glands also send hormonal messages to the liver and muscles to release their stored sugars.

When properly functioning, we should hardly know anything is wrong. If our hormonal backup system is functioning properly, our blood sugar level never gets low enough to send us on a sweet binge. Our only sense of *dis-ease* occurs if the blood sugar drops below the brain's comfort zone and ignites our cravings for sweets.

The hormonal control system often weakens, though. The problem is a common culprit: stress.

Everyday life in the 21st century is very hard on the four parts of our hormonal system that regulate low blood sugar: the adrenal glands, liver, pancreas, and thyroid gland. These components of the body's mechanism to regulate our blood sugar are often abused in modern times. They are typically too exhausted to deal with a daily diet of refined carbohydrates.

Chapter 13

Light Up Your Health

Seasonal Affective Disorder and Weight Gain

Imagine winter as a wild animal: cold nights, short days, and scarce food supplies. Unless animals migrate to balmier climates, to survive they must stay as warm as possible and burn as few calories as they can. Low activity levels, calorie-dense foods and a thick body-fat layer are animals' best winter friends—they were for our ancestors, too.

Just as hibernating animals fight the threat of winter starvation by fattening up before the coldest months, humans also evolved to prepare for the season. For us, surviving winter means eating heavier foods, limiting our daytime activities and sleeping longer.

But with advances in shelter and food production, we no longer have to rely solely on body fat and idle life-styles to endure the cold months. Consequently, what was once a survival mechanism akin to animals' hibernation is now considered a diagnosable condition: seasonal affective disorder (SAD).

Winter Weight Gain: Beyond Holiday Indulgence

Many people gain weight in the fall and winter. The days are shorter and colder, which can make outdoor exercising more challenging. Thanksgiving, Christmas, and Hanukah include great feasts filled with heavy, traditional food. Holiday parties feature tasty treats and indulgent drinks. Cookies, candies, and cakes are everywhere. For many of us, November and December are times for festive overindulgence, leading headlong into New Year's Resolutions to lose those additional pounds brought on by too much celebration.

Of course, the extra calories add up for everyone, but for some individuals, winter weight gain goes beyond holiday indulgence.

Instead, some people react to the diminishing daylight hours with depression, exhaustion, and carbohydrate cravings as a result of seasonal affective disorder (SAD). Rather than simply gaining weight from eating too many cookies and treats on too many occasions, people with SAD struggle with weight gain because their delicate hormonal balance is disrupted by winter's short days and long nights.

Definitions and Glossary (shared early to fascilitate understanding this chapter)

   Seasonal affective disorder (SAD), also known as winter depression, is a condition characterized by depresssion in the fall and winter months due to a lack of sunlight exposure. Lowered serotonin, nor-epinephrine, and dopamine levels are believed to trigger this condition, which often causes sufferers to crave carbohydrates and gain weight. additionally, people with SAD are more attuned to smells and therefore have an increased interest in foods. [1-5]

   Neurotransmitters are chemicals that control the flow of information from one part of the nervous system to another. These chemicals direct every thought, mood, and emotion. They shape our personality, as well as modulate our experience of pain and pleasure. Neurotransmitters control our food cravings, appetite, energy levels, sex drive, and our sleep.

   Serotonin is a neurotransmitter involved in many functions, including mood, appetite, and sensory perception. Low serotonin levels increase our appetite for sweets.

   Dopamine is a neurotransmitter that produces feelings of pleasure when released by the brain's reward system. Low dopamine levels can trigger cravings for sweets.

   Norepinephrine also known as noradrenaline is a neurotransmitter. Low levels of norepinephrine increase our appetite for sweets.

   5-HTP (5-hydroxytryptophan) is an amino acid precursor to the neurotransmitter serotonin. Supplementing with 5-HTP may be useful in treating depression, fibromyalgia, tension, and migraine headaches, and as an adjunct to weight loss. 5-HTP is isolated from the seeds of the West

African plant *Griffonia simplicifolia*, and is available over-the-counter in the United States. There are no known side effects; though it should not be taken concurrently with SSRI (serotonin selective reuptake inhibitor) or SNRI (serotonin norepinephrine reuptake inhibitor) medications.

Melatonin is a neuroendocrine-hormonal regulator involved with sleep inducing signals, day/night cycles, and body temperature. It also makes us drowsy and induces sleep. Produced by the pineal gland in the brain, a pea-size organ behind the hypothalamus, melatonin is often considered the "darkness" hormone since it is released in response to the absence of light. Melatonin is available over-the-counter in the U.S.

Hypericum perforatum, commonly known as St. John's Wort, is an herb that has been shown to raise the levels of serotonin, norepinephrine, and dopamine.[6-7] Since there can be interactions with some pharmaceuticals, such as SSRI (serotonin selective reuptake inhibitor) or SNRI (serotonin norepinephrine reuptake inhibitor) medications, inform your clinicians before taking.

Symptoms of Seasonal Affective Disorder (SAD) [8-11]

- Weight gain

- Appetite changes, especially craving foods high in carbohydrates

- Depression, hopelessness

- Anxiety

- Loss of energy

- Social withdrawal

- Oversleeping

- Loss of interest in activities you once enjoyed

- Difficulty concentrating and processing information

How Seasonal Affective Disorder Relates to Weight Gain

As we have discussed in previous chapters, low levels of the neuro-transmitter serotonin can trigger cravings for sweets and other dietary carbohydrates. Serotonin levels vary with the seasons, dipping the lowest during the winter months of December and January in the northern hemisphere. People with SAD have particularly low serotonin levels, so they feel energized after eating carbohydrates. Without a natural, internal source for serotonin, they lack energy, are less inclined to exercise, and are driven to continually binge on carbs. The combination of lower activity levels and increased carbohydrate consumption causes weight gain.

Did You Know?

Your ethnic background may affect your likelihood of developing seasonal affective disorder (SAD)

Research shows that in the northern hemisphere, SAD prevalence increases with a location's latitude. In the United States, 1.4% of Floridians–27 degrees latittude, 6.3% of Marylanders–39 degrees latitude and 9.7% of New Hampshirites–43 degrees latitude suffer from SAD. The further north you go, where winters are colder and darker, the more likely people are to experience seasonal depression.

But, like so much of human evolution, our experiences are not that simple or black and white.

Consider Iceland, which is *63 to 67 degrees north latitude*. From our previous analysis on latitude, SAD should be widespread throughout their population. Surprisingly, it is not. In fact, only 3.8% of residents suffer from SAD![12-14] So, how do we account for this anomaly?

Some scientists believe genetic adaptations may play a role. Historically, humans lived in proximity to where they and their ancestors were born. Without ships, trains, and planes making travel more efficient, no one had the option or ability to live far from their ancestral homes—and our genetics adapted to that reality. The Icelandic population was largely isolated for over 1,000 years, so as a people, they have spent hundreds of generations adapting to a land with long, cold, dark winters.

But for many other countries—especially the USA—people's genetics may have adapted over the ages to other climates and latitudes. If your ancestors are from areas closer to the equator than where you now live, there is a good chance you may have an increased risk for SAD symptoms.

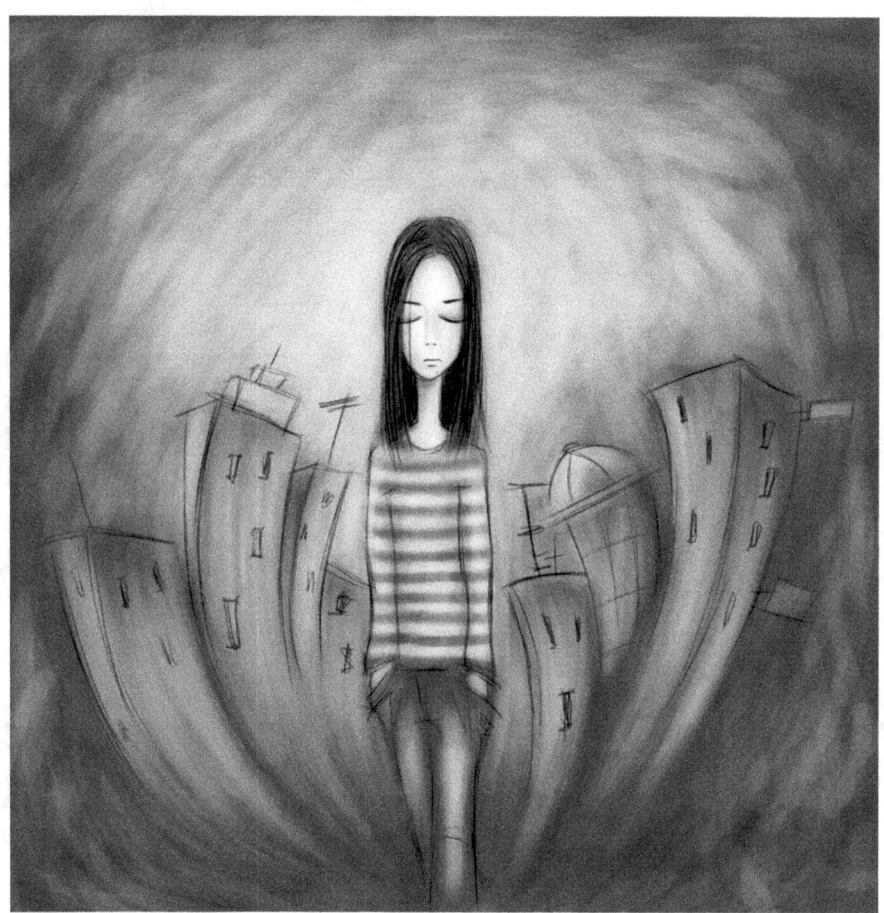

Guidance

To reduce the carbohydrate cravings SAD can cause, you must increase your body's levels of the neurotransmitters serotonin, dopamine, and norepinephrine.

To begin, there are a number of conservative actions you can try to lessen the effect of seasonal affective disorder on your weight by increasing your exposure to full-spectrum light:

- Increase your exposure to sunlight, especially in the morning; about 15 to 20 minutes should do it.

- Use a "light box" in the morning to treat yourself at home.

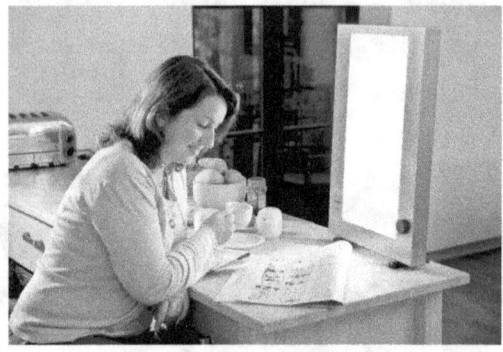

Also available are "light visors" that allow you to get your daily light treatment without having to sit or stand in one place. This is known as "light therapy" or phototherapy.

A new approch channels a bright light directly into the light-sensitive region of the brain via the ear canal. [15]

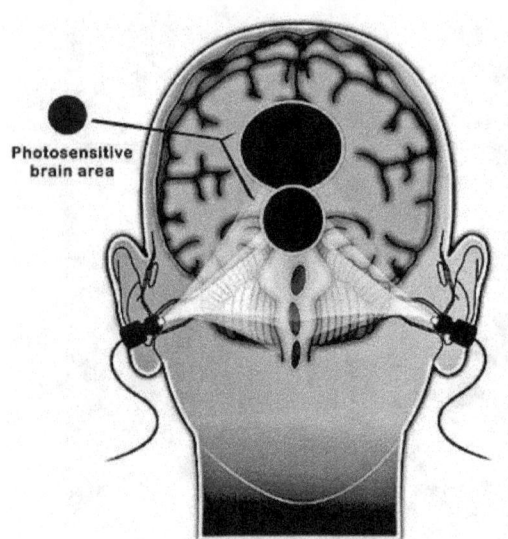

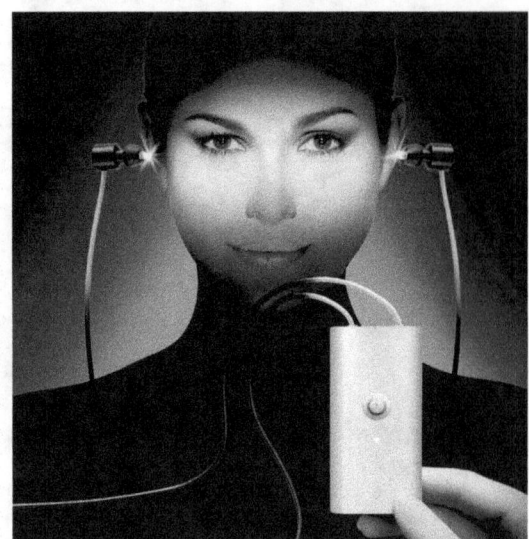

Photosensitive brain area

In addition to increased light exposure, a number of over-the-counter supplements available through your health food store may help you raise your neurotransmitter levels. Try one supplement at a time and do not combine them unless advised by your clinician.

5-HTP (5-hydroxytryptophan) and **tryptophan** raise serotonin levels and have been found to be effective in the treatment of seasonal affective disorder. 5-HTP is made from the seeds of the West African plant

Griffonia simplicifolia. It is available over-the-counter in the United States. It should not be taken concurrently with SSRI (serotonin selective reuptake inhibitor) or SNRI (serotonin norepinephrine reuptake inhibitor) medications. Atypical dose is a total of 50 milligrams to 800 milligrams of 5-HTP or 1,000 milligrams of tryptophan, in divided doses. [16]

Hypericum perforatum, an herb commonly known as St. John's Wort, has been shown to raise the levels of serotonin, norepinephrine, and dopamine.[17-18] The commonly used dose of St. John's Wort is 900 milligrams per day (given as 300 milligrams tablets or capsules, three times per day). Since there can be interactions with some pharmaceuticals, such as SSRI (serotonin selective reuptake inhibitor) or SNRI (serotonin-norepinephrine reuptake inhibitor) medications, inform your clinicians before taking.

Mucuna pruriens, an herb also known as velvet bean, cowhage, kapikachu, or atmagupta in India, can raise dopamine levels. This herb contains a precursor to the neurotransmitter dopamine, called L-Dopa.[19-20] When taking this herb, medical guidance is suggested. The correct dose varies and often clinicians start patients with a low dose of mucuna pruriens and then proceed to a higher dosage. The powdered mucuna pruriens dosage often used is one teaspoon daily.

Talking to Your Doctor

If you believe you are suffering from seasonal affective disorder (SAD), you can discuss your symptoms with your physician and ask about the appropriateness of medications that may decrease melatonin levels, such as anti-anxiety drugs and antidepressants, as well as light box therapy.

Additionally, the prescription medications, *modafinil* and *armodafinil*, are stimulant drugs marketed as "wakefulness promoting agents." These drugs increase dopamine and norepinephrine levels, and may represent the beginning of a new generation of medication to help treat seasonal affective disorder (SAD) and food addictions. [21]

Further Science:

Understanding the Science behind SAD

Several social and environmental factors have altered the quantity of sunlight many of us are exposed to on a daily basis. If you ask most dermatologists, we should adopt a "no sunlight can ever touch the skin" credo, unless you protect the skin with effective sun-blocking lotions.

While this may at first seem reasonable, the need to work, play and travel outdoors is as old as human history—and slight sunlight exposure is indeed necessary for complete health. But between today's skin cancer fears and increasingly indoor lifestyles (brought on after the Industrial Revolution), many have little exposure to natural sunlight, especially during the winter months.

Changing something as basic—and natural—as our relationship to the sun can have significant repercussions on our lives, as seen by the rise of seasonal affective disorder.

Individuals suffering from seasonal affective disorder experience a *double whammy* effect from winter's decreased sunlight: Increased melatonin levels create sleepiness and hunger, and decreased serotonin, dopamine, and norepinephrine levels trigger cravings.

Melatonin

Without adequate daytime sun exposure, the body is confused into producing excessive melatonin, a neuroendocrine-hormonal regulator involved with sleep inducing signals, day and night cycles and body temperature. Melatonin is considered the "darkness" hormone, since the absence of light causes the brain's pineal gland to release it. Although melatonin is a powerful antioxidant—which is partly why sleep is so important—too much causes chronic exhaustion.

When exposed to long nights, excess melatonin triggers an accumulation of fat, whereas levels of fat decrease with short nights. Studies also show that when scientists block a subject's melatonin receptors, the subjects lose weight.[22] Conversely, when these same receptors are stimulated for longer-than-normal time periods, the subjects gain weight.

Consequently, feeling tired and hungry all the time, seasonal affective disorder sufferers are less likely to engage in active and healthy lifestyles.

Serotonin, Norepinephrine and Dopamine

In addition to overproduction of melatonin, insufficient sunlight reduces serotonin, norepinephrine, and dopamine. When these neuromitters are lowered, our bodies naturally respond by triggering sugar and carbohydrate cravings, which boost the levels for a fleeting moment. Unfortunately, women are more than twice as likely to suffer from seasonal affective disorder, in part because they naturally have lower serotonin levels than men.[23]

The vicious SAD cycle

Combine melatonin-induced sleepiness and hunger with cravings caused by low neurotransmitter levels, and seasonal affective disorder sufferers struggle with a vicious cycle of overeating and underexercising:
- The more you eat, the more weight you gain.
- The more weight you gain, the less likely you are to exercise.
- The less you exercise, the less time you spend outdoors.
- The less time you spend outdoors in natural sunlight, the more tired you become and the more food cravings you develop.
- And so on.

But by balancing melatonin and serotonin levels, you can alleviate seasonal affective disorder's negative effects and further improve your ability to fit into your genes and cut the guilt.

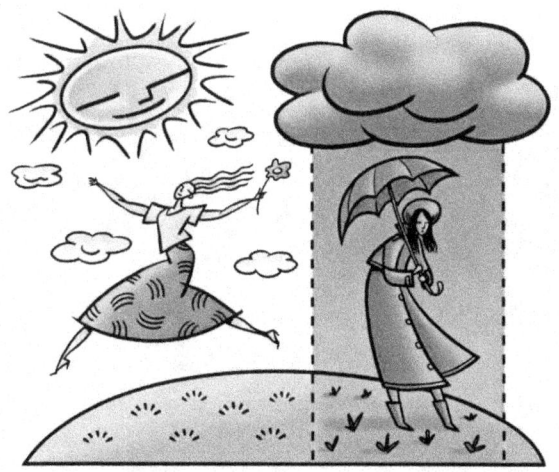

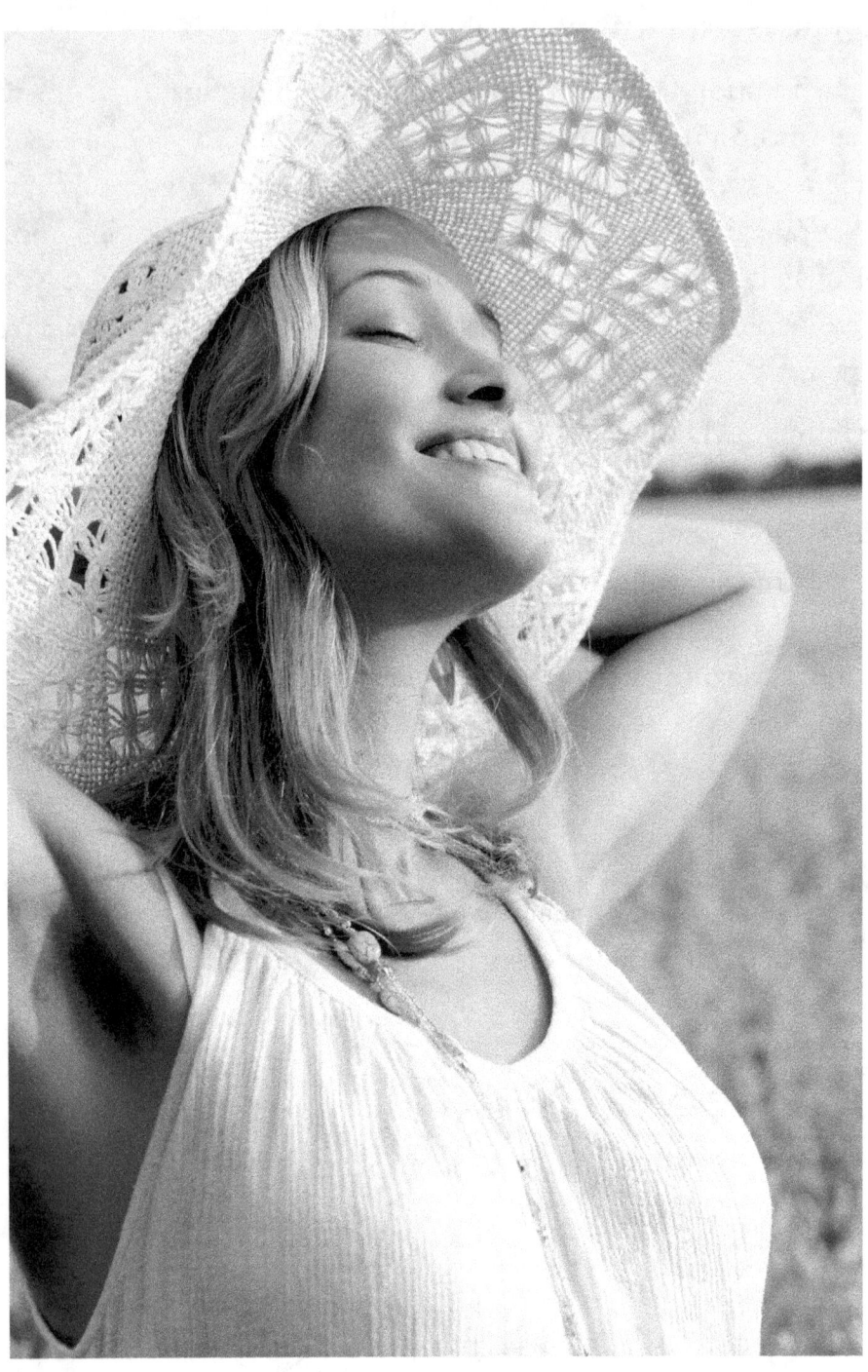

Chapter 14

Putting the Pieces Together—Looking Beyond Habits

John has been a heavy smoker since his early 20's. Every day he wakes up coughing and wheezing, and regularly feels winded when walking. He suffers from chronic bronchitis, has an increased risk of lung cancer and heart disease, and even pays more each month for his health and life insurance premiums. Multiple attempts at quitting his addiction have done little but depress John when he eventually dulls life's stresses by smoking. John is aware of the health risks and problems smoking causes in his life, yet he starts and ends everyday with a cigarette.

Anna first tried cocaine in college. She enjoyed the quick high and how the drug seemed to free her of long-held inhibitions. When she moved to a big city after graduation, cocaine was easily available. Her occasional use on particularly wild nights suddenly morphed into nightly binges. Multiple stints in rehabilitation have failed to keep her clean for long. Now in her mid-30's, Anna has lost nearly everything—a promising career, sound financial standing, and close relationships—due to her drug use, yet she continues to seek out sources for cocaine every day.

Sandy was chubby in childhood. She always enjoyed food and seemed to gain weigh bit-by-bit, while her classmates shed their baby fat. Years of over-consumption have resulted in obesity, self-imposed social restriction, hypertension, and general exhaustion pervading each day. Multiple diets—from low-carb and low-fat to fasting and beyond—have failed to help her lose weight for good. Sandy already experiences many of obesity's negative effects, and she is well aware that her life may be shortened, yet each night, she binges on chips, pizza, and chocolate to the point of being uncomfortably stuffed.

Though each individual's circumstances may be different, they all are addicted. Despite "knowing better," recognizing the consequences of their actions, and repeated attempts to quit, the drive to obtain and consume a substance rules their lives.

Whether indulging in cigarettes, drugs, or food, quitting a true addiction takes more than willpower: You must be committed to the cause and ready for the road ahead. And with the right tools, depth of understanding, and a positive support system in place, you can find freedom from the habits that hinder you from living the life you desire.

Understanding Common Cravings

Ever feel like you could: Kill for some chocolate?

Eat a large bag of chips in minutes? Finish a whole pizza by yourself ?

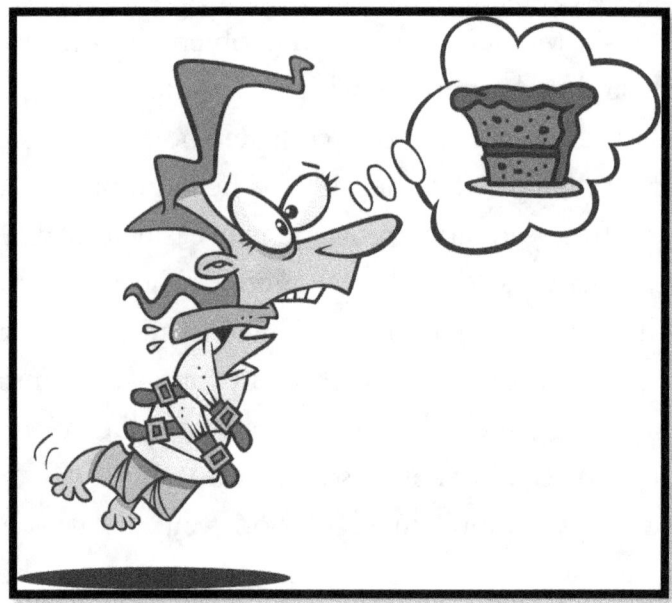

A study by the organization, *Weight Watchers*, reported that the top five foods that trigger women to overindulge are:

1. Chocolate

2. Alcohol

3. Finger foods

4. Roast potatoes

5. Desserts

What do these foods have in common?

Many of them, including alcohol, are high in carbohydrates. During challenging times, we often crave carb-rich foods because they help our body produce the serotonin, dopamine, and norepinephrine that is exhausted when we are chronically stressed.

As I discussed in "Chapter 12: A Sweet Tooth Can Be a Bitter Pill to Swallow," there is a difference between desiring a food and experiencing a visceral, desperate craving. Similarly, food addiction goes beyond merely overeating tasty food. Dr. Mark Gold, chief of addiction medicine at University of Florida's McKnight Brain Institute, defines food addiction as:

-     "Eating too much despite consequences, even dire consequences to health;

-     Being preoccupied with food, food preparation and meals;

-     Trying and failing to cut back on food intake;

-     Feeling guilty about eating and overeating."

Because food addiction can be caused by a variety of underlying factors, you can treat and cure the disorder in a number of ways. Many of the chapter topics we have covered in this book can have a direct affect on your food addictions, including:

- Omega-3 and omega-6 essential fatty acid imbalances

- Underactive thyroid

- Adrenal fatigue

- Suboptimal levels of vitamin B12

- Estrogen dominance, low progesterone levels

- Low blood sugar (hypoglycemia)

In order to truly achieve your healthy weight and fit into your genes and cut the guilt, you may have to address one or more of these imbalances at the same time to set yourself on the right path.

Additionally, *chronic pain can contribute to food addictions*. The body uses several neurotransmitters to ease pain by preventing the pain signals from traveling up the spinal cord to the brain; thus, we are not as aware of the discomfort. And what are two of the primary neurotransmitters that help block pain perceptions? Serotonin and norepinephrine!

The body therefore can diminish its stores of serotonin and norepinephrine when faced with chronic pain. And when levels of these neurotransmitters decrease, you experience less inhibition of pain signals to the brain, resulting in a pain threshold decrease and increased pain intensity. So, many people in pain "self-medicate" with carbohydrates, intuitively looking to raise their serotonin and norepinephrine levels in order to decrease pain.

There are physicians now prescribing medications to raise both serotonin and norepinephrine when treating patients in chronic pain. Interestingly, we now realize the patient in chronic pain who complains of depression is not necessarily depressed psychologically about their health condition. Instead, the pain is actually changing their neurotransmitter chemistry enough to trigger depression—and food addiction. [1]

If you suffer from chronic pain—and find yourself struggling to stop eating carbohydrate-rich foods—these two health challenges may actually be related.

But, regardless of what may be causing your food addictions, the exciting—and freeing—fact is that you now have the tools to truly address the root of the problem, rather than blaming yourself for compulsive eating.

Putting the Pieces Together

Reading back through the health topics we've addressed on this journey, did you see any patterns?

How many of these imbalances affect serotonin and/or dopamine causing you to crave carbohydrates and sugars?

As I stated in the beginning of this book, and have reinforced throughout your reading, our bodies are incredibly complex. Finding lasting health and your ideal weight depends on much more than the simple calories-in/calories-out equations so many people have preached for years. Often, the desire to eat less is actually hindered by physiological, innate cravings for carbohydrates and sweets caused by neurotransmitter imbalances. The belief that most people who overeat are lazy or gluttonous ignores the scientific fact that many individuals are not choosing to indulge, but instead, suffer from food addictions driving them to devastate their health.

Before moving forward to the next chapter of your life, however, let's review how each piece of your health puzzle connects, so you are truly prepared to fit into your genes and cut the guilt.

Balance Between Omega-3 and Omega-6 Essential Fatty Acids

Essential fatty acids are fatty acids our bodies cannot produce, so we must obtain them from food. The essential fatty acids can be divided into two main types: omega-3 and omega-6. Omega-3 fats aid the body in maintaining the cell membrane's fluidity to facilitate the production of energy from glucose, as well as the healthy development and functioning of the nervous system. Omega-6 fats make the cell membrane more rigid, and an overabundance can cause a number of disorders, including insulin resistance syndrome. Modern agriculture and lifestyles have resulted in most of us consuming far too much omega-6 essential fatty acids as compared to the omega-3 essential fatty acids. We are not genetically designed to handle the unprecedented high omega-6 to omega-3 ratios of our modern-day diet.

Biological (Physiological) Effects

An imbalance in the omega-3 to omega-6 essential fatty acids ratio results in the awful combination of *decreased energy* and an *increased appetite* for simple carbohydrates by:

- Making it harder for our bodies to transport glucose (blood sugar) into the cells to use for energy and,

- Inhibiting production of dopamine and serotonin, triggering cravings for carbohydrates.

Remember the fuel truck stranded on the highway? Just because your body has excess reserve fuel (fat) does not mean you are accessing it.

You have to balance your essential fatty acids, so you can burn your fuel instead of storing it.

Mitochondrial Production

Housed within each cell, except the mature red blood cell, mitochondria are organelles (little organs) that serve as our body's power generating factories. The human body is made up of over a hundred-trillion cells, and every cell needs energy to perform its specific functions. That energy comes from the mitochondria located within the cells. The number of mitochondria we have isn't just determined by genetics, but also by how active our lifestyles are (or are not).

Biological (Physiological) Effects

With adequate aerobic activity, we enjoy more energy and burn more fuel, because we have more mitochondria. Inadequate exercise results in fewer mitochondria and less energy and less glucose (fuel) burning.

Remember the artistic twins, Jack and Jill? Reinforce your body's innate ability to burn blood sugar and create energy by getting regular aerobic exercise.

Underactive Thyroid

The thyroid gland is the master controller of your body's metabolism. Although the gland only makes about a teaspoon of thyroid hormone per year, these hormones effect every cell in the body.

Biological (Physiological) Effects

Because the thyroid gland controls your resting metabolic rate, a thyroid performing below optimal levels can result in 500 to 600 fewer calories burned each day. Subnormal thyroid levels also decrease our serotonin levels, triggering cravings for carbohydrates. Unfortunately, excess sugar consumption suppresses thyroid function, further lowering serotonin levels and triggering more cravings for carbohydrates and sugars creating a vicious cycle. [2]

Remember the malfunctioning HVAC system (heating, ventilation, and air conditioning)? Complications can be the result of fuel shortages (iodine), a blockage (trouble converting T4 to T3) or a damaged thermostat (inaccurate testing). If you believe your thyroid is not functioning properly— and adversely affecting your quality of life— do not give up until you have explored all three causes.

Adrenal Imbalances and Fatigue

The two adrenal glands each sit atop a kidney and in response to stress, produce several hormones that influence our eating habits and fat accumulation.

Biological (Physiological) Effects

Chronic stress causes your adrenal glands to pump out too much cortisol, triggering cravings for carbohydrates and abdominal fat accumulation. If the chronic stress continues without rest, your adrenal glands just cannot pump out cortisol at the same levels anymore and you get adrenal fatigue, which can be even worse than high cortisol levels because it saps your energy, vitality, and digestive health.

Remember the glass of water held aloft? Without time to decompress between stressful experiences, your body can't continue to function properly. Allow yourself to experience the "rest and digest" parasympathetic mode, so your adrenal glands don't become exhausted.

Vitamin B12—Suboptimal Levels

Vitamin B12 is the most structurally complex and largest vitamin known, and is needed for the production of crucial neurotransmitters. Because vitamin B12 is so molecularly huge, it must be carried by intrinsic factor (IF)—a chemical made in our stomachs—in order to be absorbed through the intestinal barrier and into our body.

Biological (Physiological) Effects

Suboptimal vitamin B12 levels affect your achieving a healthy weight in two significant ways:

1. Hampering your ability to convert the T4 thyroid hormone into the active T3 form that your cells can use. Without adequate T3, your metabolism will be lowered, so your body burns less fuel (food) and stores the excess as fat.

2. Limiting your body's ability to produce serotonin and dopamine, triggering cravings for carbohydrates and sweets.

Remember the fickle and finicky Broadway actress? B12 is a powerful and important vitamin, but its requirements to perform correctly are higher than most. Don't let inadequate intrinsic factor, caused by a persnickety stomach prevent your body from harnessing B12's capabilities. Try sublingual B12 or talk to your doctor about vitamin B12 injections to ensure you actually absorb this crucial vitamin.

Estrogen Dominance

Women's bodies have naturally evolved to keep estrogen and progesterone in balance, with levels fluctuating through various hormonal stages, including pregnancy and menopause. Estrogen helps prepare the body for pregnancy by triggering fat accumulation. Whereas, progesterone helps the body turn fat into energy. By age 35, HALF of all women in the U.S. suffer from estrogen dominance (low progesterone).

Biological (Physiological) Effects

Most frighteningly, *estrogen dominance makes women 80% more likely to develop breast cancer*. This hormonal imbalance can also increase the cravings for sweets and an overall desire for pleasurable food, because estrogen is one of the hormones that enhance the effects of serotonin and dopamine but low progesterone levels decreases estrogen's positive effect on dopamine and serotonin.

Remember the musicians Estelle and Preston? Just as Estelle's individual qualities were powerful as part of a duo—but overbearing alone—estrogen and progesterone's traits are designed to work together, in balance.

Unchecked Sweet Tooth

Our bodies must maintain blood sugar (glucose) levels, because glucose is the brain's only fuel other than oxygen. As our blood sugar levels fluctuate throughout the day, a complex process protects our brain from starvation by signaling us to eat carbohydrates and sugars if more glucose is needed.

Our innate drive to maintain blood glucose levels can trigger unhealthy cravings and eating behavior when our systems become unbalanced.

Biological (Physiological) Effects

An unchecked sweet tooth has two primary causes:

1. Actual low blood sugar, which can be exacerbated by the consumption of simple, refined carbohydrates.When you eat processed carbohydrates and sugars, your body overreacts by producing way too much insulin, quickly depleting the blood sugar, thus triggering further food cravings.

2. A serotonin and/or dopamine imbalance, which can mimic the sugar cravings of low blood sugar, but is actually a result of your body searching for a quick solution to boost levels of these neurotransmitters.

Remember the importance of choosing logs, instead of leaves, to build a lasting fire? To calm a crazed sweet tooth, select the slow, long-burning complex carbohydrates found in whole foods, which offer energy and balanced blood sugar that truly fuel your body. Simple and refined carbohydrates and sugars may provide a quick burst of fire, but burn up quickly and leave you scrambling to find more fuel.

Seasonal Affective Disorder

As the daylight hours dwindle in winter, many individuals experience depression, decreased energy, and an increased appetite, which accompany seasonal affective disorder (SAD).

Biological (Physiological) Effects

Less sunlight triggers our bodies to create melatonin, a hormone associated with sleep. SAD sufferers have excess melatonin, which makes them feel exhausted throughout the winter months. Insufficient sunlight also reduces the neurotransmitters serotonin, norepinephrine, and dopimine, resulting in carbohydrate and sugar cravings.

Remember hibernating animals? Our bodies may have evolved to conserve fat during the winter months by limiting activity and increasing carbohydrate consumption, but in today's culture—and around-the-clock lifestyles—these adaptations no longer serve us well.

Ancient Chinese philosopher Lao Tzu said, "A journey of a thousand miles begins with a single step."

When you are facing the long voyage, however, taking your first step can often be the most daunting act of all, as unanswered questions loom over your resolution:

What if things don't go as planned?

Am I truly prepared for the challenges that lie ahead?

What if I fail?

Fear and trepidation are natural responses when starting on a new and unfamiliar path. But you, my courageous reader, have taken the first step toward lasting health just by traveling with me through the last 14 chapters. You have taken the challenge to reevaluate how you define well-being and now have a greater understanding of why your genetic makeup may have prevented lasting weight loss in the past. The next step may be yours, but the path to lasting health and happiness is written in your genes.

Remember the lifestyle your ancestors experienced—and how our modern lives differ from our ancient genetic survival instincts to *eat-as-much-as-you-can-now-because-I-don't-know-the-next-time-I'll-have-food.*

Be kind to yourself and bold in your choices,

Seek second opinions when needed.

Don't give up until you have exhausted your options.

And above all, listen to your body.

Best wishes on the exciting, fulfilling journey to *fit into your genes* and *cut the guilt.*

Chapter 15

New Research Currently in Development

With every chapter of this section of *Cut the Guilt* we have strived to show you how complex your body truly is—and why the simple calories-in/calories-out equation does not adequately explain many people's struggles to maintain their desired weight. As you have seen with serotonin, dopamine, norepinephrine, estrogen, progesterone, thyroid function, and more, a wide variety of hormones and neurotransmitters overlap and interact to support achieving your healthy weight. While we understand a lot about how the body functions, current research aims to discover new ways to fight obesity with scientifically sophisticated solutions, instead of the tired *eat less and exercise more* edicts that clearly are not working for many people.

Ultimately, the goal may be to create pharmacological treatments that prevent obesity—and the devastating health challenges it causes. According to the *New England Journal of Medicine*, several potential therapies are in Phase 2 and 3 clinical trials, only a few steps from becoming widely available drugs. By focusing on "a fuller understanding of the regulation of food intake," researchers are working to develop medications that "reverse the on-going acceleration of the current obesity epidemic." [1]

An article in the *Journal of Endocrinology* summarized the future direction of medical obesity research by stating:

"The brain integrates peripheral signals of nutrition in order to maintain a stable bodyweight. However, in some individuals, genetic and environmental factors interact to result in obesity. Understanding of the complex system which regulates energy homeostasis is progressing rapidly, enabling new obesity therapies to emerge." [2]

In other words, you may one day be able to take a pill that uses your body's natural chemistry to prevent unhealthy cravings and weight gain. As new discoveries occur, your toolkit for truly fitting into genes will expand.

The many topics we have discussed in this book represent today's cutting edge approach to health, but the complete story has yet to be written. Presently, the following eight hormones and neurotransmitters are being diligently studied to determine how they fit into an effective equation for lasting weight management.

The Appetite Reducers

Leptin

Leptin is a hormone produced by fat cells (adipose tissue) that sends satiety signals to the brain, letting us know when the body has consumed a sufficient amount of food. The process is designed to suppress the appetite by communicating an "I'm full" feeling when adequate calories are eaten.

Unfortunately, many obese people are leptin resistant, and their brains don't receive the satiety signal until long after that of a healthy-weight person. As a result, they overeat, unaware they should actually feel full.

Leptin is now thought to be a short term appetite balancing-hormone. It seems leptin was never meant to function for long periods of time. As stated before, there was never a need for long term obesity control in the history of humanity. Drugs that can reverse or attenuate leptin tolerance or resistance are currently a focus of pharmaceutical research. [3]

Dr. Leo Galland, a medical doctor and researcher with a special interest in alternative and nutritional therapies, published a book where he makes a convincing case that leptin resistance is mostly due to long-term, low-grade inflammation in the body. The research he references shows obesity itself, triggers an inflammatory condition in the body. Fat (adipose) cells produce inflammatory chemicals, which seem to set up the leptin-blocking chemicals. The theory is, overweight and obese people are stuck in a vicious cycle of inflammation, which triggers leptin resistance and causes them to overeat, thus gaining more weight. The resultant obesity leads to more inflammation, and on and on. Until a medication to counteract leptin resistance is developed, the solution for this obesity merry-go-round is to add anti-inflammatory foods into the diet and reduce the proinflammatory foods.

According to Dr. Galland *these foods should be* **avoided**, as they increase inflammation and contribute to leptin resistance:

- Grain-based oils with a high omega-6/omega-3 ratio, including corn oil, safflower oil, sunflower oil, cottonseed oil, peanut oil, and soybean oil. You should also avoid foods made with these oils, such as regular margarine, standard mayonnaise, most commercial salad dressings, and many packaged foods.

- Meat and eggs from *grain-fed animals*, due to their high omega-6 to omega-3 essential fatty acid ratio.

- Farm-raised tilapia and catfish, due to their low omega-3 essential fatty acid levels.

- Trans-fatty acids and partially hydrogenated oils. Avoid foods made with trans-fats, such as margarine, and deep-fried foods (French fries, onion rings, etc.). Recent regulations require manufacturers to list the amount of trans fatty acids in their nutritional content labeling.

- Refined carbohydrates, including white flour and white sugar products, processed desserts, regular soft drinks, and packaged snacks.

The following foods reduce inflammation and support healthy leptin function, and *should be* **added** *to our diet:*

- Omega-3 fats, fiber, polyphenols, carotenoids, and isothiocyanates are anti-inflammatory.

Polyphenols are found in most legumes; fruits such as apples, blackberries, blueberries, cantaloupe, cherries, cranberries, grapes, pears, plums, raspberries, and strawberries; as well as vegetables such as celery, broccoli, cabbage, onion, and parsley.

Carotenoids are fat-soluble plant pigments found in many vegetables that are highly colored red, orange, and yellow

Isothiocyanates are found in cruciferous vegetables such as broccoli, cauliflower, watercress, turnips, kale, collards, Brussels sprouts, cabbage, and radish.

- Fruits and vegetables, particularly eaten raw or lightly cooked.

Be aware that today, less than 10% of high school students eat the combined recommended daily amount of fruits and vegetables. If you have children, make sure they are eating enough fresh produce. [4]

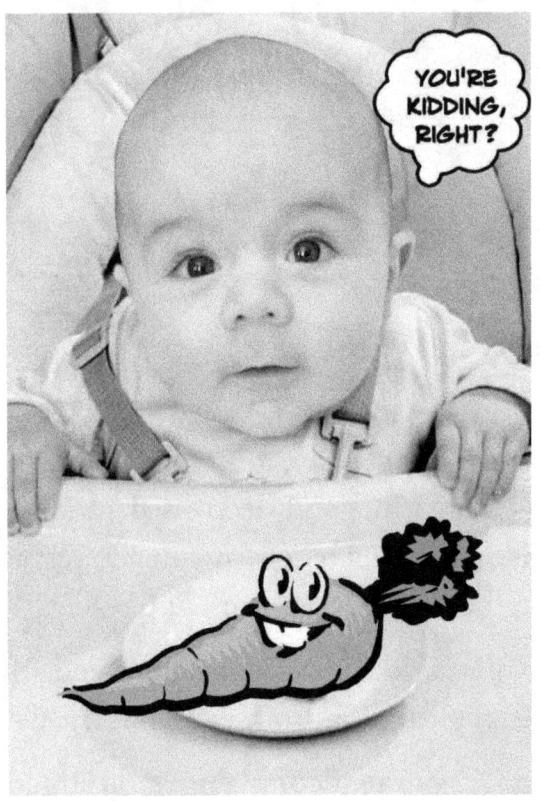

Only 22% of children ages 2 to 5 meet government recommendations for vegetable consumption, according to a 2009 study by researchers at Ohio State University.

- Fresh or frozen fish and shellfish, as they have sufficient omega-3 essential fatty acids.

- Grass-fed meat or wild game is a good choice, but if they are not available, you can eat lean meats, such as skinless chicken, and buy omega-3 eggs.

- Raw almonds, cashews, walnuts, hazelnuts, sesame seeds and macadamia nuts.

- Anti-inflammatory spices and herbs, including turmeric, garlic, ginger, dill, oregano, coriander, fennel, red chili pepper, basil, rosemary, and kelp.

- Organic oils, such as organic extra virgin olive oil and coconut oil, should be used when possible. Butter is acceptable, but the best butter choice is from grass-fed cows. A number of nationally available brands, such as Organic Valley, offer butter and heavy cream from grass-fed cows.

- Salad dressings are best when basic and homemade. Consider using extra virgin olive oil, balsamic vinegar (or lemon juice), mustard, and spices: turmeric, garlic, ginger, dill, oregano, coriander, fennel, red chili pepper, basil, rosemary, and kelp. When away from home, consider using dressings sparingly.

In addition to affecting our brain's satiety sensations, leptin plays a role in human reproduction by telling the body whether or not you should be able to conceive. Nature knows the body needs a great deal of energy to make healthy babies, and thus, women with low body fat (low energy stores), such as athletes, stop ovulating and have difficulty getting pregnant. In fact, the first-approved pharmaceutical use of leptin is for low-fat women, enabling them to become pregnant.

Pancreatic Polypeptide – Appetite Reducer

Pancreatic polypeptide (PP) is a gut hormone produced by the pancreas, in the same region that also produces insulin. Pancreatic polypeptide is released in response to ingesting food and reduces food intake. The body also makes some pancreatic polypeptide in the distal part of the gastrointestinal tract. Studies show that overweight and obese people have abnormally reduced levels of this appetite-suppressing hormone. It seems evident that the release of appetite regulating gastrointestinal peptides is disturbed in obese people; suggesting a genetic dysfunction of the brain-gut-weight-control homeostasis mechanism.[5] We call this a dysfunction in today's world; whereas for all of man's past, amassing extra fat was a positive health trait.

Current research suggests pancreatic polypeptide may have potential as a pharmacological drug for the long-term appetite suppression. [6]

Peptide YY – Appetite Reducer

Peptide YY (PYY) is a gut hormone that is released from the

intestinal tract after eating and suppresses our appetite. Peptide YY levels peak one to two hours after a meal, maintain for about six hours and are higher when fat is eaten at the meal, as compared to proteins or carbohydrates.

When peptide YY was administered to study subjects of normal weight, their food intake and appetite reduce by 30%. Unfortunately, obese individuals have lower-than-expected levels of peptide YY, which they deficiently secrete. As a result, this hormon's powerful appetite suppression is restricted. [7]

An important fact to take into account is that *stomach acid increases peptide YY levels.* As previously stated, contrary to popular belief, many people who suffer from gasric (stomach) indigestion have too little acids—rather than too much—in their stomachs. If you have indigestion, speak with your health advisor to determine if acidifying your stomach with betaine hydrochloride would be worth a try.

As research continues, there is potential for the pharmaceutical industry to develop peptide YY-based medications to treat obesity.

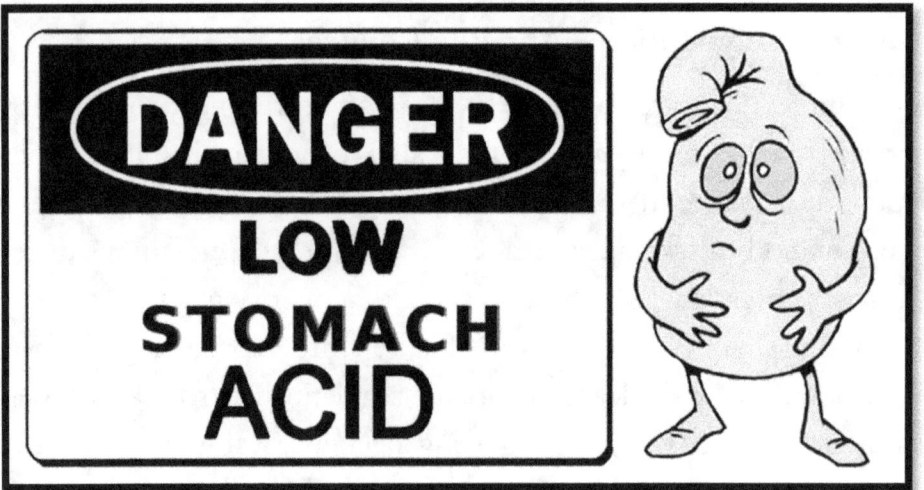

Oxyntomodulin (OXM) – Appetite Reducer

Oxyntomodulin (OXM) is a gut hormone that suppresses our appetite and is released in the small intestines in response to calorie intake. In contrast to leptin, obesity does not appear to trigger resistance to oxyntomodulin's anorectic (appetite-reducing) effects. Circulating levels of oxyntomodulin rise within 30 minutes after a meal and remain elevated for several hours. In healthy subjects, there was an almost 20% reduction in hunger and eating for 12 hours after administering oxyntomodulin to the volunteers. Pre-meal subcutaneous administration of oxyntomodulin to overweight and obese humans over a four week period resulted in a significant reduction in body weight of over 5 pounds compared to only 1.1 pounds for the placebo group. Therefore, oxyntomodulin administration resulted in an additional one pound of weight loss per week, which is better than any currently licensed anti-obesity drug.

Another benefit of oxyntomodulin was its effect on energy usage. In studies, oxyntomodulin increased activity in overweight and obese subjects back to what was considered normal or healthy levels.[8] OXM therefore has a double effect of suppressing appetite and also increasing physical activity toward normal levels. There is great potential for the pharmaceutical industry to develop oxyntomodulin-based medications to treat obesity. [9]

Cholecystokinin (CCK) – Appetite Reducer

Cholecystokinin (CCK) is a peptide hormone that reduces appetite and is released in the small intestines after eating fats and oils. The stomach stretching triggers the release of cholecystokinin. The overdistention of the stomach found in many obese people may contribute to a lack of cholecystokinin release after eating.[10] CCK slows the emptying of the stomach and partly contributes to our satiety experience by blocking the vagus nerve, also known as the tenth cranial nerve.

Because stimulating the vagus nerve promotes eating, CCK's ability to block this nerve's impulses decreases our appetite.

Studies show that as long as fat remains in the intestinal tract, the effects of cholecystokinin suppress our appetite. Therefore, if fat digestion could be slowed down, our food intake would lessen.[11]

Thankfully, Mother Nature can help support slower fat digestion. The "green" in plants comes from a substance called chlorophyll, which is found within sacs in the cells called chloroplasts. Those chloroplast sacs have walls that contain a substance that increases the time fats will remain in our intestines.

When chloroplast sac walls were added to refined food, people ate less and researchers found an increased level of CCK. The studies found it took several days for the appetite-suppressing effects to kick in, but once once they did, the chloroplast-sac-wall material was superior to the medication orlistat. Orlistat also inhibits fat digestion, but includes unpleasant side effects with disturbed bowel movements. Also, orlistat doesn't increase the release of cholecystokinin, which is the powerful appetite inhibitor we want to augment.

So, eating large portions of green vegetables with each meal is another simple and healthy way to fit into your genes and cut the guilt!

If you find starting the day with a salad or plate of kale, broccoli, green beans, and some spinach hard to imagine, don't worry. Just as you can balance your omega-3 essential fatty acid levels by taking pharmaceutical grade fish oil (instead of eating fish), there are "green" supplements you can take to increase CCK. These supplements can be taken by a capsule or in powder form and mixed into a drink. One example of this type of product is Greens Plus, but there are many others. Just ask your health advisor, visit your health food store or search the internet for *Green Superfoods*, which is a term for the category of phytonutrient-rich nutritional products derived from green plants, algae and cereal grasses. Green Superfoods contain high concentrations of natural chlorophyll.

The Appetite Increasers

Ghrelin

Ghrelin is a hormone released mostly from the stomach that travels into the bloodstream and affects the hypothalamus in the brain, stimulating the appetite to increase food intake. Studies find that obese people do not show the normal quick decrease in levels of ghrelin after eating, which results in overeating since the appetite is not satiated. On the flip side, dieting seems to increase ghrelin, which also increases our appetite and may be responsible for some of the so called "rebound" affect many dieters' experience.

Additionally, just anticipating food can increase the ghrelin levels, boosting our appetite before we eat.

Boredom can lead to suboptimal levels of the "feel good" neurotransmitter dopamine and a natural response is to elevate levels of dopamine by eating "comfort foods" such as chocolate and sweets. When our cravings arise, ghrelin is released, further triggering our appetite. The key is to understand what is happening and find creative ways to attenuate our thoughts of food, which can actually reduce our appetite.

Studies now show that taking oligofructose supplementation has the potential to promote weight loss and improve glucose regulation in overweight adults by suppressing ghrelin and enhancing peptide YY. Oligofructose occurs naturally in plants and vegetables, including onions, bananas, garlic, and chicory. Most of the oligofructose used as an ingredient is either extracted from chicory root or is synthetically manufactured. When looking for this ingredient at the store, remember it's known by several different names, including oligofructan, and fructooligosaccharide (FOS). Oligofructose is also found in natural sweetener substitutes such as Stevia.[12] Much medical research is being done in this area so stay tuned!

Neuropeptide Y (NPY) – Appetite Increaser

Neuropeptide Y (NPY) is the most potent food-intake-stimulating neurotransmitter known. Released in response to stress, and a decline in fat stores, NYP turns on cravings for food, especially carbohydrates. NPY is secreted in the brain by the hypothalamus, that portion of the brain that controls hunger, thirst,fatigue,and body temperature.

This is a key factor — stress triggers neuropeptide Y production, thereby increasing our appetites, especially for sweets. Neuropeptide Y also increases the proportion of energy stored as belly fat, which is the most health threatening type of adipose tissue.

The question arises again: Does emotional stress make you gain or lose weight? The answer is, both. Acute, short-term stresses may help you lose weight but the chronic stresses we often live with in our fast paced society, triggers weight gain, especially around your belly.

Studies suggest that long-acting, potent neuropeptide Y receptor selective blockers if developed, could be used to treat obesity. [13]

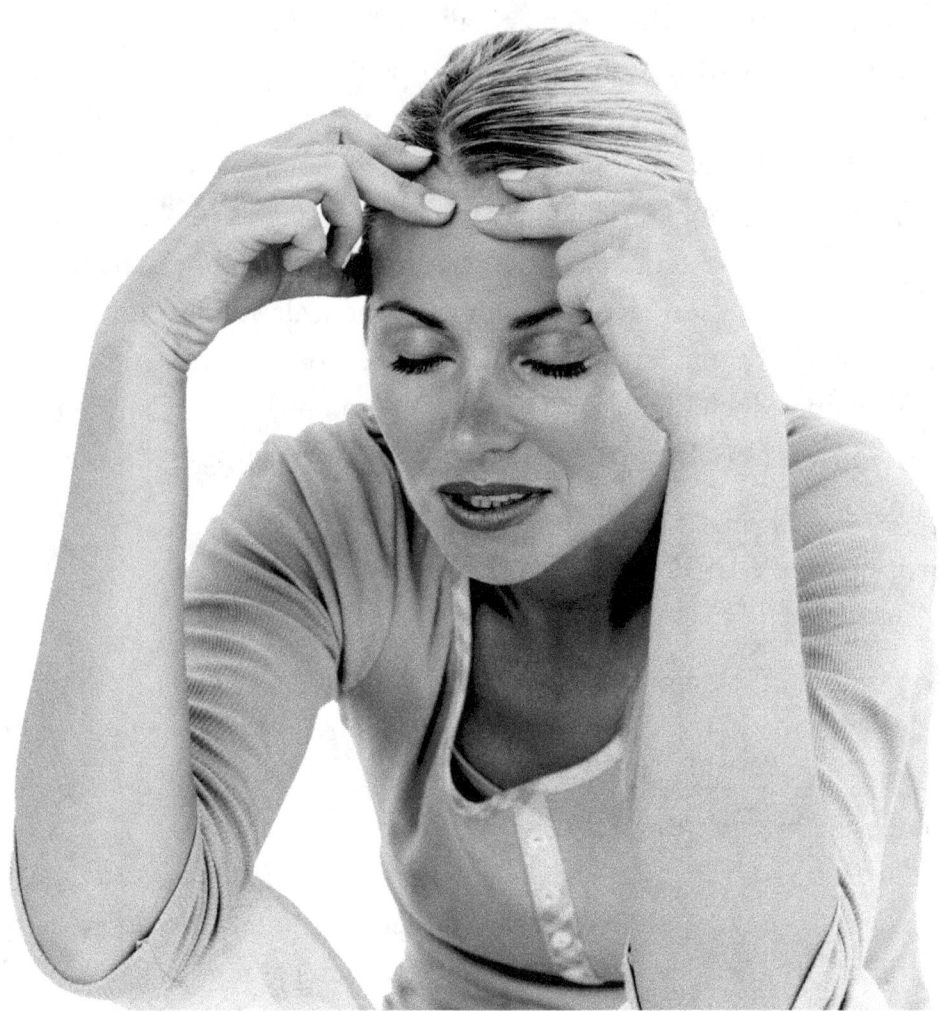

The chronic, long-term stresses we often live with in our fast paced
society, triggers weight gain, especially around our belly.

Glossary

Absent Handshake Sign is a term devised by Dr. Jason Schwartz to describe the lack of the normal "handshake position" of the hand. The normal handshake position is the palm of the hand facing the lateral aspect of the thigh and thumb pointing anterior (a forward facing direction). This abnormal hand position is present if the hand's palm faces towards the back of a person (posteriorly) and the thumb points medially to the thigh. This nonstandard hand posture requires up to 40% more energy to maintain.

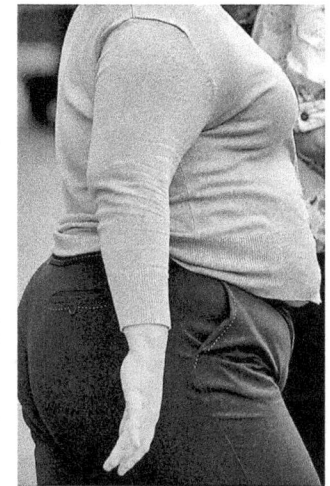
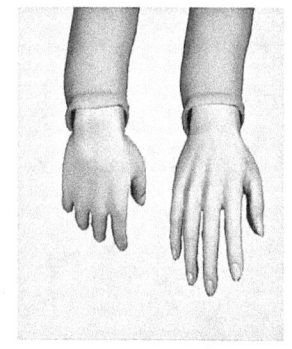
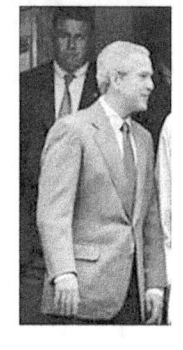
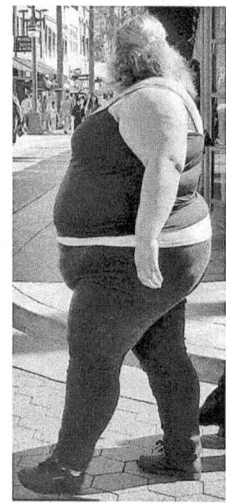

The presence of this unnatural hand position, especially if on both hands, usually indicates a weakened teres minor muscle due to a low thyroid function. Note, there can be many reasons the teres minor muscles are weak. You can injure your lower neck with resultant nerve damage. You can damage your shoulder muscles in a traumatic event. If these events are not part of the history, then the likely cause of the teres minor compromise is a under functioning thyroid gland (hypothyroidism).

Addison's disease or chronic adrenal insufficiency, is a severe deficiency of the adrenal glands' hormone production of cortisol and often also of aldosterone. Addison's disease is rare: 1 in 100,000 people.

Adenosine is a neurotransmitter and an important regulator of sleep. The commonly used drugs caffeine and theophylline (which is found in tea leaves), are both adenosine antagonist. They thus stimulate the central nervous system alleviating drowsiness and enhancing alertness.

Adipose tissue is the scientific name for fat tissue. Fat tissue insulates, cushions, and stores energy reserves. We now know that fat is also an endocrine organ effecting the rest of the body; especially the brain.

Adrenaline also known as **epinephrine**, is a hormone secreted by the adrenal glands we use to deal with stress. It gets us into the "fight-or-flight" sympathetic response. Adrenaline regulates attention, mental focus, arousal, and cognition. It decreases appetites, stops or greatly slows down movements of the gastrointestinal tract and digestive secretions. If the adrenals are pooped, low levels of adrenaline can cause fatigue, lack of focus, and difficulty losing weight.

Adrenal fatigue syndrome is when adrenal gland function is low but not pathologically low enough to be Addison's disease, a life threating condition. Symptoms commonly can include fatigue, feelings of frustration, irritability, mental depression, moments of confusion, and nervousness. The person with adrenal fatigue often is "addicted" to caffeine, carbohydrates, chocolate, and salty foods. Adrenal fatigue syndrome is also known as adrenal burnout, non-Addison's hypoadrenia, subclinical hypoadrenia, and hypoadrenalism.

Adrenal glands or suprarenal glands are walnut-sized hormonal glands that sit above each kidney. They are the body's major responders to stress. The adrenal hormones, cortisol and DHEA, are involved in carbohydrate, protein and fat metabolism and influence our eating habits, blood sugar and fat accumulation.

Aldosterone is an adrenal hormone that increases our appetite. Low levels of aldosterone from adrenal fatigue syndrome can trigger craving salty foods due to salt wasting through the kidneys into the urine.

Appetite is a set of positive sensations that make us aware that we want to eat some good tasting food. Appetite is determined by processes in the brain as well as in the gastrointestinal tract.

Barnes temperature test is an axillary (armpit) temperature test. A normal metabolism (normal thyroid gland function) should yield a basal axillary temperature, before getting out of bed in the morning, of 97.8 to 98.2 degrees F.

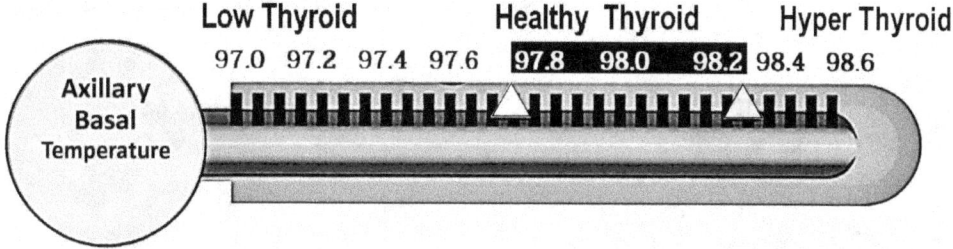

Bombesin is an amino acid peptide that decreases our appetite. Bombesin is released from the gastrointestinal tract and decreases food appetite in lean people but *not* in the obese.

Caffeine is the most commonly used drug in the world, perhaps because it raises adrenaline levels and kicks us into the flight-or-fight mode. Caffeine spares dopamine, which means it increases dopamine levels. Caffeine blocks a neurotransmitter called adenosine and this blocking of adenosine also raises the levels of dopamine. In America, 90% of adults consume caffeine daily. Often, caffeine is wrongly blamed for causing various health problems. When in fact, people suffering from malaise for various reasons, may use caffeine to try to compensate for their poor health. It is like blaming crutches for causing broken legs and sprained ankles!

Carbo-binging or **carb-binging** are terms coined to describe selectively ingesting refined carbohydrates (sugars and starches).

Carboholic is someone who consumes carbohydrates in excess, to the point of harming themselves.

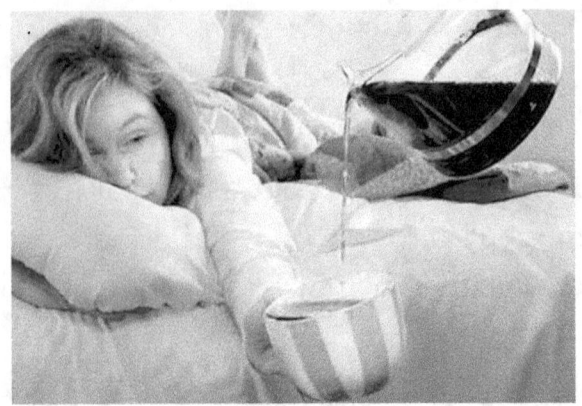

Blaming caffeine for causing many people's maladies is like blaming crutches for causing broken legs and sprained ankles!

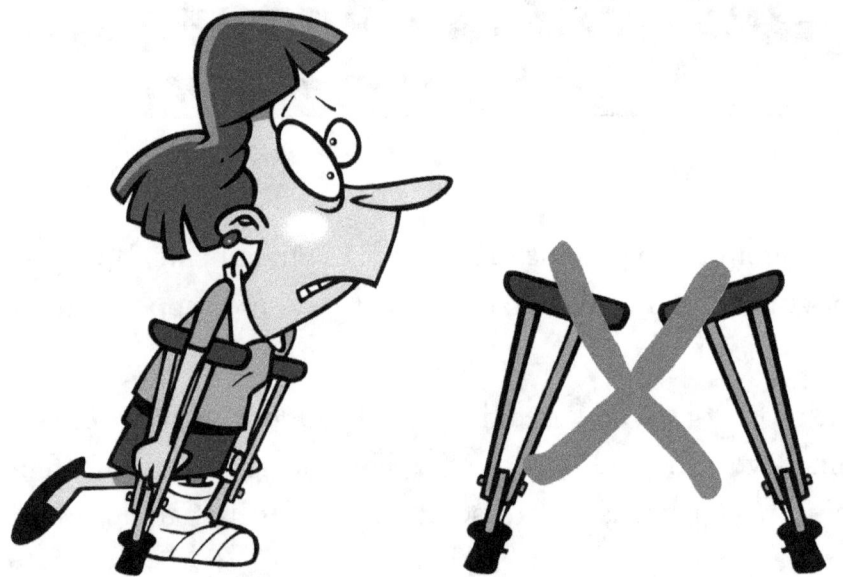

Chocolate contains compounds that are precursors to both serotonin and dopamine. Dopamine creates the "high" feeling associated with drug use, sex, eating certain foods, and even shopping. Low serotonin levels increase our appetite for sweets. In addition, chocolate contains as much as 20 mg of caffeine per ounce which also raises dopamine levels. Chocolate is also high in the mineral magnesium. Some may crave chocolate, therefore, due to needing more magnesium in their diets.

Why do women enjoy chocolate so much?

BECAUSE CHOCOLATE CAN'T GET YOU PREGNANT

Chocolate as well as sex, raise dopamine levels producing an elated euphoria !

Chloroplasts: In the cells of green plants where the chlorophyll is found, are sacs called chloroplasts that contain the chlorophyll. Chloroplast sacs have walls that contain a substance that increases the time fats will remain in our intestines; which then lessen our food intake.

Cholecystokinin (CCK) acts as a hormone and a neurotransmitter. It is released in the small intestines after eating fats and oils. CCK's actions include slowing the emptying of the stomach and reducing our appetite. Part of CCK's satiety effects are due to its attenuation of the vagus nerve (cranial nerve X). The stimulation of the vagus nerve promotes eating and therefore the attenuation or blocking of the vagal nerve impulses by cholecystokinin decreases our appetite.

Cortisol has been called the stress hormone. When the body is under stress the adrenal glands increase cortisol levels, which initially dampens hunger. Once the stress has passed our hunger hormones kick in and scream-Refuel!

Dairy - Dairy products in America are generally produced from cow's or domestic buffalo's milk. Occasionally the milk can come from other mammals such as goats, sheep, yaks, or camels.

Dairy products are treated in a very special manner by our human genetics. Dr. Alan Hirsch is a neurologist, and a psychiatrist. He is considered a leading expert on smell and taste physiology. He states, "The odor of food usually stimulates the 'I am full' signal in the brain but there is one important exception-milk. In infancy, milk is our primary food, and it promotes rapid growth in the first year of life. It appears that this is a permanent mechanism; it doesn't change with age. As adults, we can eat large amounts of dairy products without getting the, 'I am full, message'. It isn't unusual for one person to eat up to half a pound of cheese without a hint of fullness. The same is true for ice cream." (Hirsch, AR. *Dr. Hirsch's Guide To Scentsantional Weight Loss*. Rockport, MA: Element Books, 1997.)

DHA and EPA are the omega-3 essential fatty acids. DHA (docosahexaenoic acid) is an omega-3 essential fatty acid. Lower levels of the DHA inhibit the neurotransmitters dopamine and serotonin. These brain chemicals, when lowered trigger food addictions and cravings; in particular, the desire for sweets, chocolate, fatty and salty foods. DHA is also required for a healthy brain and eyes.

DHEA (dehydroepiandrosterone): The two adrenal glands release a hormone called DHEA, which helps the conversion of the less active T4 thyroid hormone to the more active T3 form. DHEA also improves energy, sleep, mental sharpness, premenstrual symptoms, and decreases body fat, and boosts muscle mass. In the United States DHEA is available over-the-counter, without a prescription.

Dopamine is a neurotransmitter that creates the "high" feeling associated with drug use, sex, eating certain foods, and even shopping. Elevations of dopamine are also connected with addictions such as nicotine, cocaine, and other substances that produce a feeling of *excited euphoria* by increasing dopamine levels in the brain. Dopamine turns on the pleasure response from foods. Low dopamine levels increase our appetite. Eating sugars raises dopamine levels.

Dopamine has multiple functions depending on where in the brain itacts. Dopamine in the basal nuclei of the brain acts to suppress unwanted muscle activity. Thus, any severe loss of dopamine causes the muscle rigidity typical of Parkinson's disease.

Eicosapentaenoic acid (EPA) is an omega-3 essential fatty acid. Among its effects on the body, it maintains the cell membrane's fluidity, allowing more glucose (fuel) to enter the cell for the mitochondria to convert to energy. EPA also inhibits platelet aggregation (thins the blood) and decreases production of inflammatory prostaglandins (anti-inflammatory).

Electromagnetic stress: cell phones, computers, microwaves, electric blankets, etc. all emit electromagnetic fields (EMFs). EMFs are invisible fields of electric and magnetic forces from the flow of current through wires or electrical devices and increase in strength as the current increases. Magnetic fields are measured in units of gauss or tesla. Most electrical equipment has to be turned on, i.e., current must be flowing, for a *magnetic field* to be produced. *Electric fields*, on the other hand, are present even when the equipment is switched off, as long as it remains connected to the source of electric power.

Both electric and magnetic fields decrease *exponentially* as the distance from the source increases.

A simple way, therefore to reduce the stress of electomagnetic waves is to use a gauss meter. The is an inexpensive tool you can use to survey nearby electromagnetic field radiation levels (EMFs) from fans, electrical appliances, wiring and power lines, from cell towers, high power tension lines, televisions, florescent lights, Wi-Fi and other common sources.

Gauss meters are available at some local hardware stores or are found through the internet.

Since Electromagnetic field energy decrease as the distance from the source increases, simply relocate the EMF emitters; even a few inches of repositioning can dramatically help reduce your exposure.

Epinephrine also known as **adrenaline**, is an adrenal gland hormone we use to deal with stress. It is a neurotransmitter and hormone essential to metabolism. It regulates attention, mental focus, arousal, and cognition. Epinephrine decreases appetites, stops or greatly slows down movements of the gastrointestinal tract and digestive secretions. Low levels can cause fatigue, lack of focus, and difficulty losing weight.

Fast foods often have a high content of salt. The craving of salty foods can be triggered by a lack of aldosterone (an adrenal hormone), which leads to salt wasting through the kidneys into the urine and hence the craving for more salt. Craving salty foods can therefore be a sign of adrenal gland weakness and is common after prolonged stress.

Flaxseed oil contains alpha-linolenic acid (ALA) which the body must convert into EPA and DHA. Flaxseed oil spoils quickly and must be kept refrigerated.

Food addiction: Dr. Mark Gold, chief of addiction medicine at the University of Florida's, McKnight Brain Institute, defines food addiction as: "Eating too much despite consequences, even dire consequences to health; being preoccupied with food, food preparation and meals; trying and failing to cut back on food intake; feeling guilty about eating and overeating."

Fructose, also known as fruit sugar or levulose, is in fruits, vegetables, and honey. High fructose corn syrup (HFCS) is a common sweetener used in the food industry. *Eating fructose doesn't trigger the release of insulin*. Insulin has a powerful appetite suppressant effect. Insulin also increases leptin release, an appetite inhibitor. Since fructose and HFCS do not release insulin, we commonly over-consume foods containing fructose, or corn syrup because satiation of our appetite from insulin is absent. The food industry claims it uses HFCS instead of cane sugar due to its lower cost. Many argue that HFCS's stimulating of over-consumption is the real reason for its use.

GABA (gamma-aminobutyric acid) is the major inhibitory neurotransmitter in the brain. Low levels of GABA are associated with fear. Elevated cortisol (stress) inhibits GABA. The herb valerian root effectively raises GABA by inhibiting the re-uptake of GABA. The active ingerdiants are *valepotriates*. This herb is commonly used in Europe. The amino acid taurine enhances the effects of GABA and typical doses are 1,000 milligrams of taurine, taken when needed.

Genes are what carries one's heredity. Current research reveals ours genes (biology) influence our lives in many more ways than previously thought—our personality, political affiliations, taste in music, and even our chances of getting divorced. [1]

Ghrelin is a hormone released from the stomach, and to a lesser extent from the rest of the gastrointestinal tract. Ghrelin travels into the bloodstream and affects the hypothalamus in the brain, stimulating the appetite to increase food intake. The anticipation of food also increases ghrelin levels and therefore boosts our appetite.

Glucocorticoid hormones are made in the adrenal glands. Cortisol, also known as hydrocortisone, is the most important human glucocorticoid. Cortisol increases our appetite.

Glucose or **blood sugar** is the principal, circulating sugar in our blood, and the major energy source of the body. It is the only 'fuel' our brain requires other than oxygen. Most cells need a transporter, insulin, to help carry glucose across our cells' membranes where it is used as fuel. Two noted exceptions to needing the insulin helper are your brain and retina; thus we get an instant brain turbocharge from ingesting refined carbohydrates.

Glutamate is the most common excitatory neurotransmitter in the brain. It is the *survival neurotransmitter*. When we are under stress the body makes glutamate at the expense of the other neurotransmitters.

Glycemic index is a numerical value given to a carbohydrate rich food based on the average increase in blood sugar (glucose) levels occurring after the food is eaten. Glucose is assigned the value of 100 and other carbs are given a number relative to glucose. Carbohydrates that quickly convert into glucose in the blood stream are given a high glycemic index value whereas carbohydrates with lower glycemic numbers, will release glucose more gradually into the blood.

Hormones are our body's chemical messengers.

Hunger is a set of unpleasant sensations which will drive us to hunt, forage or do just about anything to get some food.

5-HTP (5-hydroxytryptophan) is an amino acid precursor to the neurotransmitter serotonin. Supplementing with 5-HTP may be useful in treating depression, fibromyalgia, tension and migraine headaches, and as an adjunct to weight loss. 5-HTP is isolated from the seeds of the African plant *Griffonia simplicifolia,* and is available over-the-counter in the USA. There are no known side effects. It should not be taken concurrently with serotonin selective reuptake inhibitor (SSRI) medications or serotonin-norepinephrine reuptake inhibitor (SNRI) medications.

Hypericum perforatum is an herb commonly known as St. John's wort. This herb has been shown to raise the levels of several neurotransmitters: serotonin, norepinephrine, and dopamine. It should not be taken concurrently with either serotonin selective reuptake inhibitor (SSRI) medications or serotonin-norepinephrine reuptake inhibitor (SNRI) medications.

Hypoglycemia (*hypo* means low, *glycemia* means blood sugar) is low blood sugar.

Hypothyroid (underactive thyroid gland function) which can manifest with any of the following common symptoms: Weight gain, fatigue, depression, intolerance to cold temperatures, poor concentration, female hair thinning, coarse or dry skin, infertility, menstrual irregularities, constipation, crying for no apparent reason and an 'addiction' to exercise.

Insulin is a hormone secreted by the pancreas and released into the blood when glucose levels go up, such as after eating. Insulin, at the individual cell level, signals most cells whether to burn or store fat or sugar. Without insulin, most cells are unable to use glucose for energy. *Insulin is also a strong appetite suppressor;* thus raising insulin levels helps satiate the appetite.

Leptin is a hormone produced by fat cells. Leptin shuts down our appetite for food and the amount of leptin produced increases in obesity since it is made in the fat tissue. Obviously, for many people this particular check and balance system is not working sufficiently. We now know that obese people are *leptin-resistant.* We think people become leptin-resistant by overexposure to high levels of this hormone due to excess fat accumulation. Additionally, since insulin also increases the release of leptin, chronically elevated insulin levels due to excessive carbohydrate consumption, can contribute to leptin-resistance.

Liver is a glandular organ that secretes bile, stores and filters blood, and is involved in the conversion of sugars into stored sugar. The liver has over 500 other known functions.

Melatonin is a neuroendocrine-hormonal regulator involved with sleep-inducing signals, day/night cycles, and body temperature. It also makes us drowsy; inducing sleep. Produced by the pineal gland in the brain, melatonin is considered the "darkness" hormone since it is released in response to the absence of light. Melatonin is available over-the-counter in the United States.

Meridians are the acupuncture energy circuits or pathways that flow longitudinally, encircling the body and are generally named for the various body organs or functions in which they have a controlling influence on.

Metabolism is the term used for the process by which food is converted into energy.

Mitochondria are our body's power generating factories. These cellular power generators have their own replication machinery (DNA and RNA); so the mitochondria have the ability to reproduce and increase in number within your cells.

Mucuna pruriens is an herb that raises dopamine levels. Mucuna pruriens is also known as velvet bean, cowitch, kapikachu or atmagupta in India. This herb contains a precursor to the neurotransmitter dopamine, L-Dopa. Mucuna pruriens is available over-the-counter in the United States.

Natural thyroid medications including these brands, are examples of thyroid medications that contain a mixture of the thyroid hormones: T4 (thyroxine) and T3 (triiodothyronine) in proportions of 80%—T4 and 20%—T3: (Armour® Thyroid), (Nature-Throid™) by Forest Labs, (Westhroid™) by Western Research Labs, and (Qualitest) by Time Caps Labs.

Neuropeptide Y (NPY) is the most potent neurotransmitter food intake stimulator known. The sympathetic nervous system innervates fat tissue and releases NPY at the nerve ending, which causes fat to accumulate. NPY turns on the cravings for food, especially for carbohydrates. Chronic stress, triggers NPY production. That means *long-term stress, triggers our appetites, especially for sweets*. NPY is also released in response to a decline in fat stores.

Neurotransmitters are chemicals controlling the flow of information from one part of the nervous system to another. These chemicals direct every thought, mood, and emotion. They shape our personality, as well as modulating our experience of pain and pleasure. Neurotransmitters control our food cravings, appetite, energy levels, sex drive as well as our sleep. Over 100 different neurotransmitters have been identified.

Norepinephrine (NE) a.k.a. as **noradrenalin,** is a hormone that increases our appetite for sweets. When under stress, our level of norepinephrine rises, which mobilizes stored fat for use as fuel. Norepinephrine acts as a neurotransmitter and a hormone. In the peripheral nervous system, it is part of the fight-or-flight response. In the brain, it acts as a neurotransmitter regulating normal brain processes. Norepinephrine is usually excitatory, excitatory, but is inhibitory in a few brain areas and *aides in the reduction of pain*. Norepinephrine is important for attentiveness, emotions, sleeping, dreaming, and learning. Norepinephrine also is released as a hormone into the blood, where it causes blood vessels to contract and the heart rate to increase.

Obesity is defined as being 30% or more above your healthy weight. Today 34% of adults in America are classified medically as obese.

Omega-3 essential fatty acids:
- Anti-inflammatory (decreases production of inflammatory prostaglandins)
- Make the cell membrane (plasma membrane) more fluid to facilitate the transport of glucose into the cell to be converted into energy
- "Thin the blood" (inhibits platelet aggregation)
- Are brain food
- Can be an antidepressant as potent as *Prozac*®

Omega-6 essential fatty acids balance the omega-3 EFAs. Omega-6 makes cell membranes (plasma membranes) more resistant to allowing your fuel (glucose) to enter the cell to be used for energy. If too much omega-6 is present, the glucose "bounces off" our cell membranes and gets deposited as fat. Omega-6 EFAs also "thicken the blood," and promote the inflammatory process. Omega-6 fats are found in grains and the animal fat of animals fed grains.

Overweight is defined as being 10% or more above your healthy weight. Currently more than 65% of adults in the United States are overweight.

Oxyntomodulin (OXM) reduces hunger and is released in the small intestines in response to calorie intake.

Oxytocin is a pituitary hormone that reduces the appetite. It is stimulated by dopamine and promotes sexual arousal, feelings of emotional attachment, and the desire to cuddle. It's released from the posterior lobe of the pituitary gland in the brain.

Pancreas is a gland near the stomach that secretes insulin and digestive juices (enzymes).

Pancreatic Polypeptide (PP) is released in response to ingestion of food and reduces our appetite. Pancreatic polypeptide is a gut hormone produced mainly by the pancreas in the area that also produces insulin.

Parasympathetic nervous system is part of the autonomic nervous system. The "rest and digest" parasympathetic nervous system is concerned with keeping the body's energy use low and involves the *3 D's: Digestion — Defication — Diuresis* (urination).

Parasympathetic activity is illustrated, for example, by a person who relaxes after a meal. In the state of parasympathetic relaxation, blood pressure, heart rate, and respiratory rates are low, but the gastrointestinal tract is active. The parasympathetic activity also *induces gastric (stomach) acid production.*

Peptides are short strings of amino acids linked by peptide bonds. Amino acids serve as the building blocks of proteins.

Peptide YY (PYY) suppresses our appetite. It is released from the intestinal tract after eating. Peptide YY peaks one to two hours after a meal and maintains that level for about six hours.

Progesterone ($C_{21} H_{30} O_2$) is a hormone produced in the ovaries after ovulation, and to a much lesser extent, in the adrenal glands. During pregnancy a large amount of progesterone is made by the placenta. *By age 35, fifty percent of women in the U.S. have an unhealthy deficiency of progesterone.* Be aware that many physicians and even medical writers incorrectly believe that synthetic progestins, such as those in birth control pills and the medication Provera ($C_{24} H_{34} O_4$), are actually the same as progesterone ($C_{21} H_{30} O_2$). This confusion is so pervasive that progesterone is blamed, due to misunderstanding, but without evidence, for the sins of Provera® (medroxyprogesterone acetate).

Progestins (progestogens or gestagens) are a classification of chemicals. Technically, natural progesterone is in the chemical group called progestins; but many progestins are not progesterone. Progestins are often incorrectly called "progesterone", even in scientific papers!

Perhaps, it's like saying since apples and kiwis are both classified as fruits, that apples are the same as kiwis; which of course is false.

Many mistakenly believe that synthetic progestins, such as those in birth control pills and the medication Provera®, are actually the same as progesterone. Perhaps, part of the confusion is this…

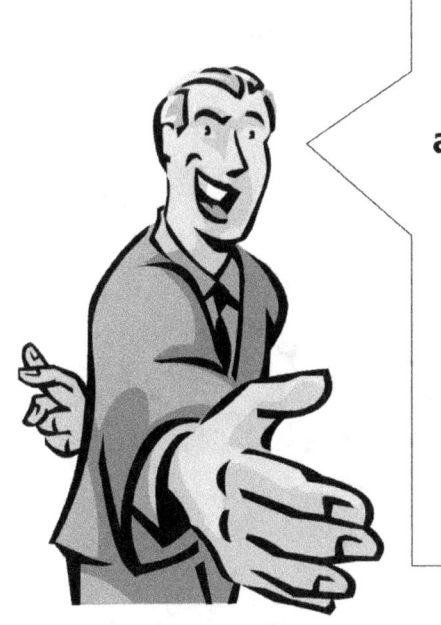

Take it from a drug rep., that so called "natural progesterone" stuff is really about the same as our Provera®.

Whether they call them progestins, gestagens, progestagens, or progesterone, they're all related.

Yes doc, it's all very confusing to me too…

Prometrium® (progesterone) ($C_{21} H_{30} O_2$) is a prescription oral capsule form of bioidentical progesterone.

Provera® ($C_{24} H_{34} O_4$) is a synthetic progestin. Be aware that many physicians *erroneously* believe that synthetic progestins, such as found in the medication Provera®, are progesterone ($C_{21} H_{30} O_2$).

Pupil dilation test (Rogoff Sign test) can be used to screen for adrenal fatigue syndrome. To perform this on yourself, a flashlight and a mirror are needed. Dim the lights. Face the mirror, and shine the light into one eye. If after 30 seconds the pupil (black center) starts to dilate (enlarge), adrenal fatigue syndrome should be suspected.

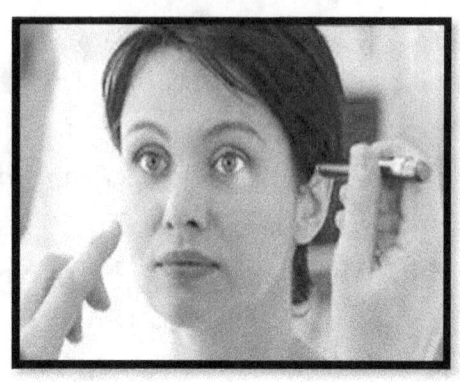

Why does this happen? During adrenal insufficiency, there is a suboptimal level of sodium and an abundance of potassium in the body. This mineral imbalance causes an inhibition of the sphincter muscles of the eye. These muscles normally initiate pupil constriction in the presence of bright light. However, in adrenal fatigue syndrome, the pupils actually dilate when exposed to light.

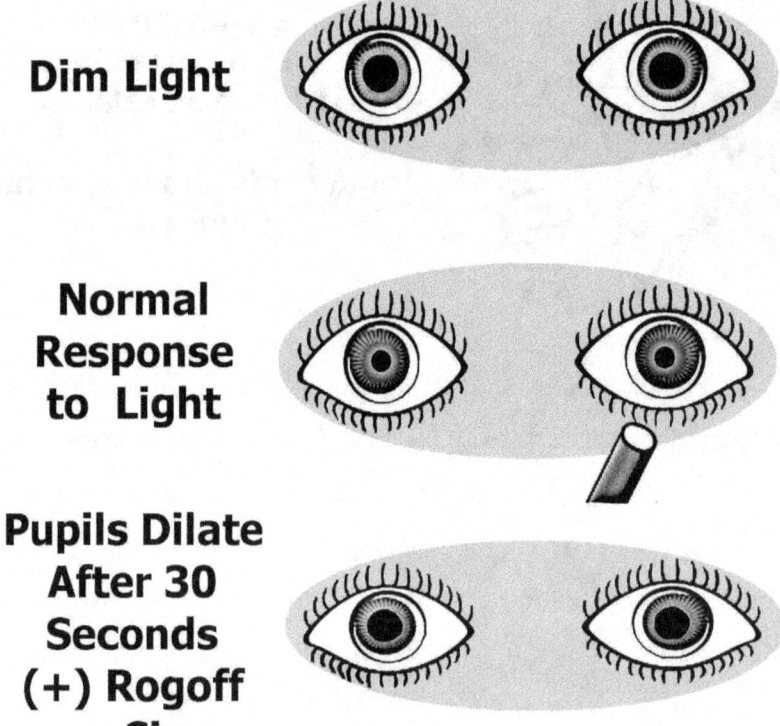

Dim Light

Normal Response to Light

Pupils Dilate After 30 Seconds (+) Rogoff Sign

Ragland's sign ("Blood Pressure test") can be used to screen for adrenal fatigue syndrome. The equipment needed is an accurate blood pressure kit. To perform this test, take your blood pressure while supine (laying face up on your back). Then, stand up and immediately take your blood pressure again. Your systolic (first) number should have risen 8 to 10 mm. If the number dropped, you may have adrenal fatigue.

Resistin is produced by adipose (fat) tissue and increases insulin resistance. Insulin resistance can deny glucose from entering our cells and the cells' energy power plants, the mitochondria; instead the glucose gets stored as fat.

Satiety is the "I am full" feeling and is regulated in the brain by the satiety center, technically known as the ventromedial nucleus of the hypothalamus.

Seasonal affective disorder (SAD), also known as winter depression, is a condition characterized by depression in the fall and winter months in the northern hemispheres, due to a lack of sunlight exposure. Lowered serotonin, dopamine, and norepinephrine levels are believed to trigger this condition, which commonly causes sufferers to crave carbohydrates and gain weight.

Often suffers of SAD may be helped with the use of a "light box". Also available are "light visors" that allow one to get a daily light treatment without having to sit or stand in one place. This is known as "light therapy" or phototherapy. A new approch channels a bright light directly into the light-sensitive region of the brain via the ear canal.

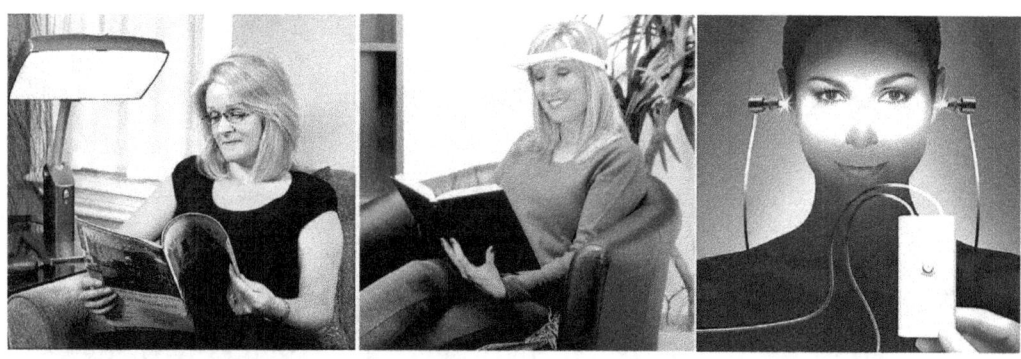

Serotonin is a neurotransmitter involved in many functions, including mood, appetite, and sensory perception. Adequate levels of serotonin turn off our appetite. Low serotonin levels increase our appetite for sweets. Women make about seven times less serotonin in their brains then men do do and this may explains why women crave sweets more than men. The reasons may involve the fact that the female body has a lower percentage of muscle mass and therefore can make and store less serotonin than the male body.

Sucrose is the organic compound commonly known as table sugar, white sugar, or processed sugar. The common source of commercially produced sucrose is from harvesting and processing sugar cane and sugar beets.

Sympathetic nervous system is part of the autonomic nervous system. The "fight-or-flight" sympathetic nervous system responds to survive "emergencies." The sympathetic nervous system is involved with the 4 *E's:* Exercise—Excitement—Emergencies—Embarrassment.

The sympathetic nervous system's activities are illustrated by a person who is threatened; thus the heart rate increases, breathing is rapid and deep, blood sugar levels rise and gastrointestinal functioning decreases. The body shunts blood from the gastrointestinal tract to the muscles, heart, lungs and brain to maximize the effectiveness of our emergency survival mode.

Synthetic balanced thyroid medications are thyroid hormone preparations that have both T4—thyroxine and T3—triiodothyronine combined, which is similar to the composition found in (Armour®). One synthetic T4 and T3 combined medication is (Thyrolar®).

Synthroid® is a synthetic medication containing only T4 (thyroxine). Other medications with only thyroxine (T4) include: Eltroxin®, Levothroid®, Levoxyl, Oroxine, and Unithroid®.

T4 or **thyroxine** is a thyroid hormone. T4 is *not* easily used by our body's cells. Instead, our bodies convert T4 to the more active and utilizable thyroid hormone, T3. These medications only contain thyroxine (T4): Synthroid®, Eltroxin®, Levothroid®, Levoxyl®, Oroxie, and Unithroid®.

T3, **triiodothyronine** or **liothyronine sodium** is the active form of our thyroid hormones. These medications contain only T3—triiodothyronine: Cytomel®, Tertroxin®, Triostat®, and Cynomel®.

TSH (thyroid stimulating hormone) is made by the anterior pituitary gland in the brain and stimulates thyroid gland secretion. *It has an inverse relationship with the thyroid hormones.* Abnormally low levels of thyroid hormones will trigger high levels of TSH in the body's attempt to 'wake-up' the thyroid to work harder and produce more thyroid hormones. A key point to remember is that the pituitary is much more sensitive to the thyroid hormone T4 than the rest of our body's tissues and therefore, TSH blood tests are *not* an accurate way to determine proper doses of T4 medication.

Traditional Chinese medicine (TCM) is commonly called acupuncture. Traditional Chinese medicine includes the use of herbs, diet, lifestyle modifications, mental and emotional well-being, traditional Chinese manipulation (which is similar to chiropractic adjustments or osteopathic manipulation), and acupuncture with needles, pressure, electricity, heat, or cold laser.

Tryptophan is the stuff serotonin is made from. It is an essential amino acid, and amino acids make up proteins. When under stress and/or inflammation is present in the body, you make less serotonin from your tryptophan.

Vitamin B12 (chemical name—cyanocobalamin) low or suboptimal levels of vitamin B12 are now a pandemic due to common problems with intrinsic factor (IF), also known as gastric intrinsic factor, which attaches to B12 and allows B12 to be absorbed into the body via the small intestines. Unlike many vitamin deficiencies, low vitamin B12 is often caused by suboptimal stomach function, rather than failing to ingest sufficient doses of the vitamin itself.

Suboptimal levels of vitamin B12 can affect your achieving a healthy weight in two significant ways:

- Hampering your ability to convert the T4 thyroid hormone into the active T3 form, that your cells can use. Without adequate T3, your metabolism will be lowered, so your body burns less fuel (food) and stores the excess as fat.

- Limiting your body's ability to produce serotonin and dopamine, triggering cravings for carbohydrates and sweets.

Low vitamin B12 concentrations are associated with cognitive impairment in older people, even in the absence of anemia. [2]

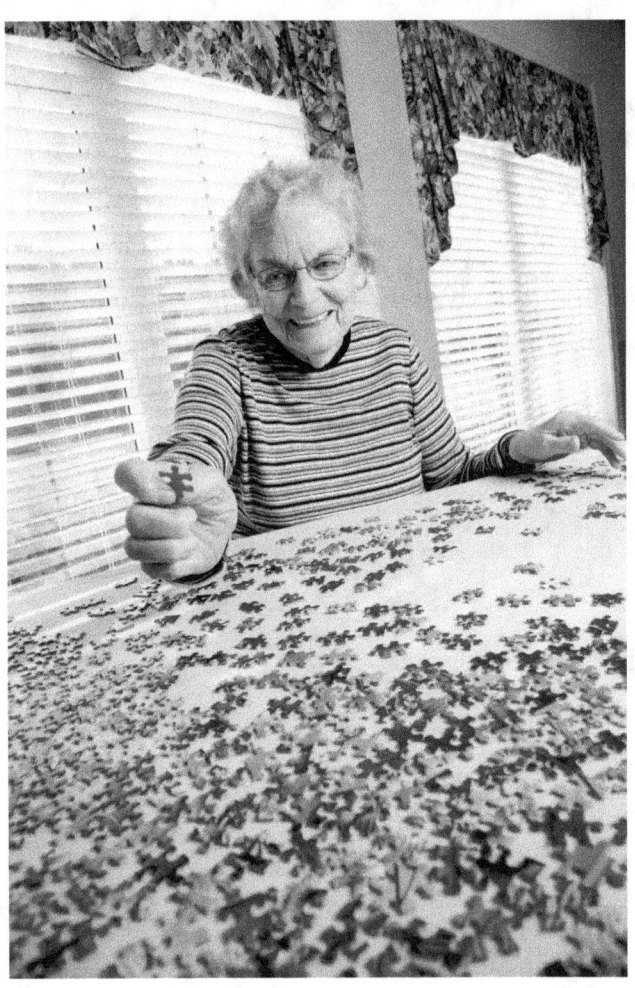

Half of people in their 50's, 60% of people in their 60's, and 70% of people in their 70's have low vitamin B12.

Section 2

Using *Psychology* (Nurture) to Show You the Power to Change Your Eating and Weight

Acknowledgments

Within every problem is a gift waiting to be discovered. I'm fortunate to have had the experience of struggling with the problem of an eating disorder in this lifetime—and experiencing the blessing of overcoming it.

Exploring eating disorders gave me more than answers about why it happens. I've discovered solutions that address and alleviate the problem at its source. As a result, I live by these spiritual truths every day. This experience has given me the impetus to share these truths and insights with others by writing this book.

So many shining stars helped me write this book, both directly and indirectly. First, I'd like to thank my pre-publication editor, Coleen Rehm. Without her knowingness, endless patience, and dedication to her profession, I could never have written this book. She is a bright shining star of God who has catapulted me into new awareness. I'd also like to thank my longtime friend, Denise Nearing for referring me to Linda Anderson who ultimately directed me to Coleen.

Many writers inspired me at the 2000 ECK Writers and Creative Arts Conference in Montreal. Thanks to Vicki Williams who graciously offered to read the first rough draft. I'd like to extend my warm gratitude to Rainbow Sally Glassburn, who gave creativity and love, and Beverly Bowles who helped me stay balanced. Many thanks go to my assistant Marty Rapert who did whatever job I needed done.

Gratitude goes to my family: first to my love, Jeff Lang who nurtured me with back rubs to help release stress from typing at night and on weekends. To my oldest daughter Danielle Crouch, who helped me enter the manuscript into the new computer. David Scarpa helped pick out and set up my new notebook computer. Thank you to my youngest daughter Shannon Crouch for her continued love notes that helped uplift me. Love and thanks also to my Mom and Dad, Sue and Weldon Fuller, and Grandma Nettie and Grandpa Frank Fuller and Grandmother Susie Matthews and Grandfather Edward Matthews for their gifts of many challenges, which have been transformed into polished diamonds in my life.

To Margo Maine, Ph.D., for her words of wisdom at EDAP's Eating Disorder Conference. Also to R.D. Longacre, Ph.D., who took time to show me that getting started is easy with an outline of my first draft at the International Hypnosis Conference in 1996. And thanks to everyone who said, "Go for it!" in response to this dream. All of you were so precious in this incredible process.

Special thanks to the DCT Team 2 Crystal and Megan for their care in loving my book in the publishing/designing process and Lee Sanderline, publishing consultant.

Special thanks to Harold Klemp who has given me spiritual support and inner guidance for many years. Without him, I wouldn't be here today.

Thank you all and I love you.

I have changed the names of the people in the stories throughout this book to protect their privacy. Any resemblance to any person, living or dead, with these same names is purely a coincidence.

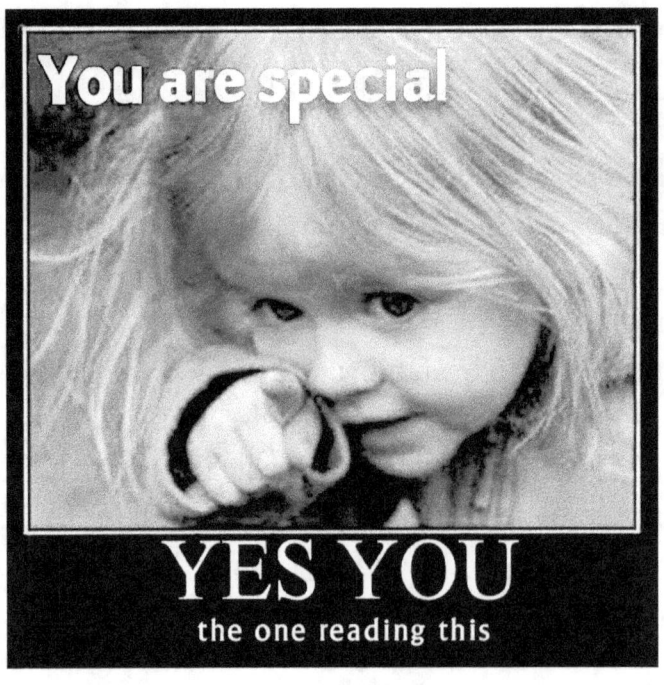

Hope for Your Healthy Eating Journey

It is a hot, steamy day in Stuart. The wind blows off the St. Lucie River. Faintly I hear the clang of sailboat masts anchored a few hundred feet off the seawall near my office. The phone rings. A woman we'll call Annie is looking for a Psychotherapist/Life Coach, but she is hesitant to tell me her full story over the phone. I continue to talk with her, hoping to get a feeling for what she expects from therapy. Although I get all kinds of calls and requests, I never know how the conversation will go. I only know that if I can help, I will do so.

Annie explains that she's feeling desperate. Her weight has ballooned to more than 180 pounds. "I don't know what to do," she cries.

I listen, then explain that my specialty is eating disorders. I offered her a consultation to determine the next step. I am rarely refused, for what I offer is hope.

Annie arrives and when she sits down I notice she's nervous. Her body is visibly tight and guarded. she twists slightly away from me as she answers my questions. Her whole demeanor shouts low self-esteem and I detect an undertone of hostility, possibly due to her inner turmoil and struggle. Yet, I know she is vitally open to what I have to offer for she has shown an incredible amount of determination and courage by simply being here. From this I know our mutual adventure in the process of healing has begun.

We'll follow Annie's quest to weight balance success throughout some of this book so that you can use her experience of the journey as a "road map" for what you might find along the way. (Annie's road map has components which can help bulimics, anorexics, food addicts, and compulsive overeaters. Plus all techniques have been clinically researched. I know what works because I have recovered from depression, anxiety and eating disorders.)

The Importance of Having a Star to Guide You

When I was growing up in the Puget Sound area, I had a life-changing experience as an eighth-grade student. In an assembly of eight hundred, I viewed a film that showed a street corner filled with businessmen dressed in dark gray suits. As they crossed the street in unison, the announcer's voice asked,

> *"Do you want to be just another gray-suited person conforming to the masses? Or do you seek a different kind of truth?".*

This message is powerful. Even today it stands out as inspiration for everyone to go beyond what is known and commonly accepted. It inspires valuing and honoring what is unique and authentic for you as an individual. It implies finding a higher spiritual perspective to guide your life—one that is true to you.

On a personal level, it also confirmed my inner desire to make a difference in this world by following my heart and creatively blazing new trails. The realizations born from this experience became a pioneering vision—a star to guide me throughout my life.

The inspirational vision of a guiding star came from one of my closest mentors—my mother. When I was 13 years old, she gave me a framed poem entitled, "Ideals Are Like Stars" by Helen Steiner Rice.

The poem spoke to me about keeping morals, standards, and ideals high, as well as living a life based on truth. Steiner Rice's poem compared ideals to the stars in the sky, in that we can always reach for them and they will be there for guidance through dark times. By aligning my heart with high ideals, my life would also shine like a star. These thoughts and principles laid a firm foundation for me in my youth, inspiring and guiding me through some difficult teenage years.

Later when I divorced and went back to school for my master's degree, my mother sent the framed poem to me. I hung it in my office when I entered the business world for the first time at the age of 45. Every time I read that poem, it acted as an inner, guiding star to lead the way.

Each time I connected with its inner strength, I found I had vision and roots.

Each time I set a goal, it was the absolute highest and purest I could set in light of the principles of this guiding star. Having a star to guide you is like having the Source of All Love bring you a fuller, more loving heart. Having an inner star for guidance led me to a purer awareness of love.

In this world, mentors, images, and the written or spoken word can be guiding stars to help everyone move through difficult life transitions. The simple act of reading this book can act as an inner star to guide you. Practicing the principles found within these pages can help navigate and smooth out the shoals of diet myths. You'll find anchor points of rest and reflection throughout these chapters as you voyage toward successful weight balance. In time you'll find hidden attitude keys which (when exercised) can unlock untold spiritual gifts hidden in the treasure chest of your life experiences.

This book can be an inner star to guide you when you regularly practice the techniques, exercises, and visualizations. In time, these components will help you tap into the pure love that already exists within you. This love burns with an eternal flame and can act as a guiding star or a lighthouse beacon, as you journey toward a more peaceful, contented life.

Take Inventory of Yourself and Societal Attitudes Before Beginning the Journey

Many twists and turns convolute the path and the process when healing eating and weight issues. Each person's journey is unique, but certain behavioral similarities are fundamental at the start for nearly everyone who is affected.

Why?

This may surprise you, but the sociocultural roots of diet and weight issues are hidden deep in plain view. They are found in the often unspoken and generally accepted expectations we hold about the world in which we live. These expectations are primarily determined by the combined attitudes of people who comprise this culture and society.

It is personally surprising to find out how deeply entrenched these sociocultural systems are to each of us.

> *Yet, taking stock of the conscious and unconscious influence these expectations hold on us individually is the first step to freeing ourselves from them forever.*

To find out for yourself how immune or immersed you are in these biases, complete the *Checklist for Eating and Weight Issues* quiz by answering "yes" or "no" to the following questions. The results may surprise you, but they can also act as a catalyst and a wake-up call.

Checklist for Eating and Weight Issues

Have you ever:

(1) thought constantly about food or talked incessantly about dieting?

(2) felt overwhelming emotional stress?

(3) felt depressed with low self-esteem over several weeks, months, or longer?

(4) felt out of control?

(5) believed that all it takes to conquer weight issues is willpower?

(6) tried to restrict your diet to lose weight gained from overeating?

(7) felt guilty or ashamed about your eating habits or patterns?

(8) started eating, then found you couldn't stop?

(9) eaten so much at night that you could hardly get up in the morning?

(10) experienced relationship or family problems because of over-eating, dieting, bingeing or purging?

(11) held high expectations or standards for yourself and others?

(12) told family what you think they want to hear about your eating habits, rather than the truth?

(13) maintained a lower or higher than average weight?

(14) gorged yourself, then used exercise, vomiting, or laxatives so you wouldn't gain weight?

(15) placed overt importance on your physical appearance?

(16) admitted physical appearance is of ultimate importance to your family and/or yourself?

(17) experienced swollen glands from vomiting?

(18) experienced menstrual irregularities?

(19) felt compelled to monitor what you or your children ate?

If you answered yes for one to five of these questions, then you've found this book at a good time. If you answered yes to five to ten questions, it's a wake-up call. Pay attention to the warning signs of weight issues now and begin seeking help. Implementing this book is a good first step.

If you answered yes to 10 to 15 questions, consider employing the help of a qualified therapist as you use this book, for the sake of your health and wellbeing.

If you or someone you know can answer yes to 15 or more questions, it's time for immediate action or a personal intervention. You can call the National Eating Disorders Association (NEDA) at (800) 931-2237 or contact *www.NationalEatingDisorders.org* for referrals and help. Your life or the life of someone you love may be at stake.

You will find hope, help, and the answers you seek by using this book and by contacting NEDA like millions have before you. In my heart, I know you will.

The Preliminary First Steps to Healing

The first step on the journey to healing is to take an inventory of where you are in relation to societal attitudes about food and weight. This you've already done by completing the *Checklist for Eating and Weight Issues* quiz. The next step is to make a commitment to become actively involved in the techniques, exercises, and process of actually living the principles outlined in this book.

> *Once you make the commitment to "walk the walk,"*
> *your life will never be the same again.*

As a good faith measure of your commitment, write down in your own words how you intend to implement the wisdom contained in this book through your actions every day.

I am willing to _____

_____.

Now that you've taken inventory and affirmed commitment to your goal, it's time to set the proper pace.

The Importance of Setting the Proper Pace

For me, finding solutions took many years of clinical experience and documentation. To my surprise, most of the wisdom and love came from the past seven years of practicing true inner balance.

If you're like I was in the beginning, you'll want all this wisdom as fast and as soon as possible. However, getting it fast can leave you with a case of spiritual indigestion, which will put you off the material indefinitely and ultimately defeat your progress. A ravenous style of questing can shock and overwhelm your body, mind and emotions. A better and more balanced way to absorb this information is to allow yourself to learn by reading a chapter and then taking some time to merge its principles into your life.

Another way to proceed is to begin an ongoing series of book discussions that meet once a month with friends in your home or others interested in weight balance success in a private room at a local library. This pace allows you to devote a month of practice to the exercises and techniques in the book, sharing the harvest of wisdom you've gained from your collective learning experiences with the group. The exercises and techniques contained within these pages are surprisingly powerful when combined with this type of group support system.

Move gradually to each chapter, reviewing it nightly or weekly while continually doing the exercises that speak most pointedly to you or draw your attention. Most exercises or techniques can be done at least once. However, you can use them as many times as you want as you progress through subsequent chapters.

> *Give yourself a natural time boundary, or pace, in which to digest, review, and sustain your growth. This is the most loving action you can take for yourself.*

Routinely making new mini-goals or purpose statements for your weight balance success helps keep the adventure fresh and exciting.

You can return to any section in this book at any time and use it as a steady reference guide for change. The continual process of taking action, following through, and manifesting change empowers the divine you (Soul) to creatively transform any arena of your life.

The Next Step to Manifesting Your Goals

My golden invitation to you throughout this book is to explore with a light heart and a sense of freedom. Only you can make this grand adventure happen in the most enjoyable way possible. It all starts now when you turn the page with the expectation of being open to a new level of weight and balance success.

We'll begin by exposing and dispelling the social and personal culture surrounding eating and weight issues, exploring the validity or rhetorical hyperbole of these myths in depth throughout Chapter 16.

Part 1

Steps Toward Your Freedom and Taking Control of Your Eating Issues

Chapter 16

Overcoming the Eight Diet Myths That Can Bind You

The Diet Myth

Remember when you used to get the newest diet book in your hands, literally hot off the press? Guaranteed, it says. Guaranteed to work or your money back! "This time it's going to work," you think. "I just know it. It says so right here in print. Guaranteed!"

Although you've been here many times before, you still think this time is going to be the last, so many feelings are wrapped up in this moment. It's almost magical. A confluence of emotions race through you as you simultaneously experience the thrill of hope, success, approval, attention, and a feeling of rightness with the world. This time you know deep in your heart that you will do it right. "I'll be beautiful," you think. And then you're lost in a dream—a diet dream.

This is the basis of the insidious diet myth. We're led to believe that all our problems will be solved, all our dreams will come true—if only we diet. Even the word *diet* conjures up seemingly magical wishes and promises. Among these are hopes and dreams of future success about everything from beauty, self-esteem, feeling all right, being a good girl, as well as approval from others. But the diet myth is not magic. It is a lie.

Because it is silently sanctioned by society and tied in with equally misleading myths about being overweight, the diet myth continues to pervade society and is impervious to criticism. The combination of myths about dieting and the causes of overweight weave invisible threads that have the potential to knot up years of your life and wreak a megaton of damage to your health and well-being with time.

What's most frustrating is that one person can't change these societal beliefs (which are imbued as if they were the truth) for everyone. But one person *can* change their personal relationship to this propaganda for themselves—largely by seeing the diet myth for what it really is, gaining a truer understanding of its fallibility, and altering their response to it.

Seeing the Reality of the Diet Myth for What It Is

The reality is this: diets promising fast results create false hope.

Women have been bound by this false hope for a hundred years or longer and now men are starting to buy into it. The truth is we have been and continue to be sold a misleading bill of goods that perpetually doesn't deliver on its empty promises.

For too long, myths about diet and overweight issues have been accepted as fact. Now you can free yourself and understand your feelings of hopelessness, confusion, and frustration—but *only* by first exposing the myths in their entirety. No more dieting to be beautiful, feel good enough, or feel better about yourself. No more dieting to gain the approval of family, society, or others. No more instant, dieting solutions to make everything better.

Take a deep breath now and bring yourself back to the present. It's time to take a gentle step across the realm of diet dreams. Take a gentle step toward real success with the secrets of weight balance contained in this book. Are you ready? The secrets are waiting for you.

The One Essential Quality to Develop for Weight Balance Success

One quality that you can develop, which will guide you through the misinformation of the dieting myths, is awareness.

With awareness the secrets to successful weight balance will unfold as naturally and effortlessly as turning the pages of this book.

Finding my own awareness took years of digging. I first learned to dig for answers as a child of eight. One of my favorite things to do was to dig to the secret China Smuggling Caves from my Puget Sound backyard. I remember being outside, endlessly digging with a shovel in the backyard. My mother called me tenacious for I rarely gave up on what I wanted to accomplish or know. I wanted freedom even then and my spirit knew it.

Unfortunately only three years later I mistakenly applied my tenacity to my first diet. In 1957, I lost 16 pounds one summer at the age of eleven. I used my creative thinking to make up a diet. At that time, I'd encountered the concept of calories. I reasoned if I ate less, then I'd lose weight. Thus my first starvation diet was born. Believe it or not, I'd reward myself with an ice cream bar as needed. Does this sound familiar? That was my start on a dangerous cycle of dieting.

Later in life when I was in my late twenties, I disliked the ways I reacted to unhappiness by starving myself and calling it "my diet." In my thirties, I became worse. The more I tried to find answers in diets, the worse my unhappiness became. By the time I was in my forties, I was on the verge of self-destruction.

What I learned from all this is it never works to diet—never !

What I found is that diet myths can be hypnotic in their persistent calling. I could not stop until I got to the bottom of the myths. It took me nearly thirty-three years to uncover the deceptions and discover the real answers I've found in weight balance.

Although my digging and searching certainly took me into the abyss of dieting, I wouldn't change one thing about my journey because each painful stumble and fall taught me more. Even though following each diet myth led me to another dead end, I would always discover a new direction or a new lesson to be learned. The uncovering process seemed like walking in a labyrinth for decades at the time, but with awareness I found freedom at the end.

The most important key I learned was this: *those who have found the way are best at showing others the way out.* Pathfinders who have been there before can map the invisible threads and untie the binding knots of diet myths. You too can chart your own personal journey.

In my practice I recently helped a formerly diet-bound woman let go of cravings, yo-yo dieting, and leave depression behind by using the processes explained in this book. We cleared myth after myth with these non-prescription techniques. All the while she was able to release the issues that kept her diet-bound. She is now off medication for depression and eating healthfully, with no cravings or compulsion to overeat. She's feeling good about herself and moving forward into a new career, loving herself and her life. *You can do it, too.*

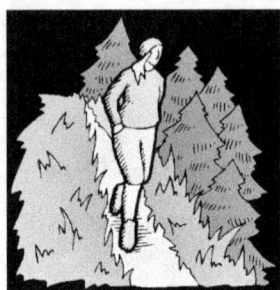

Pathfinder

Understanding the Roots of "Genetic" Societal Beliefs

Diet myths are a collective group of family experiences, which turn into beliefs and are then handed down for generations, in a metaphorically similar way that genetic traits are handed down. Through family connections, everyone has generally accepted myths. They are often built upon a consensus of group responses to life experiences and group wishes, rather than true wisdom. In accepting and embodying diet myths, false knowledge is distorted as truth and passed on for generations.

One example of this is reported in Ellen Ruppel Shell's book *The Hungry Gene*. The chapter called "Spammed" highlights the disastrous effects of group consensus on diet after World War II.

Natives on a tiny South Pacific island of Korsrae were influenced by the perceived status of eating imported American fast foods. In time, their diets evolved from ones based on island-grown whole foods (fresh fish, breadfruit, mangoes and papayas which had kept their ancestors healthy for millenium) to ones based predominately upon canned Spam®, turkey tails, sodas, and beer.

Most of the children now have abscessed teeth and the adults expect to die in their fifties from diabetes, hypertension, and heart disease as a direct result of eating the imported foods. The nutritious breadfruit, mangoes and papayas that once ensured native good health now rot on the ground.

The Difference between Knowledge and Wisdom

The best education combines knowledge and experience, and bears fruit in hard-won personal wisdom.

We understand experience. But knowledge and wisdom are often confused in relation to diet myths. Knowledge can lead to wisdom when it is combined with awareness—when an individual is open to change with additional information and experience. Wisdom is the culmination of vast stores of knowledge based on experience (yours and others). It grows out of logical thinking, helping you understand how to make the best use of your knowledge and experience for the highest good of yourself and the world around you.

How do you take experience and knowledge to the level of personal wisdom? One way is by combining them with the practice of the techniques, exercises, and activities shared in this book. By digging at the logic and psychology upon which most of the diet myths are based, you'll discover true human needs are buried there. With awareness, you'll understand better the true source from which diet myths spring and the real reasons why they seem so irrefutable. Using that understanding with this book, you can expand your viewpoint to allow for the whole truth.

For example, you may discover when people hear you are on a diet, they are proud of you and you feel happy. You may realize the reason for this is the basic human need for love, acceptance, and approval.

Later when you're off the diet, you may find yourself defeated. The instant success is gone and you're still unhappy, only now you've added even more weight than before, due in large part to an unbalanced diet regime. Your needs haven't changed. Only now you know the truth about the diet myth—that it's all a lie. Now you're ready to take personal knowledge and experience to a higher level of weight balance wisdom.

You're now on the threshold of freedom from diet myths. The success you desire is just around the corner. Are you ready for the truth?

Here are eight diet myths that bind the heart, which we'll explore in the rest of this chapter.

Myth 1: If I diet, my bad feelings will go away.

Myth 2: Dieting will make my world all right.

Myth 3: Dieting will make me beautiful.

Myth 4: Dieting will give me self-esteem and acceptance.

Myth 5: A diet makes me feel like a good girl.

Myth 6: Dieting will make others proud of me.

Myth 7: Dieting is just for a little while, then I can enjoy eating again.

Myth 8: Diets will work like magic to make life better.

Myth 1: If I Diet, My Bad Feelings Will Go Away.

In this myth, the idea is that going on a diet will make you feel good. The practical explanation is your attention is hooked into believing the myth and you expect to feel good *after* the process of dieting. How many times have you heard in conversations around you that being overweight isn't natural and a shame? The silent implication is "You need to lose weight."

You may then think, "If I lose weight, I'll be perfect. If I'm perfect, then I'll feel good. My feelings of shame, guilt, and frustration will go away as I lose weight. If only I could fit into a size 12, 10, 8, or even smaller. It will solve all my problems."

Once again, your attention is key. Placing your attention on a positive expectation works instantly to elevate your mood. However, what is *not* talked about is the reality of no attention put on how to get in touch with the healthy self-esteem required to get there. Without it, the emotional challenges of low self-esteem will always recur for you to deal with, even when you lose some weight. We'll explore some successful ways to use your attention for weight balance success in more depth in Chapter 21, under the subheadings *Practical Tools to Find More Answers and The Butterfly Technique*.

Sizing of women's clothes is often confusing.
Over the years, many brands have changed measurements
so that a woman who previously wore a size 12 can now wear
a size 10 or a size 8; a practice known as *vanity sizing.*

Vintage Sizes	12	14	16	18	20	40	42	44
Bust	30	32	34	36	38	40	42	44
Waist	25	26	28	30	34	34	36	38
Hips	33	35	37	39	41	43	45	47 1/2
POST 1970's ⬇	MODERN			⬇		VANITY SIZING		⬇
Modern Sizes	4	6	8	10	10	14	16	18
Bust	30	34 1/2	35 1/2	36 1/2	38	39 1/2	41 1/2	43
Waist	25	26	27	28 1/2	29 1/2	31	32 1/2	34 1/2
Hips	35 1/2	36 1/2	37 1/2	38 1/2	40	41 1/2	43	45

Myth 2: Dieting Will Make My World All Right.

It's easy to get caught in this myth. You may hear from family and the media that being fat is wrong. What is their definition of fat? Does their definition really apply to you? You may get caught into their judgment and then assume you are fat. This is also a situation of low self-esteem.

The next thought that accompanies this low self-esteem is, "If only I could lose weight, I'd be a better person and then my world would be all right." People at work will be more accepting of you, you reason. Mom, Dad, or husband will take the pressure off you. Yet life has a funny way of putting something else in our path to help us learn the truth. Discovering the truth will lead you to unshakable self-esteem.

> *Dieting myths based on misinformation that doesn't address personal well-being and self-esteem are quick fixes that only delay learning the real secrets to weight balance freedom.*

One patient told me she lost weight consistently for two years. She started a new life, fell in love, and married for the second time. After her wedding, she began gaining weight again. When I saw her, she wanted to lose the weight one more time. Her first purpose and primary reason for coming to see me was to lose the weight. Yet I soon discovered she was deeply depressed with serious thoughts of death.

When we talked further, she realized dieting never worked. Dieting in the past for her was up and down, and she always gained back more weight than before, *after she stopped dieting.* What was most shocking was her description of the diet she used to maintain a size 10 figure. She ate a salad a day. Sometimes she'd order a hamburger, which she'd then take home and eat only the meat patty. That's all she would eat—*daily.*

I asked her, "How do you expect to live if you starve yourself to reach a size 10 again?"

She told me, "Well, my husband bought me some expensive size 10 dresses. I have so many of them I want to be able to wear again." From her regime of starvation dieting, she weighed 135 pounds when they first met. It was the first (and only) time in her life that she was ever that thin.

She was on the road to discovering that proper weight balance meant giving her body the nutrients she needed. *Most importantly,* that meant eating three balanced meals a day. Other steps would follow on her road to healthy, active, balanced living. What she didn't yet understand is that her attention was still fixed on *starving to reach a size 10,* primarily in order to please others. Yet, living in more balance would eventually make her life all right and her weight would effortlessly reach just the right size. See Chapter 22 under the subheading, *The Tinsmith's Escape and Moving Past Blockages and Denial,* for more on this.

Myth 3: Dieting Will Make Me Beautiful.

How many of us have bought this myth? Remember how beautiful Marilyn Monroe was? She was a size 14. Now think of Twiggy in the 1960s. All of a sudden, television and fashion latched on to something new. A new image for women, only the new image seemed to say starving, deep-sunken eyes and a childlike figure are sexy.

This myth took only thirty-odd years to develop and take hold. It encouraged women to believe dieting to the size of a pubescent child is beautiful. Thus was born the myth dieting will make women beautiful (while displaying a child's figure as the ideal). But this myth leads to deprivation and inner dissatisfaction. I personally wonder who designs advertising based on this myth—pedophiles? I apologize for the shocking candor of this statement, but examining this question is the first step to discovering ways to disallow others outside of yourself from having this much control. We'll explore the power of asking the right questions in Chapter 18, under the subheading of *Learn How to Ask the Right Questions to Get Answers.*

At the pace of today's world, a myth can develop quickly. Each decade of communication builds upon group responses and group wishes ingrained by the previous one. In recent years designers have shown the heroin-chic look (a skin-and-bones image of near-starving models that appear drug-addicted).

This myth shows once again how corrupt images can have power over us, instead of empowering us to feel beautiful. Remember the saying, "Beauty is in the eye of the beholder?" An image of child addicts begins with subconscious general acceptance. This spells disaster with fatal consequences to generations of women and girls, for these distorted symbols of beauty subconsciously program or brainwash society into accepting the image or myth as truth. Decades later, fashion cycles back in again and the myth becomes even more deeply entrenched because it was so easily and unconsciously accepted the first time.

How do we, as women, want to respond? You can make a better choice right now. You can empower yourself by saying aloud, "I choose to break my old paradigms about dieting right now."

Myth 4: Dieting Will Give Me Self-Esteem and Acceptance.

What a powerful illusion! This myth is like a dark, dirty window that hides endless, black, fearful, trapped feelings. A myth as dismal as this one leads to the false expectation that dieting can give you lasting self-esteem and self-acceptance. Yet, you end up failing each time—feeling you have no willpower, thus little self-esteem and low self-acceptance.

The truth is that this myth takes your real will away. It actually cuts you off from others while cutting you off from your own heart, separating you from your dreams of feeling good about yourself by perpetrating a lie—that the means to accomplish whatever you want is outside of yourself. It cuts you off from true self-acceptance, which is integral to real willpower. You end up paradoxically lonely and unhappy with yourself and your life.

> *Realize this right now: any mistake can be good when it helps lead you to learn more about truth and your true self. Truth is like a clean window that lets in light and allows you to see more clearly.*

The truth is this: *nothing* and *no one* can give you self-esteem and acceptance—only yourself. Real self-confidence and self-esteem always comes from within. It's a gift you give yourself with the help and grace of God. It comes in part from the experience of continually seeing yourself with all your strengths and courage clearly from the inside out. We'll explore this in depth in Chapter 24.

Myth 5: Diets Make Me a Good Girl.

This is what I call the "Parent Myth." Can you hear one of your parents in the background of your memories saying, "Be a good girl. That's right"?

Remember wanting attention from Mommy or Daddy? Your father may not have been around much of the time. When he was, he might have been tired from working all day. Do you remember him, off in the distance, too far away to talk to or reach? He may have been in his favorite chair watching television, but you weren't able to talk to him. He may have seemed just too distant. All you may remember is trying to be a "good girl." It's as if the voice of your parents is inside your head, saying "Be a good girl." All you wanted is to be noticed or acknowledged in some way.

If you combine this myth with the one that says dieting will make me beautiful, you might guess what your parents meant when they said be a good girl, which could lead to the birth of another myth—Dieting Makes Me a Good Girl.

With the 20/20 vision of hindsight, you can see the many sides of the myth involved with Dieting Will Make Me a Good Girl. You may think that what you originally thought was the truth, yet the key is to look at the bigger picture and begin to see more.

To enhance your ability to see the bigger picture, I'll share the story of three blind men and the elephant. To find the essence of the elephant, each blind man felt a different part of it and described it to the others. The blind man at the tail described the elephant as a thin, long rope-like animal that hung in the air and moved side to side. The blind man at the elephant's ear described the elephant as a large flat creature that moved like a sail. The third blind man said the elephant was thick like a trunk of a tree since he only felt the elephant's leg. Which blind man was correct? Having a limited piece of truth or awareness can be misleading.

In connection to the myth of Dieting Will Make Me a Good Girl, those with sensitive natures and the very young will have a tendency to accept hand-me-down beliefs easily, taking on the beliefs of others as if they were the truth (though they are illusions).

> *As you read this book, the truth for your success will become clearer as you develop more compassion and understanding for yourself.*

You already have the ability to recognize illusion. You do so every time you watch a movie. You *know* it's just a movie. The aware part of you knows you're not only just watching a movie; you're also in a theater and you'll leave the theater after the movie is finished. The aware part of you recognizes the bigger, whole picture of life, not just a single part.

In a similar vein, your awareness has the ability to easily see through all the dieting myths listed here and any new ones you can imagine. You'll find out more and explore this amazing ability you already possess in Chapter 21 *(Tips for Getting Unstuck and Moving Beyond Discouragement)* and Chapter 25 *(Visit a Museum Technique).*

Myth 6: Dieting Will Make Others Proud of Me.

This story, from the American West, is about an eagle's egg that was placed in a hen's nest by a Blackfoot Indian brave. When the egg hatched, the eagle was raised as a chicken. It grew up believing it was a chicken. It pecked and scratched in the dirt, just like the other chickens. Fully grown one day, it saw a beautiful eagle soaring high in the sky. The eagle asked the old grandmother chicken about the beautiful bird that soared in the sky. The grandmother chicken said to stop wondering about things that weren't chicken business. So the eagle continued to scratch in the dirt and the grandmother chicken was proud of the way he listened to her.

Dieting often keeps you occupied with "the chicken business" of making others proud of you. This myth is a trap to keep you with your head down, busy pecking at the same useless diets which predominately define womanhood and keep you from fully realizing your full purpose and potential in life.

Now is the time to accept responsibility for being yourself and not react to other people's experiences, myths, emotions, or efforts to control you. This act is being the cause in your life (the source of true self-confidence), not the effect of others' attitudes and beliefs (a slave to myth). With full understanding of this knowledge, gained from reading Chapter 25 you can reach for freedom and be released from diet myths.

Myth 7: Dieting Is Just For a While, Then I Can Enjoy Food Again.

How did this myth become truth for so many women? I hope you question what we have heard as truth from advertisers for years from the point of view that diets never work. I had the misfortune to buy into dieting myths from age 11 to age 44—especially the myth telling me "dieting is just for a little while, then I can enjoy food again."

With this myth the focus is on food constantly. Too busy thinking about what we can and cannot eat, there's no time or energy left for building self-esteem or fully living life. By buying into this myth I found I never truly enjoyed food for thirty-three years.

The empty promise that I could eventually enjoy food again never happened for me. I experienced anxiety associated with the act of eating and preparing food, which only increased every year or two.

From my experiences, I came to realize truth comes on many levels. Others may have different views based on their family values and beliefs. For example, some families believe dieting promises that preach: fast, easy, weight loss or your money back. For those who believe it, their imaginations have created desire on a low level of reality. The key is to recognize how this type of thinking catches your attention but never works because the physical world in which we live runs on certain universal laws which are as immutable as the Laws of Physics. We'll explore these more fully in Chapter 23.

Secondly, this myth of *Dieting Is Just For a Little While, Then I Can Enjoy Eating Again,* can be viewed through attitudes. This myth puts you face to face with a choice between two statements. One says, think about dieting for a short time and the other says, then you can enjoy food again. The truth is dieting never works *when you go back to eating in the old ways.* Weight naturally comes back again with old eating habits, especially when it's combined with a lethargic metabolism which is often the legacy from most diets. An attitude adjustment about the kind of results you want— short-sighted or longer lasting, healthy ones—will help alleviate this situation. We'll explore this further in Chapters 18 and 19.

Myth 8: Diets Will Work Like Magic to Make My Life Better.

The greatest enemy of truth is the myth of how things seem to look versus reality. To illustrate, think about the following question: is a glass of water half empty or half-full? Which is true? In some cases, both answers are true. The only difference is in the point of view or attitude, and *that* can make all the difference in the world, as shown in the following story.

Two women were having soup at a luncheon counter. One ordered a cup of soup and the other ordered a bowl of soup. One woman looked at the cup and bowl and said, "I believe the cup and bowl have the same amount of soup in them."

"Nah!" said the other. So they asked the waitress to bring two empty glasses. They poured the soup from the cup into one glass and the soup from the bowl into the other glass. Both were exactly the same amount. The first woman said, "See, you're paying more for a bowl and you aren't really getting more soup."

The second woman got irritated and said, "I don't care. I want the bowl of soup."

We often determine the value of what is advertised by its appearance and presentation. If diets say you can lose weight in a hurry, then it's magically believable. The image is an illusion to get you to buy the false promise of the quick fix, which only looks good on paper. We'll cover and explore better ways to use your resources for weight balance success, which ties into attitude and viewpoint in Chapters 19 and 20 (Understanding Your Personal Cycles Technique).

All the diet myths you've read about are one illusion after another. Psychologically true. Yet in Chapter 2, Dr. Schwartz states, "research shows the obstacles most people face on the road to achieving their healthy weight are rooted in biochemical and physiological causes." Now is the time to reaffirm the commitment you made from the writing exercise in the introduction. Use it as an opportunity to carry you further into the next chapter as you discover five-plus passkeys for weight balance success.

Reach for your star to guide you.

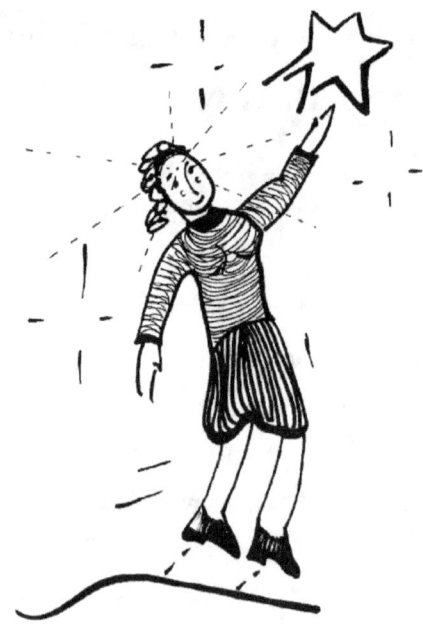

Chapter 17

Five-Plus Keys to Your Healthy Diet Success

Tips for Breaking through the Mind Traps that Bind You

In an article from *Treatment Today* (reprinted in the October 1998 issue of *Reader's Digest*), Robert Epstein, a professor at the University of California, and his students surveyed more than 2000 years of self-change techniques.

I've distilled the results of his study and analysis into the following five principles. Adopting this approach is the easiest and fastest way to change your personal habits and start using this book for weight balance success.

> *When you take action and apply these steps to your life and personal situation, you join countless others who have reaped the benefits in effective results. Everyone who has tried them is heartened by the powerful way they work to manifest positive change.*

Passkey 1: Set Up Your Environment for Success.

I accomplished writing this book, even after working 60-hour weeks, simply by putting my word-processor within two feet of my bed. When I returned after 12-hour counseling days, it's the first thing I saw. My love for getting this book to you was all the additional motivation I needed to write daily. Changing your environment to facilitate positive change is a powerful catalyst for success.

People who change their eating habits by growing fresh herbs or vegetables in their dining room or kitchen windows illustrate one way to set up your environment for success. With fresh herbs growing so close, it's easy to reach for them to perk up meals with color and delicious, just-picked goodness and flavor—instead of reaching for canned goods, a high-calorie snack, or a frozen entrée that you can pop in the microwave oven.

The power of *changing your environment for the better* has proven results. Many psychologists first rediscovered and taught this technique in the 1960's with excellent results. I suggest you give yourself this gift by saying, "OK, I'll do that." Only *you* can do this for yourself.

In another example, one woman wanted to attain more balanced eating by learning ways to put more love into her meals, instead of stuffing the food down quickly without gentle thoughts. She started to change her environment by buying place mats in her favorite colors. Every time she looked at the place mats on the kitchen table, she was uplifted. She also purchased a set of whimsical yellow dishes that make her smile as she prepares food. By setting up this environment change, she harmonized her meal preparations and eating rituals with the power of loving attention.

Nothing is more powerful and simple to do: change your environment in loving, thoughtful ways and life will start to change in response to this. Where will you put this book so you'll remember to give loving, thoughtful attention to the success of your weight balance dream?

Passkey 2: Commit to New Behaviors by Writing a Positive Purpose Statement.

I know what you're thinking. You'd like to put this one off. You could put the book down and forget to read more right now. Or you could conveniently "forget" a written commitment was even mentioned. However, if you really want to harness the power of the subconscious and make it work for you, it's necessary to make your goal concrete in the physical world first by writing it down.

When you write down your purpose statement and accept this technique, it will help make your endeavors effortless. You'll enlist the help of your subconscious and your weight balance ventures will be easier. It's all in your attitude, for the attitude you choose to hold makes all the difference in your behavior, the results, and the ultimate outcome.

In my practice, I show patients how effortless change can be. First, I ask them what they specifically want to change. Second, I help them state it in positive words. Third, I help them write it down. For example, when people want to lose weight, their purpose statements need to reflect this in a simple way that's easy for the subconscious mind to understand.

I'm sure you've heard most people only use three percent of the total brain consciously. The subconscious comprises the other 97% of the brain. This part of your brain controls success through creativity, image, and the unspoken communication between the conscious and subconscious minds. By learning and utilizing the techniques outlined in this book, you'll harness the full power of that extra 97% to aid in effortlessly reaching your goal.

Many steps exist in reaching any goal. To be successful, each step or part of the process needs to be predetermined and then accomplished one stage at a time. Keeping your goals in mind while taking one step at a time eventually allows you to accomplish your dreams.

Likewise the process of weight balance needs to be examined and understood as many small steps on the journey to achieving your goal. Part of the process is learning to value the small steps along the way as you develop patience with yourself and others, while giving yourself permission to keep moving toward success.

Let's take a look at how to write a positive purpose statement. The following technique will lead you specifically through the steps of how to do it. (A positive purpose statement is the foundation for successful change. If you try to include diet myth misinformation into your positive purpose statement, it will undermine your well-being and the effectiveness of your purpose, delaying your ability to attain real weight balance results and success.)

Making a Positive Purpose Statement-Your Map to Your Destiny

This is the foundation of your success. It's relatively simple to manifest what you want in your life, but it's important to be clear, specific, and put it in writing. Again, a positive purpose statement is a golden key to unlock successful change for you by enlisting the help of your subconscious mind.

The following steps will take you past the conscious, judging part of the mind that prevents progress or change. Please take your time with this exercise. It works if you take your time. For clarity in this example, we'll use the positive purpose statement Annie chose for herself.

1. *Write on an index card, "I want to be successful and learn the weight balance secrets. I am on my way to being successful and learning them."*

2. *Think of a symbol that you see often or every day, such as your watch or your keys.*

3. *Close your eyes and place your attention upward to the center of your forehead. This is where insight occurs in your mind.*

4. *Imagine someone or something you love. Imagine the love you feel is filling and overflowing your heart.*

5. *Now conceive of a favorite sound. Take your time and imagine listening to that sound.*

6. *Next conceive of a favorite healthy smell.*

7. *Finally conceive of a favorite healthy taste.*

8. *Now silently remember the exact words of your purpose statement and your symbol. Give yourself time to let it integrate by quieting your mind. The action of doing this is the secret key to getting the subconscious on your side.*

Passkey 3: Self-Monitor Your New Behavior.

Research over the past twenty years shows that self-monitoring is the final step that works to change behavior. Nothing is simpler to do. To self-monitor, find a time best suited to your schedule and use it to read and practice what you learn from this book. Maybe it will be only 30 minutes a day or an hour. Keep track of the time you spend reading and practicing the techniques in this book by documenting it on your calendar or making notes about it in your journal every day.

These three powerful techniques are the first steps to attaining non-prescription diet success. The techniques, visualizations, and exercises in the remainder of this book will help ensure your continued success.

How to Effortlessly Stay Powerful in Attention and Attitude for Continued Success

Like learning to ride a bike, the process of weight balance begins as a mechanical one. First you learn to pedal, and then you learn to steer, and then you learn overall balance, all at the same time. By practicing putting them all together as often as it takes, you eventually get all the pieces of the process happening easily, effortlessly, and simultaneously. Once this happens, you start having a great time and feeling free.

Once you've mastered riding a bike, you don't need to think about the pedals, balance, or steering. You just do it! It's the same with the weight balance secrets. First learn the steps, then practice them, and finally they just flow together effortlessly. You don't have to think twice about how to do them. You just do it!

Two More Keys to Weight Balance Freedom

The two final passkeys to weight balance success, however, are not as mechanical as pedaling, steering, or balancing a bike. These two keys cannot be learned by drilling yourself. That's because they are of a spiritual fabric. The two keys vital to your success are attention and attitude. If you forget to use one or the other, nothing you or I can do will make the principles in this book work for you. It's like leaving off the handlebars of the bike and still expecting it to navigate.

Lacking correct attitude and attention, you'll just be going through the motions of trying yet another diet book. Poor attitude or improper attention leads to boredom and discouragement, which can lead to disillusionment that convinces you to stop reading this material and quit doing the recommended techniques, visualizations, and exercises. When attention and attitude are mixed well with the correct practical steps, you will attain weight balance freedom. If you have trouble with this section of *Cut the Guilt*, it will usually be with one of these three keys: attitude, attention, or practice. Commit to using and studying this book with real interest, practice the techniques and the results can be outstanding. This is just one way of working with the "as if" principle. Acting "as if" is simply (1) believe the change has already happened, (2) release it to your Higher Power, and then (3) take responsibility to do the actions, habits, and behaviors that make it real for you in this physical world.

> *A word about your Higher Power: It is simply what you want it to be. For some people, this is God or the Christ Consciousness. It can also be the highest part of you (divine Soul), nature, or even divine love. Base your interpretation of this on what's most comfortable for you.*

Be sure to turn the results of your situation over to your Higher Power (another attitude key). Then, put in the effort to read this book and practice its techniques. It may take many steps before others recognize changes in you, but each step brings you closer to your dream of success.

Mastering the Subconscious Using Visualization

The following visualization exercise for success is designed to help you move beyond the conscious mind using pleasant images and thoughts that appeal to your senses and the right side of the brain. It works for two reasons. First, by connecting you to pleasant colors, shapes, sounds, and memories, it helps bring all your positive energy to the experience, setting you up for success.

Second, it's a master key. Think of your mind as metaphorically well-guarded between the conscious and subconscious. Security between the two requires confirmation of identity or authorization before access is allowed. The master key for entry just happens to be encoded in an exciting memory, colors, shapes, sounds, smells and tastes that I refer to in the visualization. Ensure the success of your master key by using an exciting memory as well as color, shapes, sounds, smells and tastes that are memorable and pleasant for you in the following exercise.

A Visualization Exercise for Success

1. *First close your eyes and look up to the center of your forehead. This is where insight occurs in your mind.*

2. *Now remember a happy time in your life when something really exciting or thrilling was happening. Tune in deeply to the memory and pause for a moment. What thrilling or exciting event is happening? Notice the details in the experience. See the shapes and colors around you. Hear the sounds. Notice the air has a particular scent to it. Describe it to yourself. Notice a taste in your mouth and describe it to yourself.*

3. *Next, conceive of yourself doing this visualization exercise daily. Think of a time when you can relax to do this visualization undisturbed for five minutes each day. Finally, see yourself in a location in your home, doing this exercise, and feeling excited about it. Give yourself this gift: Commit to take the time each day to do this visualization exercise.*

A Simple Way to Release Excuses That Controlled You in the Past

First and foremost, remember that you are a spiritual being. Your inner, spiritual Self is the true Self that always is. Between every excuse, action, or feeling of doubt, exists a silent space where you can be your true Self. Think of the relationship that your mind, body, and emotions have to your true spiritual Self as being like a car that needs an excellent driver to take care of and properly operate and maintain it.

Another way to look at your true spiritual Self is to view it as true attention. Other names for attention could be awareness or viewpoint. Being aware of where and how you focus your attention is finding your true, authentic Self. Think of this Self as beautiful, light, flowing, fexible and yet extremely disciplined—like an ice skater or a dancer.

Go ahead and do the following exercise to get in touch with your true Self, either upon awaking or just before falling asleep. You can choose to either play the recording or simply run through the steps of this visualization exercise in your mind as you follow it.

First of all, your physical body will fall into a deep relaxation. Your thoughts and personality will quiet down to a restful state. By the count of ten, you'll reach a deeply relaxed state of consciousness. Following this, you'll have an experience as your true Self. When you are finished, you'll awaken feeling refreshed, alert, and good.

Sometimes the Hardest Thing and the Right Thing Are the Same.

Touching Base with Your True Self

1. *Begin by saying, "I am going into a deep relaxation state to experience my true Self by counting from ten down to one".*

2. *Begin counting down now, saying each number upon your exhale. 10 . . 9 . 8 . . deeper and deeper . . 7 . . 6 . . that's right, deeper into relaxation . . 5 . . even deeper . . 4 . . it's safe to have your experience . . 3 . . relax deeper . . 2 . . let everything go . . and . . 1 . . That's right, you're completely relaxed.*

3. *Visualize yourself in a perfect garden, a place you may have visited before, seen in a picture, or just created right now. Perhaps it is an expansive area of lush green grasses with rose arbors, purple clouds of lilacs, flowering pink cherry blossoms, and ponds with banks of brilliant wild flowers. One area might host a thick, round lawn of chamomile flowers. Make your garden as simple or complex as you like.*

4. *Place yourself in the garden after you have completed visualizing it. See yourself take a walk, smell the flowers, or gather a bouquet. At one point, you decide to rest on the inviting chamomile lawn. As you sit, notice the fruity aroma and breathe it in deeply. Chamomile, known for its ability to soothe the nervous system, lets you relax even more. Sink into the yielding perfume and softness of the lawn. Look down at your true Self and note what you see, sense, or hear.*

5. *Feel vibrantly refreshed and energetic. Do something fun: run, swim in a nearby pond, or dance among the flowers. Hear your favorite music. Bring others to your experience. Have an adventure.*

6. *When it is time to come back by the count often, you'll easily remember the feeling of your true Self-experience. Feel free to return at a pace that's comfortable for you . . . 1 . . . 2 . . . 3 . . . 4 . . . 5 . . . 6 . . 7 . . .8 . . 9 . . . 10. Welcome back.*

Write down what you experienced as your true Self. Next time you practice this visualization, you will experience even more of your true Self.

Now let's move your attention to three different reasons you have for continuing to read this book. For example, remember when you first thought about buying this book. Consider when you'd like to read this book tomorrow. Next, imagine yourself balanced and at a healthy weight, feeling good about yourself. Can you do that? The part of you that remembered, thought, and imagined, is *your true spiritual Self*. Write down three reasons for continuing to read this book.

(1) _____

(2) _____

(3) _____

Getting Ready for True Success

True success is right around the corner. It's your privilege to discover it for yourself. How do you do this? First, by looking with a true heart at the automatic excuses you normally use to avoid following through on your intentions. What are your most frequent excuses? If you can write them down this will lead you to the next step. Take a moment to write them down.

(1) _____

(2) _____

(3) _____

Ask yourself, do I really want to be stubborn, tied fearfully to my excuses? Or do I want to experience freedom and success

> *By distracting your attention from these excuses and asking questions about a possible scenario of freedom and success, you set up curiosity about an alternate future.*

Like a story that's only half-told, once your curiosity is engaged, you've just got to see how the story ends. It's on this principle that you, as your true spiritual Self, can start and proceed toward success.

Using your curiosity right now means being willing to put the book down for five to ten minutes to do the next exercise. This exercise will teach you how to get ready for true success. Find a quiet place where you can lean back right now for ten undisturbed minutes.

A Loving Technique

1. *Close your eyes and place your inner attention on an imaginary spot between your eyes. This is where insight occurs in your brain.*

2. *Next silently ask to connect to your Higher Power, as you know it. Some people believe their Higher Power is God; others experience their Higher Power as the highest part of themselves. Choose whatever truth is best for you and connect with it while doing the exercises, techniques, and visualizations in this book.*

3. *Next, pick a word that means or feels like love to you. It could be the name of a loved one or a beloved pet. If it's the right word, you will feel love. This is the most important indicator and part of this technique.*

4. *Say or sing the word to yourself for five minutes. Most people who do this are at first surprised to find out how long five minutes takes. You might set a timer or your watch if needed.*

5. *Your mind may be actively running thoughts in your head, like monkeys doing tricks. Just let those monkey-like thoughts run by as if it was a television program. You'll soon become bored with them and your mind will calm down shortly.*

6. *Notice your breathing as you sing your love-word, and notice how your body begins to calm down.*

7. *Next ask yourself, what is a balanced, healthy weight for me? Trust yourself to know exactly what is best for you as a healthy weight. Use the space given at the end of this chapter to write that down now. The sentence starts with "I am on my way to _____." For one person the statement might be "I am on my way to being (fill-in-the-blank) pounds." For another, the statement might be "I am on my way to being a size (fill-in-the-blank)." What's important is that it's your purpose statement, you write it down, and you accomplish it in small steps.*

> 8. *Go to the last page in the chapter now and write down what you received. Be bold enough to push through any hesitancy or lethargy you may feel about doing this right now. Just do it to ensure your continued success.*
>
> 9. *Close your eyes again and sing or say your love-word three more times. Fill yourself with love and contemplate the weight you wrote down. Explore how comfortable you are with it as you imagine how you will feel at that weight.*
>
> 10. *Next, imagine a symbol that represents your purpose. One symbol that works for some people is a rainbow. Another symbol is a sunrise or a rose. Trust yourself to know exactly what is right for you to choose as the symbol of your success. Make it personal and meaningful for you. Pick one symbol and when you sing your love-word, imagine your symbol too. Again, use the space at the end of this chapter to write down the symbol of your success. When you are finished, close your eyes and sing your love-word three times. Say to yourself, "It is blessed in love; it is filled with love; it is finished in love." Take three deep breaths and open your eyes.*

Annie, a compulsive dieter, chose a white dove to represent herself on the way to eating healthfully in just the right amounts to fit into a size 16. She is on her way to seeing herself at this goal, *walking more and loving it* with joyful feelings—the way she feels when she laughs. This is a beginning step for her on the way to her destination of weight balance.

If you skimmed through this part of the book without using the tape or doing the exercise, I urge you to stop and carry through with it right now.

> *Know that there is no right or wrong way to do it. Like making bread, you can stir it any way you choose, just as long as you stir it and get the job done.*

Just do it now. Go to *Guidebook Questions to Contemplate and Journal* in this chapter. As you go through each item, write down what you receive.

The importance of doing this exercise and carrying through by writing it down cannot be emphasized enough. Think of it this way: What if you were baking some wholesome bread for your family and later discovered you forgot to put in the leavening agent?

Would the bread rise?

It probably wouldn't turn out as well because you forgot one of the most important ingredients.

> *The techniques, exercises, and activities in this book are clearly the metaphorical leavening agent that brings healthy weight balance success.*

Guidebook Questions to Contemplate and Journal

1. What do I want? I want _____

2. Now rewrite what you want and make it failure-proof. For example, if you wrote, I am on my way to losing ten pounds, rewrite it as "I am on my way to being lighter and lighter as a size (whatever size is healthy for you while discounting the weight

3. Now write the purpose statement again. Start your sentence by writing the exact wording, "I am on my way to being _____" and finish the sentence with your exact written purpose statement from the first question. Write it in the blank lines provided.

   _____
   _____
   _____

4. My personal symbol of success is _____

   _____
   _____

To review:

1. Commit to singing your love song to yourself each day at the same time daily.

2. Imagine yourself seated comfortably and relaxed, doing that now. See yourself in the room where you'll be.

3. Change something in your environment to help you remember to do this for yourself. Tell yourself, "I deserve to do this for me."

4. Think of a beautiful sound. Then imagine a wonderful smell and think of a favorite taste and color.

5. Now close your eyes and sing your love-word to yourself as you imagine your loved one, the beautiful sound, the wonderful smell, a favorite taste, and let go as you accept love flowing to you. Briefly record your experience in your journal.

6. Did you use feelings to describe your experience? Did you use thoughts to describe your experience? Did you describe how your body felt doing this? Rewrite it again using feelings, thoughts, and body sensations.

7. Remember to (a) set up your environment for success, (b) commit to new behaviors by writing a positive purpose statement, (c) self-monitor your new behavior, and (d and e) focus your attitude and attention on your commitment.

When Beginning Something New

When you first try something new, it's natural to have mixed feelings about it. Often inner conflicts are revealed. For example, sometimes when people try these techniques for the first time, they write, "I felt I was doing it wrong. My body couldn't relax." It's okay if this was your experience. It's fine for a first step. As a springboard into the next chapter, try the following journal activity.

Think of an area of your life occupied with inner conflicts. This can be any situation you've had mixed feelings about. Next, write down your feelings about the situation. For example, confusion and anxiety are two emotions that can revolve around inner conflicts.

Now draw a picture of those feelings. You can pretend you don't know how to draw when doing this exercise. Draw a funny stick drawing or doodle your feelings. This will help you release them by engaging the subconscious mind.

Lastly, make a positive change in the picture. It's all right for the drawing to turn out any way it does. If it makes you feel better, then you've helped give a voice to some of the inner conflicting feelings you have about the situation. This activity helps clear away some feelings (by using the unlimited perception of image and the nonjudgmental aspects of the right brain to get them down on paper,) so the logical verbal language centers of the left brain can eventually express what you feel through journal writing.

Where do these conflicted feelings come from? What's the true meaning behind them? More importantly, what can we do about them? We'll explore these questions and more as we discover ways to break through the emotional traps that bind us in Chapter 18.

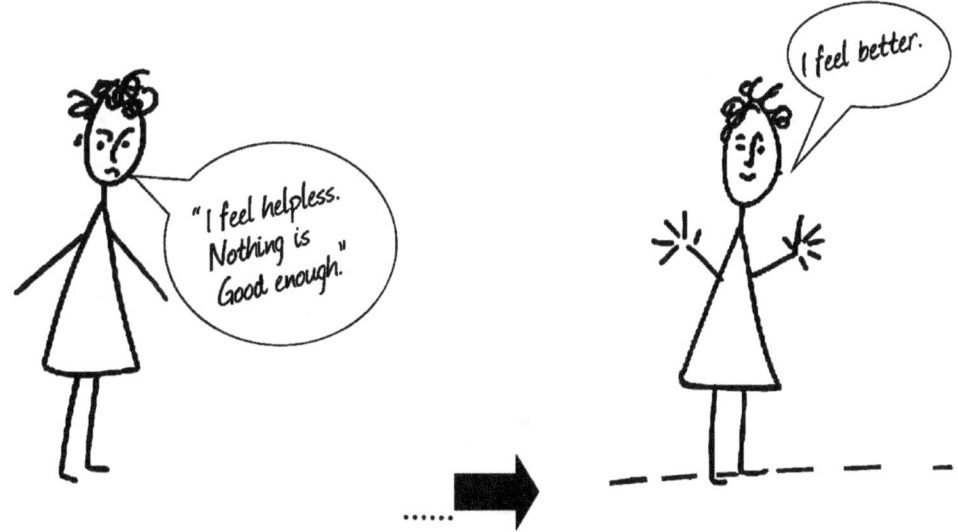

Make a postive change in your drawing.

Chapter 18

A Deeper Understanding of Society's Diet Programming Trap

The Diet Paradigm on a Social Level: More Than Fifty Years in the Making

Annie wondered aloud about how the diet paradigm had gotten the firm hold it has on society today. Let's examine recent history by scanning aspects of the last fifty years.

During World War II, the threat of European-based dictatorships splashed across the headlines of nations. The people of the world perceived the dictators in power as domineering and manipulative of others. Many feared for their lives and faced the real possibility of the total annihilation of their people. In the United States, mothers supported the war effort by working in factories.

When the war ended, a great publicity effort turned women back to their homes so jobs would be freed up and available for the men returning from overseas. The homemaker role was glorified and best epitomized in the new television shows of the day, such as "Father Knows Best" or "Leave It To Beaver."

The widespread influence of television shows like these began to indoctrinate girls from the baby boom generation from a very early age by encouraging them to strive for the 1950s ideal: picture-perfect life situations and personal appearances that mirrored what they saw on these television programs.

The reality behind the scenes was that families struggled to live up to the two-dimensional, superficial images of the happy households they saw on television. This resulted in denial and stuffing real emotions to keep up the appearance of the television families, breeding personal confusion and resentment among family members for being unable to attain this perfect image and unable to express their true feelings about it

The long-term result of denial and swallowing real feelings within the family unit is that the situation continued to worsen in subsequent decades. Family members erupted in negative, self-defeating behaviors, such as overeating, out-of-control shopping, alcohol and drug abuse, and escapism into even more hours of television viewing. All this simply supported more living-in-denial to avoid addressing real-life problems and issues. Who would guess that generations of loss during the Great Depression and two World Wars would predispose the people of this nation to become willing participants to television's hypnotic influence and the sedative world of entertainment it offered?

Not only did television distract and entertain us, it even told us which products to buy, eat, use, and wear. The idea of molding every woman to a feminine ideal helped divert everyone's attention and placed more importance on consumerism to uphold outer appearances. Who could have predicted that the influence and manipulation of trends through image would spread so far, so fast, and so thoroughly and that our future would be altered forever by television?

Baby Boomers in the Cross Hairs

The years 1951 to 1957 focused on rebuilding the economy and the world after the war. In November 1957, a monthly general interest magazine named *Cosmopolitan* focused on the question "Are Teenagers Taking Over?" For the first time in history, teenagers had money to spend. Since their parents had lived through years of lack during the Great Depression, they wanted to give their children more of the good life, the things they never had.

The New Yorker picked up the trend that month and printed, "These days, merchants eye teenagers the way stockmen eye cattle." During this time teen magazines became an important influence and element of teen subculture

By 1960, more than a dozen magazines had slanted their marketing toward teenage girls. By the end of 1963, the British Invasion and the musical revolution began making a mark internationally.

Teenagers expressed their natural rebellion through new fashion standards when Mary Quant defied the status quo with the Mod look and the mini-skirt. *Seventeen* magazine then featured them. Soon more teen magazines began to feature these fashion trends.

As a natural part of the rebellion experience and wanting their own identity, teenagers looked for a new image. Initially Twiggy was discovered for her face but was considered too skinny to model. However, her popularity increased by 1966. I remember the influence Twiggy had on me when I modeled for the January issue of *Seventeen* that year. I lost weight until I was below 100 pounds in order to feel thin enough. Other girls and women copied Twiggy in the decades that followed.

The 1962 release of Rachel Carson's *Silent Spring* inspired the ecological, back-to-nature, co-operative movement, which grew in the 1970s when certain segments of the US population began to express renewed interest in health, nutrition, and organic foods. A portion of the general public recognized the relationship between mind, body, Spirit, and the quality of the food we ate.

But the Twiggy image of thinness still equaled "health" in the mind of mainstream fashion magazines. The voluptuous image of Marilyn Monroe as the feminine ideal was gone and so was acceptance of flesh in commercial images.

Overtly critical judgment of others tracked the trend of thinness. Already beautiful models' good looks were further enhanced with photographic touch-ups. Plastic surgeons plied their craft of body sculpting in their quest to perfect their conception of what the feminine physique should be. Eventually, mass consciousness working through mass media led to more emphasis on controlling the feminine mystique with outward perfectionism being the driving behavioral force and primary goal.

Yet despite this, the consciousness movement grew, bringing with it the energy of cooperation and compromise. Those who were interested in spiritual matters began deep explorations within to find the most basic values of their innermost selves. Awareness about how the modern world had systematically polluted the air, water, and land grew. In the arena of diet, investigation into what advertising influences had done to corrupt the mind/body image and glimpses of how they had directed the feminine body ideal became conspicuous.

Exposing the Illusion

The struggle to be free of the mass-marketed illusion is a process similar to what the butterfly goes through when freeing itself from a chrysalis. What I strive to do in this section is shine light on how the diet paradigm evolved—with the intent of helping readers break free of the illusions it casts.

To further expose the illusion for yourself, take time to leaf through a fashion magazine and view present-day advertising images while keeping the previously mentioned history in mind. Notice what kinds of bodies top fashion designers employ to display their creations. Ask yourself: Which movie stars have had ribs surgically removed in order to permanently alter their waist measurements? Who is surgically altering other body parts or areas in order to appear slimmer, tighter, or forever young? Digital computers and retouched photographs improve images, magically giving models fuller breasts. Undoubtedly, healthy-looking, athletic images of women abound, but they fall mainly on the low-flesh side.

Where is acceptance of variety and individual beauty?

> *What do natural, healthy women need to do in order to value themselves for what's inside?*

The answers to these questions can lead to a deeper awareness of who you really are and where you stand on the topic of buying into the Hollywood or Madison Avenue images for women.

This advertisement in *Seventeen's* 1966 issue in which I modeled— started me down the road of sugar addiction. I followed the ad's recommendation of eating sugar. A New York City corporation—Sugar Information, Inc. revealed sugar is low in calories and would give me the energy I needed to keep dieting and remain popular. Modern media acknowledges "that they sell more than products... the images in advertising affect the reality of our lives." – *Slim Hopes*, Advertising and the Obsession with Thinness by Jean Kilbourne, www.mediaed.org.

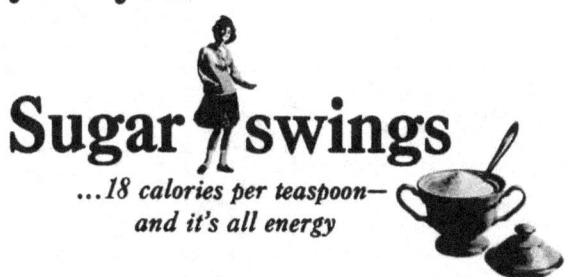

There is one sure thing that will separate a "wallflower" from the wall–and that's vitality. So if you're dieting, we suggest you keep some sugar in your life.

No other food supplies energy so fast–or satisfies hunger so fast–with so few calories. At only 18 calories per teaspoon, sugar actually helps you reduce by keeping your vitality up, and your appetite down.

The phone's ringing. It's probably for you!

Sugar ❦ swings
...18 calories per teaspoon— and it's all energy

Sugar Information, Inc.

An advertisement in *Seventeen's* 1966 issue in which I modeled.

How the Dieting Cycle Begins on a Personal Level

A little girl, about seven or eight years old, wants to get parental attention in the worst way. She wants to be noticed, soothed, or protected from the emotions of her childhood psyche. She wants to be closer to her parents, but how?

Maybe she sees her mother enjoying something, eating a meal or preparing breakfast on the weekends. Her father might be relaxing with a beer or cocktail. Maybe he takes his little girl for an ice cream during a special time when she gets to go with Daddy. Maybe the special times she remembers sharing with her mother were surrounded by food experiences.

It's possible that as the little girl grows up, classmates tease her for being fat. Or maybe she just has self-conscious feelings about plumpness because Daddy talks disparagingly about obese women or criticizes her mother for putting on weight. Maybe the remarks from her father or the teasing of her classmates provoke an angry response in the little girl. What does she do?

Since little girls are taught it isn't nice to express or feel anger, this little girl learns to swallow it. Yet the hostility flashes deep inside her for a moment before it's swallowed. The hurt and betrayal she feels may also be swallowed so fast that they're nearly forgotten. And almost without a thought, the swallowed anger seems to magically go away.

Yet the result of swallowing anger (or any other strong emotion for that matter) is that eventually it comes out sideways in unconscious, uncontrolled behavior. The primal feelings of anger and betrayal that are swallowed become scattered through the subconscious, resulting in confusion. What happens to the little girl?

She grows up and—like Annie—thinks it's paramount for her to focus on the feminine diversion of diet worries or the hunt for the perfect body. This is how the personal dieting cycle is born.

The Wisdom of Honoring Your Emotions

Emotions are often misunderstood. They are seen as negative outbursts that are best repressed. But strong emotions can be a way for your intuitive self to get your attention when you're in the midst of a situation.

> *Your intuitive self uses emotions to flag a situation and bring it to your attention, so that you can take a deeper look at the truth.*

A heightened sense of awareness can help you discern what's happening on a deeper level, so you can make the best-informed decision about what's right for you in that situation.

Once you listen to the deeper truth underneath your emotions, you'll know what the truth of a situation is. Then you'll be calm and relaxed, responding from your true Self when choosing your course of action. Emotions can be important intuitive indicators that help you evaluate situations—*but only when you stay in touch with and honor your true Self from moment to moment.* The important thing is not to hold on to, or stay stuck in, any emotional state but simply pass through it to the higher ground of a greater understanding of what is true for you.

This can only happen when we first acknowledge the emotions within ourselves and see them for what they truly are—indicators—instead of denying, ignoring, squashing down, or swallowing how we really feel.

What to Expect When You Take New Actions

It's normal to feel conflicted and uneasy when you start to take new actions in your life and break old habits or thought patterns. Many people know the best course of action to take to improve their lives (such as reading and applying the principles in this book). But knowing and doing are two different things. When they do take action, it often causes the reverse of what they expect to happen. Instead of everything getting better, they may feel empty, hurt, angry, or aggressive inside.

The truth of it is this: first it gets worse and then it gets better. If you don't fight or repress your feelings, but rather accept them as a natural part of the process, you'll be on your way to dealing with your emotions in a healthier way sooner.

It's relatively easy for someone who doesn't know this to go back and get stuck in the same old habits and patterns when they're in doubt. Yet it's all a matter of breaking through the illusion of childhood loss and fear.

When you let go of a past habit or way of being, you may experience the change as loss. But by knowing what to expect emotionally at the outset, you can calmly reassure yourself that there is nothing to fear. Unlike others who get caught up in doubt, you know your purpose and goals. You can stay centered and clear while focusing on learning more skills and tools from the techniques offered in this book.

Remember first and foremost, you are a tremendous spiritual being. You can decide to take new, positive actions with the expectation that you'll feel sad or empty at times, knowing this will pass as part of the process of letting go. It doesn't matter if the change is large or small; the process of letting go is the same for both.

For example, when we experience the death of a loved one, religious rituals help us accept, let go, and cope with it. We attend funerals to help us surrender to the reality and assist us in fully accepting what has happened. Friends and family show support and sympathy for us. Crying at funerals helps release some of the grief by giving it a voice.

Our physical bodies and emotions need to be honored similarly in any letting go process. This honoring process helps empty and clear out old behavior patterns and ruts in our thinking. Support from friends also helps with this process. Just remember that emptying out the old makes room for the new, allowing more space for success to develop and grow.

Feelings Are a Golden Key

Not being fully connected to your feelings or misperceiving thoughts as feelings can create more confusion and miscommunication within you. The following activity shows one way to get better acquainted with your emotions. The goal is to become friends with your feelings, instead of treating them like the enemy. Even if you think you already know what you feel, try this exercise. You might be surprised to discover something new about yourself.

Look over the following *Emotions Awareness Chart* with the idea of befriending your emotions. When making new friends, we often make plans to spend time together. So spend some time doing the following: At the end of each day, at the same time every day, check off all the emotions you felt during the course of that day. After a while, you'll become more adept at recognizing and differentiating them. This is a first step to more fully recognizing your feelings, which can lead to building greater awareness. When subtler feelings emerge, add them to the list.

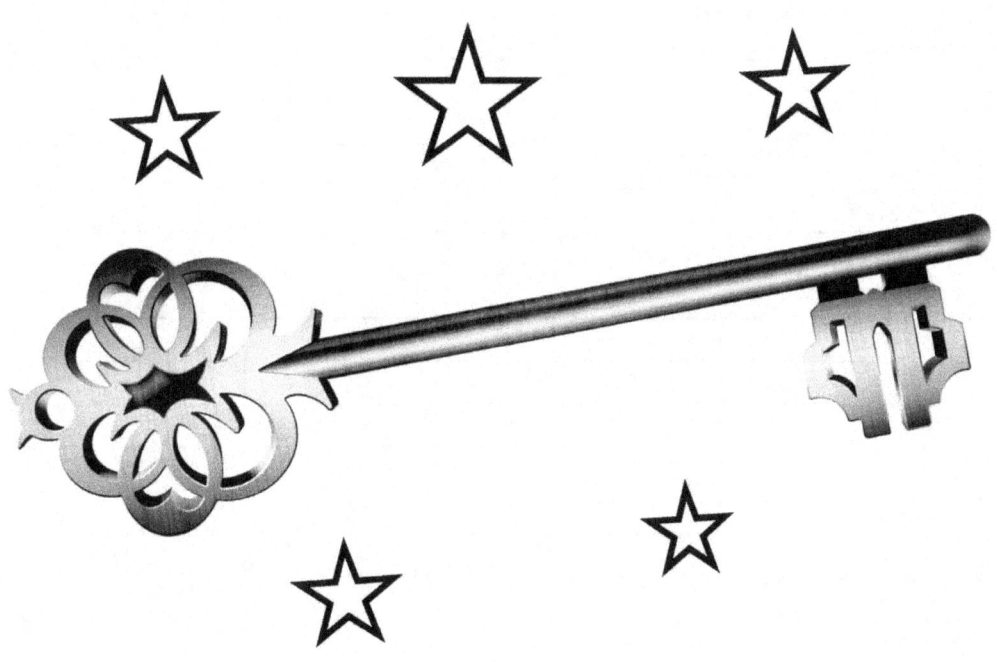

Feelings Are a Golden Key

Emotions Awareness Chart

	Monday	Tues.	Wed.	Thurs.	Fri.	Sat.	Sunday
Annoyed							
Angry							
Aware							
Hurt							
Interested							
Used							
Withholding							
Repressed							
Willing							
Lust							
Content							
Threatened							
Scared							
Brave							
Safe							
Sad							
Self-Punishing							
Sincere							
Numb							
In Balance							
Unloved							
Loving							
Helpless							
Hopeless							
Complete							

At the end of the week ask yourself, what did I learn from my emotions? What greater truth were they trying to bring to my awareness?

For example, sometimes you can plumb the depths of your emotions (like anger) and find beneath it a real human need. One such need is the need to have more love in your life. Moving through anger and other emotions to acknowledge the deeper needs underneath brings you to the source of your truth and the cause level of your misgivings. Acknowledging and addressing the deeper truths and causes of your emotions (a need for love) has the potential to permanently alleviate anger at the source.

Be sure to write down the answer to the question "What did I learn from my emotions?" in your journal as a simple way to record your changing awareness and document your quest for the truth in writing. In a month, re-read your entries to review your progress.

If you'd like, draw a picture in your journal that represents the emotions you experienced that day at the end of each day. Lastly, be sure to make a positive change in the picture just before you finish it.

Three Myths Society Holds about the Cause of Obesity

In Chapter 16, we explored the eight myths individuals hold about dieting. Society also holds three stereotypical myths about the causes of overweight, which are then projected upon anyone who is considered fat or the least bit heavy for their height. They are, as follows:

Myth 1: Just eat less and lose weight.

Myth 2: Just exercise more and lose weight.

Myth 3: Just use more willpower (to eat less and exercise more) and lose weight.

Once we explore these in detail, you'll see why they're myths.

Myth 1: Just Eat Less and Lose Weight.

This myth assumes that people who are overweight or obese eat large amounts of food. Sometimes this is true, but not always. More often than not, many people who are perceived as fat eat less than their thin counterparts and still can't seem to lose weight, no matter how little they eat. What's really happening here? Why doesn't eating less work?

The answer is not necessarily in how much you eat, but in the quality of what you eat and in what proportions. Too many times people who struggle with weight issues miss essential macronutrients (proteins, carbohydrates, and fats) or micronutrients (vitamins, minerals, trace elements and enzymes).

The key is *not* necessarily in counting (and restricting) calories in foods you eat, but rather in *maximizing nutrition* in the foods you eat. Many people today are literally starving from lack of proper nutrition due to diets based on modern-day, highly processed foods. Most of these foods are so low in essential nutrients that they put people who base their diets on them within flirting distance of deficiency diseases.

Cutting back further on nutritionally inadequate and deficient foods only serves to slow and eventually shut down the body's natural ability to metabolize foods and effectively burn calories. In effect, the body switches to starvation mode.

Instead of burning stored fats, it begins to cannibalize itself by breaking down precious muscle tissue (protein) for the nutrients and amino acids that are crucial for life. Since retained muscle mass naturally and metabolically burns more calories than fat (even in resting states), losing any muscle mass further impairs the body's ability to metabolize nutrients and burn calories.

In the cannibalizing process, the body will pull vitamins, minerals, and other elements from the bones, muscles and other tissues if it's not getting them from food sources in the diet, leaving dieters prone to osteoporosis and other degenerative conditions and diseases.

The answer is not in restricting foods or eating less. Restricting only leads to panic and binge eating, which is a natural response to starvation or lack of any essential nutrients.

> *For those who do tend to overeat, their behavior can also be viewed as nutrient starvation, as well as the mind game a chemical imbalance from lack of proper diet can play on people. The feeling of being out of control and acting out on it through uncontrolled eating, are signs of lack of nutrition and nutritional starvation just as much as they are characteristic of deeper emotional issues with regard to food.*

As an example, I'd like to share the story of Ann. "Look at me," she said. "I can stay on a diet and I've quickly lost thirty pounds in just a few months."

Yet Ann didn't realize that once she reached her goal, she'd throw out restrictive dieting and slowly start eating the way she used to eat. When you restrict your food, your natural instincts tend to want to binge or balloon out of control, to save the body from what it perceives as famine. This ballooning effect can be gradual as in Ann's story: a little ice cream treat one day, a double cheeseburger for lunch, and a rich dessert that night. Soon all the weight she lost comes back gradually and then some. What is the philosophy behind the balloon effect?

When you pinch the middle of a tube balloon, it simply balloons out in other directions. So restricting food only results in closet eating, binge-eating, or spending more than the overeater can afford for food after strict deprivation diets. The cycle begins to spin out of control because no amount of willpower to restrict or eat less food will work to sustain life over the long haul.

This may run its course in weeks, months, or years, until the next time you gather together the impetus to restrict your diet again. The "less food" concept leads not to permanent weight loss, but to yo-yo dieting, repressed anger, and a state of perpetual weight gain because of a chronically lowered and sluggish metabolism that tries to survive on nutritionally deficient foods.

How can you combat this? Choose to let go of the myth that eating less is the answer to your weight problems. In the beginning of Chapter 19,

I'll share a resource that will help you customize your diet to your own nutritional needs, help stop cravings, as well as ensure optimum health, high energy, peak athletic performance, basically a way to stay young at any age.

Myth 2: Just Exercise More and Lose Weight.

The flip side of the eat-less myth is the exercise-more myth. The truth is that if you're not getting enough nutrition, exercise can be deleterious to your health. A metabolism sluggish from improper diet will not easily jump-start just because it's coerced with exercise. Many times the body will pull magnesium from the muscles and calcium from the bones when driven by exercise, causing even more of an imbalance and ultimately leading to more serious conditions, such as osteoporosis.

If you've been sedentary for some time, you may want to ease back into activity. It's important to do just the right amount of the right form of exercise initially to enhance your health and condition. Your overall weight can unconsciously pull you, like gravity, into the same old patterns of inactivity so it can take an effort to get started. Here's a gentle way to start manifesting a safe, gradual change into more activity.

Try this one half-hour before a meal: Choose to eat a healthy appetizer (a healthy complex carbohydrate, such as a glass of fruit or vegetable juice, some raw vegetables or fresh fruit; or a healthy protein, such as a few ounces of cheese or yogurt with a handful of raw nuts or seeds).

Then take a short walk around your home or office (six to eight blocks for a fifteen-minute stroll). Do this gently to begin erasing past habits of inaction. Start with one fifteen-minute walk per day and gradually increase it to two. Strive to reach the goal of walking for fifteen minutes before every meal. As you gain fitness over time, gradually increase your pace to a brisk walk and increase the number of blocks that you walk to ten to twelve each time.

This simple activity has the effect of jump-starting your metabolism over time. Since your ability to burn calories is already enabled by the brief exercise, when you return and sit down to eat you'll automatically process the meal much better and burn calories in your fat storage more efficiently.

If you combine exercise with a meal plan that focuses on foods geared to your metabolic type, you'll see even faster results in your quest for weight balance. (See Chapter 19 where we'll explore more on metabolic typing, and you can check out *The Metabolic Typing Diet* by William L. Wolcott with Trish Fahey.)

If you like the results you're seeing and feeling with mild walks before meals, in a month or two you'll easily be able to add a mild workout or two during the week. On one day of the week, try some easy cardiovascular movement, such as moving to music for 20 to 30 minutes.

Engaging in light weight-training two days later can help strengthen your bones, further reducing the potential threat of osteoporosis. An inexpensive way to weight-train and build your upper body strength uses water-filled plastic bottles for inexpensive weights. To avoid potential injuries, increase the amount of water in the bottles gradually over time as your strength increases.

I would be remiss if I didn't address those people who fall at the *other* end of the spectrum however—those who exercise to the extreme as a way to burn calories and keep weight off, as shown in the following story about Diane.

Diane is a typical dieter although her eating and exercise routines are fanatical. She would exercise morning, noon, and night in order to facilitate binge eating. Although her whole life is built around accommodating her eating and exercise habits, she doesn't see how much it affects her emotional state, relationships with family and friends, job performance, or what she does in her spare time (when there's spare time left after excessive exercising and overeating).

Diane bought the myth of exercising more to lose weight because of a fantasy. Primarily, she wanted to look like her favorite ultra-thin model. At first glance, the myth of exercising more to lose weight seemed to satisfy her in that this is what she believed she needed to do to attain her desired results. Soon Diane was on her way to becoming her model-thin fantasy.

Diane's thoughts and attitudes were not grounded in the real world when she was binge exercising however. Her daydreams progressed to fantasizing about getting revenge, winning, and being on top of the world. For a little while, Diane pretended that her dreams and fantasies would come true, until the pain of overeating and excessive exercising brought her back to the present. The reality is that Diane had to cancel a date she was looking forward to once again, because she binged and then exercised herself into exhaustion. She wound up being too sick and too tired to go on her date. This happens more often than Diane allows herself to acknowledge.

Yes, regular exercise is healthy for everyone. It's when the will or ego starts manipulating how much you exercise, how long you exercise, or how often you exercise that problems can surface. Thirty minutes of specific body exercises or aerobics a few times a week are good for your health and cardiovascular system.

A healthy self-esteem goal for your exercise routine is good health and a stronger body (not necessarily to lose weight). You can choose to be healthy, strong, and maintain a balanced weight with exercise and eating right.

An additional 30 minutes of walking at the end of the day is relaxing and one of the best ways to keep your body moving and healthy. Think about inviting a friend or spouse for a relaxing walk along the beach, down city streets, or around the local park in your neighborhood. Who would you love to share this with? Who might you meet and what might you see? What natural adventures can you have during this time?

Now shift your perspective and think about *having* to take a walk, from the viewpoint of thinking you have to exercise more. Think of forcing yourself to walk from fear of not losing weight or fear that someone will once again comment about your weight.

Worse yet, you might be angry about those comments and you don't even recognize it. You might be so used to denying anger that you don't know when it's healthy to express it. It's natural to be angry with anyone who makes snide comments about your appearance. You might be seething deep inside, yet you don't even recognize that you are angry because you automatically channel your anger and energy into exercise. Allowing old attitudes and stubborn behaviors to take charge and entice you to binge with exercise is hostility turned upon yourself—self-punishment by exercising to the extreme. Choose instead to think of exercise as inviting and relaxing.

Make a choice and choose to let go of past behaviors and attitudes today. Embrace choosing to trust in positive outcomes and choosing to trust yourself. We'll explore this concept of trusting yourself and positive outcomes more through an exercise in Chapter 21.

Myth 3: Use More Willpower (to Eat Less and Exercise More) and Lose Weight.

The third myth combines the first two myths and just adds willpower. If the first two myths didn't work alone or together, they won't work when combined with more willpower.

This myth emerges when people feel hopelessness, helpless, useless, and don't know consciously what to do with their power. Many of them automatically act in ways to exert control over their bodies. When you're feeling out of control and panicked, more willpower isn't going to push back tides of past controlling behavior. More willpower can't hold back the tides of emotions, especially the anger and hurt that led to overeating and comfort foods. Willpower can't hold back the illogic of societal beliefs and myths.

The myth that you need more willpower over your food or your behavior is completely misdirected. This is comparable to the way that you can only hold your breath for so long before you have to take the next breath.

The instinctual urge to breathe is the same as the urge to eat. Both are vital for life. The instinctual subconscious can drive you to eat when your anger is so repressed that you're about to self-destruct. More willpower, or control in any way, only heightens repression and the urge to eat. More willpower just doesn't work.

What *does* work is building up your self-esteem so that you feel more adequate and more encouraging of yourself, so that you have the inner power to make different behavioral choices that set you free. You *can* choose to release old, controlling, willful ways and make new choices. We'll explore the fact that you have a choice in how you respond in more depth in Chapter 21.

Later in this chapter, I'll give techniques for recognizing and addressing feelings before they get the better of you behaviorally. You'll learn ways to release controlling behavior, rather than trying to exert more control over yourself by using more willpower. Reading and practicing the interactive exercises included in this book will give you more trust in yourself, your body, mind, emotions, and Divine Spirit. Developing a deep level of self-confidence and trust is key to your weight balance success.

The eight myths from Chapter 17 and these three myths are worth noting because they are potentially dangerous in any combination. Why? Because when taken together, they collectively and progressively lead to more serious eating disorders, such as compulsive overeating, bulimia, and even anorexia, as well as long-term nutritional deficiencies.

Compulsive Overeaters, Bulimia, and Anorexia Defined

According to the National Eating Disorders Association, five to ten million women and girls and one million boys and men in the U.S. suffer from some type of eating disorder. Many will die from serious complications arising from this behavior. Most people have no idea how dangerous this slippery slope can be in progressively leading to serious conditions that permanently undermine health.

Compulsive Overeaters & Food Addicts are those who continually overeat. There is no brain-stopping inner mechanism that communicates it is time to stop eating. Dinner could continue on into the evening with late-night snacks and even getting up to eat in the middle of the night. The word "compulsion" is used in the same way the word "addiction " can be used to describe this out-of-control type of eating.

Bulimia Nervosa is a serious eating disorder characterized by secret cycles of bingeing and purging. Bulimia nervosa can cause death. The three primary symptoms are (1) eating large amounts of food in a brief period of time, (2) feeling "out of control" and (3) an inability to feel fullness or hunger. Some kind of purging or a combination of the following usually follows eating binges: self-induced vomiting, laxative or diuretic use and abuse, fasting, and obsessive or compulsive exercise. Those afflicted with bulimia nervosa also possess a blown-out-of-proportion worry about body weight and shape. This condition is serious, yet treatable.

Anorexia Nervosa is a serious eating disorder characterized by self-starvation and excessive weight loss. Anorexia Nervosa can cause death. The five primary symptoms are as follows:

(1) rebelling against sustaining a bottom line normal weight for their height, age, activity level, or body build;

(2) extreme fear of weight gain;

(3) a prevalent fear of feeling fat, even when there is much weight loss;

(4) loss of menstrual periods in women and girls who have reached puberty; and

(5) extreme worries about body weight and shape.

Anorexia nervosa is most simply, self-starvation. It results in the highest death rates of all eating disorders.

The Difference between Dieting and More Serious Eating Disorders

What is the difference between dieting and bulimia? Bulimia Nervosa is all of the following:

- recurrent binge eating (rapid consumption of large amounts of food in a short period of time)

- feeling lack of control over eating behavior during a binge self-induced vomiting, use of laxatives or diuretics, strict dieting or fasting

- vigorous exercise in order to prevent weight gain

- and persistent concern with body shape and weight.

Please note that dieting and bulimic behavior can lead to anorexia.

In contrast, dieting is recurrent restriction of calories in order to lose weight. Usually dieting is followed by gradual or quick weight gain. Feelings of depression and other negative emotions are common to both Bulimia Nervosa and dieting. Simple dieting *can* progress to more serious eating disorders that affect brain function (depression) due to inadequate nutrition for extended periods of time.

When to Enlist the Help of a Therapist

When you have been unsuccessful using the exercises in this book, or are feeling blocked, defeated, totally hopeless or helpless, look for a therapist who specializes in eating disorders, *not* weight loss. A therapist who knows eating disorders is like a good coach who has the resources to pull together a winning team. Your body, mind, and spirit can be brought together to learn more balanced eating with the help of this professional.

What can you do to help a friend or loved one who is having dieting problems? Read as much as you can about eating disorders. Continue reading this book. Know the difference between fact and truth versus the myths about weight loss, diets, and exercise. Be honest and talk openly about your concerns with the person who is struggling with eating disorder or body image problems. Avoiding this subject or ignoring it completely is counterproductive. Be caring, but firm.

Mention the situation to someone else who cares about your friend. You can help by telling family, a counselor, teacher, or any other trusted adult. Remember that you can't force someone to change or to reach out for help, but you can share your honest concerns and the information you've found about where to find help. Ultimately, your friend needs to take responsibility and action for his or her problem and behavior.

Finding a Gentle Coach/Therapist to Show You the Long Term Way

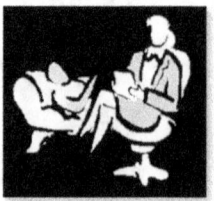

It's scary just to think about finding a person whom you can trust with your inner most thoughts, doubts, and fears. Most of us don't want anyone to know these things about us. You may think, "I'd rather forget they ever happened." That's easy for you to say, but another thing to really do it. Those thoughts of the past are stored in the basement of your mind. When it gets too full these garbage thoughts start coming up the basement stairs. Then what do you do?

A person with an eating disorder will eat over it, starve over it, purge over it, over-exercise, but never really deal with it and get over it. Now is the time to discover a new way of handling it. The "stuff" we stuff can be a whole lot less scary when we decide to process and deal with it.

Have you heard the following spiritual axiom: "When the student is ready, the (spiritual) Master will appear "? Often the only prerequisite to this happening is hitting bottom. By hitting bottom I mean you get sick and tired of being sick and tired on every diet available. It's when you are ready to try anything that the advice and guidance of a skilled therapist who has experience in eating disorders or healthy eating can help you the most.

From my experience, here are a couple ways to find a therapist. Ask around among your friends and find out if they can recommend someone from personal experience. Another great idea is to call 800-931-2237 and ask for local therapist recommendations from NEDA. It's like a gift from heaven to find a therapist you can trust.

Forty-three Symptoms to Heed

The following questionnaire, *Self-Inventory for Dieting*, can be copied for multiple use. It will help you determine if you are suffering from a serious eating disorder or if you're experiencing any dieting symptoms you need to heed. You'll zero in on specific areas and chart how severe they are for you each time you take this inventory. It takes only two minutes to complete and is the first step to understanding what to do next.

Directions: Put a 0, 1, 2, or 3 in the space to the right of each symptom on the following list. Use the number that best describes how much each symptom upset you in the past week using the following scale: 0 - not at all, 1- sometimes, 2 - many times, 3 - most days.

You may take this inventory more often than once a week. If you take the test when you are feeling anxious or before or after an eating binge, make a note of this to the side of your results and write down whatever else was happening in your life. Take this inventory also when you're feeling at your best. By comparing the results during your best and worst times, you can get a better idea about your range of symptoms and the life events that trigger more symptoms.

Keep at least a weekly record of your progress while reading this book. Record and date your answers on a separate sheet of paper (numbered 1 to 43) in your journal, instead of using the spaces to the right of the list, if you choose.

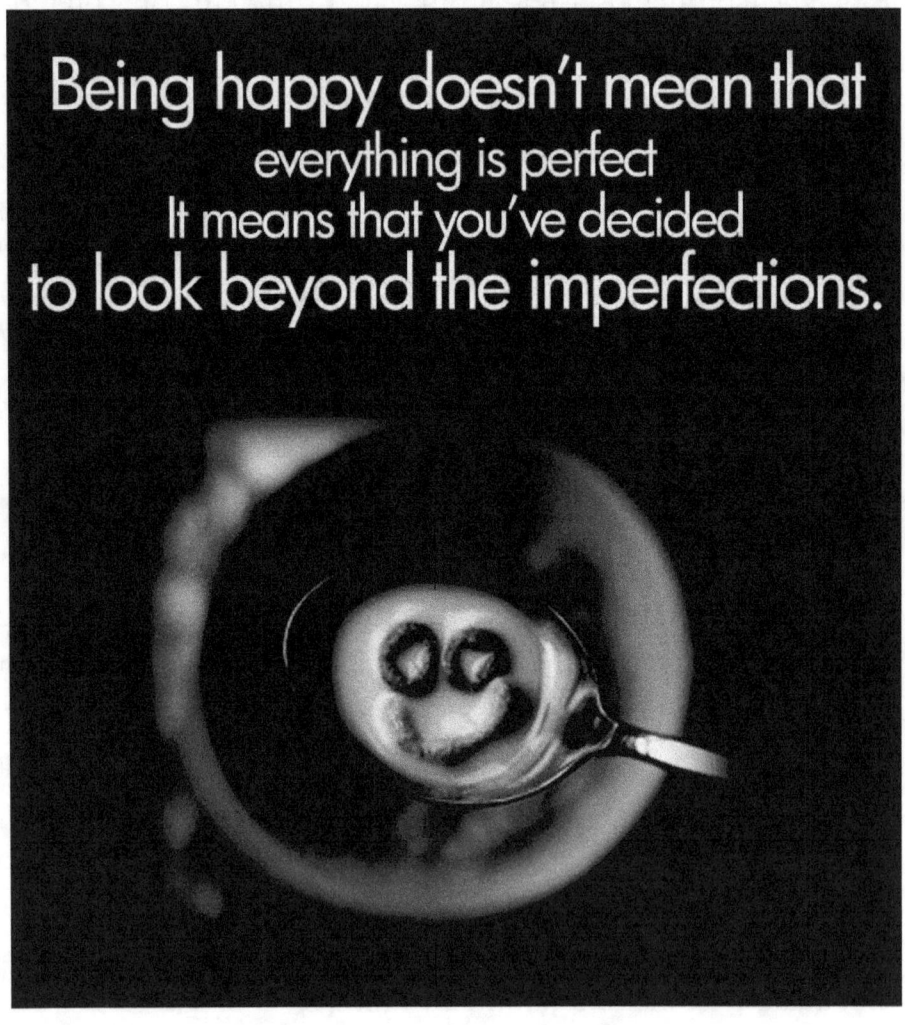

Self Inventory for Dieting

Category 1: Dieting

____ 1. Do you have a problem with food?

____ 2. How often do you binge?

____ 3. Do you often make special trips to get binge foods?

____ 4. Do you have special foods?

____ 5. Do you feel urgency as you eat or binge?

____ 6. Do you feel out of control when it is all gone?

____ 7. Have you gained weight in the past year?

____ 8. Do you exercise for longer than an hour per session or per day?

____ 9. Do you try to control your binges?

____ 10. Do you use pills or chemicals to stop yourself from bingeing?

____ 11. Do any family members have what you would consider a food problem?

____ 12. Do you think you have emotional problems?

____ 13. Do family members think you have an emotional problem?

____ 14. Have you ever considered suicide?

____ 15. Did you seek professional help?

____ 16. Does your relationship with food affect your job?

____ 17. Does your relationship with food seem to affect your relationship with your boss?

____ 18. Does your relationship with food seem to affect your relationship with family (husband, boyfriend, mother, father, sister, brother, children)?

____ 19. Does your relationship with food seem to affect your relationships with your friends?

____ 20. When you're eating, do you find you want to be alone?

____ 21. When you're eating, do you find you want to be with people?

____ 22. When you're eating, do you find you want to be with people you trust?

____ 23. When you're eating, do you find you want to be with strangers?

____ 24. When you eat, do you find a quiet place?

____ 25. *When you eat, do you find a noisy place?*

____ 26. *When you eat, do you find that the place doesn't matter?*

____ 27. *Do you use laxatives?*

____ 28. *Do you purge?*

____ 29. *Do you purge more than once after a meal?*

____ 30. *Do you ever use any medication to induce vomiting?*

____ 31. *Have you ever had problems stopping the regurgitation effect?*

Category II Anxious Thoughts

____ 32. *Difficulty concentrating*

____ 33. *Fear of going crazy*

____ 34. *Fear of passing out*

____ 35. *Fear of being alone*

____ 36. *Fear of criticism or disapproval*

Category III Feelings

____ 37. *Feeling confused*

____ 38. *Feeling guilty and blaming yourself for everything*

____ 39. *Feeling weak and a loss of motivation*

____ 40. *Feeling angry*

____ 41. *Feeling hopeless*

____ 42. *Feeling helpless*

____ 43. *Feelings of hate for your body or behavior*

Add up your total score and record it: _____ **Date:** _____

Total score	What it means
0-5	No problem
5-12	Edging toward a problem
15-29	Mild problem
29-45	Medium problem
46-89	Severe problem
90-125	Extreme problem

How reliable is this inventory? If you track it weekly, look for a small change of one, two, or three points from week to week. This small change is a big step in your journey of feeling more balanced. Keeping track each week will help you learn to value and sustain each small step in building a new you. This inventory will help you chart your course to peace and balance.

Remember only you can choose to get better. Choose to monitor your progress as you read this book and do the exercises. As your totals go down, you make progress. Stay committed to the journey, even when your totals go up or stay the same. Keep saying to yourself until you believe it to the core of your being, "I choose to trust in positive outcomes."

To review:

1. Commit to singing your love song from Chapter 16 at the same time every day. Briefly record your experience in your journal.
2. Did you use feelings to describe your experience? Did you use thoughts to describe your experience? Did you describe how your body felt doing this? Rewrite again using feelings, thoughts, and body sensations.
3. Review the Emotions Awareness Chart and check off the emotions that you experience daily. At least once a week, write in your journal what greater truths your emotions brought to your awareness. Review your entries at least once a month to self-monitor your progress.
4. Take the Self-Inventory for Dieting at least once a week. Chart and review your totals at least once a month to see if certain life events trigger more symptoms. Strive to reduce your exposure to the stress of these events, when possible.
5. Must read "Hunger—Friend or Foe?"- Section in Chapter 2 and "A Sweet Tooth Can Be a Bitter Pill to Swallow" in Chapter 12.

Now that you've gotten an understanding about diet cycles and gained some techniques for breaking the emotional traps that bind you, let's explore the power of asking the right questions to get the real answers you seek in the next chapter.

I'll also highlight books you can use as references to help you fashion a customized eating program which will give you optimum health and peak athletic performance while getting rid of food cravings, deprivation, and helping prevent and reverse disease. All this can be found in Chapter 19, as well as finding the inner resources you already possess to better channel your energies toward weight balance success.

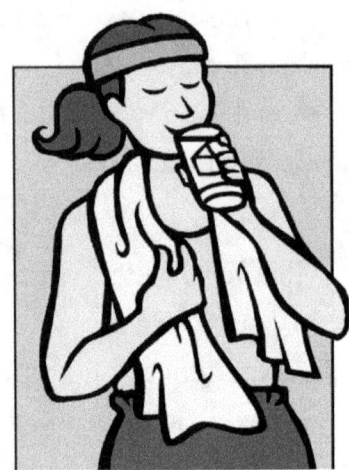

Choose to Be a Healthy Woman

Chapter 19

The Power to Ask the Right Questions to Get Answers You Need

Freeing Yourself to Make Mistakes

The following story about Tina shows how making mistakes can work as wake-up calls to inspire a change for the better. When combined with awareness and asking the right questions, these mistakes can lead you to turn your life around.

Initially Tina sought help from a counselor for an eating disorder. "I'm here because of my weight and being so tired," Tina told the counselor. "This is a serious problem for me. I've gained 40 pounds, largely due to the fact that I can't sleep through the night. I get up and eat and then I'm so tired the next day that I can't work well. I can't stay awake in the evenings and I usually fall asleep at 8:00 p.m. each night."

The counselor asked Tina many questions and found she was depressed and had repeated thoughts of her husband dying. Tina told the counselor that each time she came home from work, she binged on snack foods and couldn't stop until she went to sleep. She found all of this was causing her to become more distant from her husband. She and her husband both wanted her to get these issues addressed, and it was her husband who suggested that she seek treatment under his HMO plan.

The counselor thought about Tina's problems and how she could address them under the guidelines of the HMO plan before recommending that Tina see a psychiatrist to get evaluated for medication.

"If you are experiencing tiredness, sleeplessness, weight gain, anxiety, and repeated thoughts of your husband's death," she said gently, "I'm sure a psychiatrist can work with you to relieve the depression and insomnia."

Tina kept seeing her counselor during this time. The medication from the psychiatrist gave her more energy, however her sexual interest and sexual feelings went numb. This disturbed Tina since this was the one area of her life that she hadn't had problems with previously. Needless to say, Tina wasn't happy with the medication.

After two weeks she returned to the doctor and told him about the loss of sexual feelings. "The medications still aren't helping me sleep. I still wake up several times a night."

"Here's another prescription plus an additional one which will help you sleep," said the doctor. Tina hesitated, but said, "OK."

"Take these two new medications with what you're already taking for the next two weeks, then come back to see me," he said.

Tina took the combined medications, but they were a hassle. Each day Tina came home from work, she fell asleep on the couch by 6:00 p.m., and yet still awoke at 3:00 a.m. She could hardly finish her work the next day due to being groggy and tired. This didn't make sense to her because these were the issues she was paying the doctor to address. On top of everything else, her sexual interest disappeared completely. This was most disturbing to her and her husband.

The next time Tina went to the doctor, she mentioned falling to sleep early, grogginess, tiredness, not sleeping through the night, and the complete loss of sexual feelings. "The medications make me groggy during the day. They don't seem to help," she said.

"Here, try this prescription instead. Also, these will help you sleep. Remember it takes time for your body to adjust. Come back and see me in three weeks," he said.

Tina wanted to tell the doctor what she thought of the medications but held back, figuring she needed to give the doctor's advice a little more time. She hesitantly filled the prescriptions, then went home and started taking the new medications.

From this point on, her life was a mess. She looked terrible and every time she took the medications she felt worse than ever. Her husband was worried. He tried talking to Tina, but she was so groggy that she couldn't listen. Her husband took time off from work one afternoon to cuddle and be romantic with Tina, but nothing happened. It was the worst situation

Tina could imagine.

After more than three months of prescription changes, Tina had a shelf full of pills and was no closer to a good night's sleep. She talked to her counselor and told her that she'd had it. "I've never taken medications before, and now I have three prescriptions I take twice a day. When I showed up for my last appointment, the doctor's office was locked so I went home and called."

"The receptionist who answered the phone rudely asked, 'Didn't you get the message that the office is moving? Well, there was a sign in the window.'" She told Tina that the doctor's office would call to set up another appointment. That was two weeks ago and Tina hadn't heard from them since.

Tina steamed with frustration and anger as she talked to the counselor. Eventually, Tina concluded that she wanted to wean herself off the medications since they only caused more complications and sexual dysfunction.

A week later she returned to her counselor and said, "You know, I am much happier off the medications. I feel alive."

"I am happy to hear this," the counselor said. Tina and the counselor continued their work on Tina's underlying feelings of guilt that had led to the bingeing and depression in the first place. Tina was pleased and relieved with what she had learned. She returned home and reconnected with her husband.

From that moment on, Tina and her husband became allies, working together to ask the right questions. Eventually they discovered through the Internet that Chronic Fatigue Syndrome (CFS) is often misdiagnosed as depression. Tina's husband saw the information first and said, "This sounds like you, Tina."

They found dietary and supplement recommendations for CFS from books at the local library as well as Web sites dedicated to CFS on the Internet. When Tina applied the suggestions for dietary and lifestyle changes, her health improved.

Tina and her husband discovered through this experience that they were relieved to be free of the side effects from the medications. Subsequently they developed a stronger commitment to living more balanced in every aspect of their lives. Through Tina's determination to ask the right questions and practice awareness, she addressed the underlying cause of her tiredness as CFS and treated it at the source. With proper diet, nutritional supplements, lifestyle changes and time, Tina eventually alleviated all her symptoms and gained true permanent weight balance. Ultimately Tina felt better for having made the journey—and survived the worst it could get.

Leave No Stone Unturned in Your Quest

One resource that is often overlooked in the search for weight balance success is a thorough check-up by your family, internist, or general physician. A complete physical examination and full blood work done by your physician or a qualified nutritionist who knows what to look for can often isolate developing underlying medical conditions that can potentially cause unexpected weight gain (CFS, fibromyalgia, diabetes, and arthritis, to name only a few).

Some other possible causes of weight gain are head injuries, food allergies and sensitivities, candidiasis, thyroid conditions, hormonal imbalances, as well as interactions between herbs, over-the-counter and/or prescription drugs and medications, or cortisone (steroid) drugs.

In *The Food Allergy Cure,* Ellen Cutler writes, "Reports of food allergies began to appear in Europe in the early 1900s, and since the 1940s these allergies have been recognized by doctors around the world. Doctors estimate that up to two million people in the United States are affected by food allergies."

The symptoms allergies present include the following: hives, eczema, asthma, gastrointestinal disturbances (diarrhea, cramping, nausea, swelling, gas, even colitis), headaches, migraines, attention deficit hyperactivity disorder, cold and canker sores, recurrent ear infections, arthritis pain, fatigue, premenstrual and menopausal symptoms, infertility, *obesity, bulimia and other eating disorders.* Other medical reasons may cause these complaints; however Cutler says if you have already explored these possibilities and your physician cannot explain the symptoms, your might consider being tested for food allergies. Some of the most likely culprits for food allergies are refined carbohydrates (pasta, breads, and pastries), chocolate, and sugar, among others.

Cutler has developed a protocol, outlined in *The Food Allergy Cure,* that clears allergies from your system. It's a comprehensive approach for retiring allergies and the food cravings, weight gain, and depression that often accompany them for good. This book is worth checking out if you suspect that you have allergies or food sensitivities.

A Most Important Tool for Regulating Weight Balance

A change in eating habits, patterns, and foods can always dramatically affect weight gain at any age.

It's appropriate to look at whether you're getting the right foods (macronutrients) in the proper ratios for your metabolic type. One of the most powerful tools for regulating your body's ability to metabolize food is proper nourishment-basically food choices geared to your individual needs.

Isolating the root cause of what accelerated the weight gain in the first place and treating the originating offender is often the first step to reversing obesity. When you combine this tactic with eating a diet that's perfectly attuned for you metabolically and getting proper exercise, you'll attain steady, lasting results in your quest for weight balance success.

A Crucial Reference for Weight Balance Success

The most important weight balance tool you'll need is a comprehensive guide to nutrition and the proper foods. This guide can serve as a foundation resource for your eating patterns for the rest of your life. *The Metabolic Typing Diet* by William L. Wolcott with Trish Fahey, is by far the best system I've found for customizing food to your individual nutritional needs.

This definitive work is based on more than seventy years of comprehensive research, pioneering effort, and discoveries from various physicians, biochemists, dentists, physiologists, clinical nutritionists, and psychologists. Its dynamic, groundbreaking technology teaches you how to metabolically fine-tune your diet to meet your unique nutritional needs.

Providing you with the tools to understand, address, and speed up your metabolism through the foods you eat is only the first step. Metabolic typing also gives you the ability and flexibility to adjust your diet with great precision and accuracy as your metabolism shifts throughout your life. You can achieve and maintain your ideal weight with no feelings of deprivation and be free of food cravings and hunger forever with this cutting edge approach. This simple, user-friendly book is the last one you'll need on how to eat well to stay well. It boosts your immune system, naturally conquers indigestion and fatigue, prevents and reverses chronic illness while helping you overcome depression, anxiety, and mood swings. Metabolic typing is considered the "missing link" in modern nutrition science today.

Your quest for weight balance begins when you integrate and synchronize the truth about food from *The Metabolic Typing Diet* with the techniques, exercises, and visualizations in this book. Take the Metabolic Type Self-Test on page 135 of *The Metabolic Typing Diet*, start applying its principles, and you'll begin feeling and looking better today.

Another must-have book for your personal reference is Julia Ross' *The Diet Cure,* which offers specific recommendations to natural supplements that will supply your brain with nutrients needed to eliminate food cravings, depression, low energy, anxiety, and sleeplessness. Ross also lists interventions for other physical problems and gives step-by-step solutions. Be sure to check out the Amino Acid Therapy Chart for balancing brain chemistry in her book.

Cut a Striking Figure and Look Thinner

When many people are asked why they want to be thinner, three reasons come up often. They are (1) to be healthier, (2) to be more physically active throughout life and (3) to look better in clothes. Granted, being thinner doesn't necessarily guarantee being healthier or more physically active, but looking better in your clothes can begin right now, even *before you lose a single pound!*

In *Flatter Your Figure,* Jan Larkey shares a fun way to "figure out your figure" which uses no measuring tapes—just two sticks, a string, and a friend. Not only does she help you discern why some clothes look great on you while others make you look 10 pounds heavier, her style guide helps you find the most flattering styles-and pinpoints which ones to avoid for your specific figure challenges.

Camouflaging figure problems is only the first step to looking the best you can be, according to Larkey. Her book covers everything from basics to accessories. It explores how to use fabrics and prints and gives special strategies for appearing thinner or taller. *Flatter Your Figure* is a personalized guide for women to coordinate the most flattering ensembles from their wardrobes. This system engenders the utmost confidence in knowing that your figure assets are accented always.

How you look in clothes also depends on getting the best fit and the right size. On page 9 of *Fitting Finesse* by Nancy Zieman is a method for determining your correct size by taking one simple measurement—your front width measurement. Zieman includes a front width fitting chart and complete detailed directions for getting an accurate measurement. (Ask a friend to help you with this).

Zieman notes, "You may be pleasantly surprised by the results of the front width measurement. It is very common for someone who has been sewing with a size 20 in order to fit her bust to find out she is actually a size 16."

Although *Fitting Finesse* is written primarily for home sewers, Zieman's recommendations for measuring your figure will help you determine the right size and right area of the store in which to shop the next time you're looking for clothes. Her additional trouble-shooting methods and tips for sizing up the tailoring will come in handy when you're checking the quality of your potential buys in the fitting room as well.

Height and Weight Proportionate

A better determinant of your ability to maintain health and remain physically active throughout your life is finding out if your height and weight are balanced in proportion to each other. Have you heard of BMI (Body Mass Index)?

Body Mass Index specifically relates your height in proportion to your weight. Many BMI calculators can be accessed on the World Wide Web through your favorite search engine. One such online calculator is at www.halls.md/body-mass-index/bmi.htm.

First type in your height in inches and your weight in pounds. Then click on "calculate." This body mass calculation is based on the ratio of weight (in kilograms or pounds) to height (in meters or inches) squared. For **most** people, this number falls between 20 and 25.

The calculator not only gives you a body mass ratio number for your current weight to height, it also provides a zone of weight for your height. If your ratio is far less than 20 or far greater than 25, a bit of weight balancing by using this book and *The Metabolic Typing Diet* can help you move closer to an ideal zone.

Please note that the BMI range can give you a ballpark of weights that might be best for you—in other words, those that can help provide optimal health and strength to personal weight—but do take the BMI calculator with a grain of salt. Since it does not measure body fat and does not take into consideration activity levels, life styles, and healthy eating patterns, as a measure of obesity and overweight, it can be flawed.

Instead of trying to hold your weight too firmly to it, use it as a general rule that can be helpful for gauging the ballpark. The cut-off points can be arbitrary, because if your weight is above the 25-29.9, you can still be in a range that is normal and healthy for your individual metabolism. According to Glenn Gaesser, Ph.D., weight levels above these are *not* unhealthy when you practice a regular exercise routine and eat a healthy, balanced diet.

Those who have been overweight and sedentary since a young age may need to start slowly with the exercises recommended in Chapter 19 to bust *Myth #2: Exercise More and Lose Weight.*

One additional element to take into consideration when fine-tuning the weight balance estimate that's right for you is a basic test to determine whether you have a small, medium, or large bone structure.

Measuring Your Bone Structure

Encircle the bony part of your wrist with the longest finger and thumb of your other hand. If your finger and thumb overlap, you're small-boned. If they just meet, your medium-boned. If they don't meet at all at the boniest circumference of your wrist, you're most likely large-boned.

Establishing Realistic Goals

Big-boned people feel healthier and stronger at heavier weights than small-boned people of the same height do. In addition, men are healthier at heavier weights than women of the same height mostly because of muscle mass (since men are generally more highly muscled than women are).

Muscle weighs more than fat, so it makes sense that anyone (male or female) who is well-muscled will be healthier (as well as more fit) at a heavier weight. Muscle also burns fat, so developing more muscle increases your fat-burning capacity.

The right weight for you is a judgment call you can make based on your personal observations about yourself and what you know feels best for you. Please try to take every personal factor (including age) into consideration when determining your best balanced weight and be sure to practice understanding, compassion, and benevolence with yourself.

One quick note: It is generally agreed that carrying extra weight around your abdominal area is a sign of more serious health concerns. If your waist measurement is about ten inches less than your chest/bust measurement, you're in the healthy zone. When your waist measurement starts to inch toward equaling or exceeding your chest/bust measurement, it's time to take immediate steps toward a healthier diet and weight balance, ideally using *The Metabolic Typing Diet*. Also read Chapter 9-*Over Stressed & Over Weight*.

Learning How to Ask the Right Questions to Get Answers

After you read and apply the principles in *The Metabolic Typing Diet*, you'll want to further develop your ability to ask the right questions. Be aware that the answers can come from many places. Within every question is an answer waiting to be discovered.

When Carol stumbled upon this concept, she began asking questions right and left. Some of her favorite questions evolved out of her goal statement of "I want to achieve a healthy weight." She turned this statement into a series of positive questions such as, "How do I learn to eat in a balanced way to maintain my desired weight?" Carol chose questions that began with the words what, where, and when, such as, "What is balanced eating?" and "Where do I find the support I need to maintain more balanced eating?" Carol let her mind follow the clues generated by these questions, similar to following clues in a mystery. Carol found the answers she sought in the library, at the bookstore, at a local health center, and even through the Yellow Pages.

Carol decided to have some fun, so she called whomever she thought would have the answers from the listings in the Yellow Pages. Some people were helpful; others weren't. Carol ended up with notes and more phone numbers to call. She picked a good day to follow the trail to answers. She expected it to be an unexpected adventure and it was! Carol found four personal trainers near her home and one nutritionist that day. She was able to make appointments to interview them later that week.

Harnessing the Power of Your Dreams

Another way to get answers is to ask questions in a dream as illustrated in the next story. Toni, a woman struggling to lose weight, had a dream where she met a famous diet authority as he lectured in a mall. Toni stopped to listen and asked him, "How do I lose weight?"

The answer she received was, "It must be from the inside out." This answer came from her Higher Power through her inner wisdom and it pulled at her heartstrings for it meant a lot to her. On one hand, Toni wanted to lose weight; on the other hand, she was pulled by what she loved to eat. What decision would she make? To gain the result she wanted, Toni needed to decide what to release from her life. Those of us who want to lose weight need to ask positively turned questions that will ensure balance.

Even when using an excellent resource such as *The Metabolic Typing Diet*, initially we may be pulled by food cravings because we've built a dependence upon them or we are allergic to them. We need to ask ourselves, "What do I need to keep in my food plan and what needs to be released?"

Foods Can Be Your Best Friends

Foods can rejuvenate and help shape your body. In *The Metabolic Typing Diet,* turn to the list of foods that are right for your metabolic type. Here's a fun, healthy foods exercise.

Find a quiet time and a quiet place. Close your eyes and remember a time from long ago when you felt wonderful and excited. Take your time with this. Remember what you were seeing or experiencing. Remember your feelings of excitement, openness, how energized you were with youthful energy and adventure. Let these feelings fill your heart.

Now open your eyes and switch your attention to the list of foods that are right for you. Still embracing your feelings of excitement, openness, and adventure, ask which ones you would be willing to include more of in your lifestyle. Marrying your feelings to your intentions may entice better eating habits, which lead to a more shapely body and better health for you.

A Helpful Natural Aid for Weight Balance, Enhanced Mood, & Sleep

If you're accustomed to a diet based largely on refined carbohydrates, fruits, and sugars with very little emphasis on protein or fat, chances are you may be unconsciously using food to stimulate serotonin production in your brain (in an attempt to use food to make you feel good).

Abusing your body by eating refined carbohydrates and sugars without the proper balance of vegetables, proteins and fats can seriously compromise your health and bring on diabetic and pre-diabetic conditions with time. It is also predominantly responsible for weight gain due to increasing fat reserves.

This type of eating pattern is also subconsciously addictive. It's relatively easy to become addicted to your own body chemicals (serotonin, adrenaline, among others) and subconsciously repeat certain behavior patterns, such as binge eating of refined carbohydrates, in order to stimulate serotonin production. Anyone who has eschewed a balanced diet in favor of one based largely upon sugars and refined carbohydrates is familiar with the food "high" or "rush" that can result.

You can address your serotonin needs without resorting to stressing your body by abusing food. Simply take 50 to 800 milligrams of 5-hydroxytryptophan (5-HTP)—an over-the-counter amino acid-once a day to elevate your serotonin levels without compromising your eating habits. Although, over-the-counter, it should not be taken concurrently with SSRI (serotonin selective reuptake inhibitor) or SNRI (serotonin norepinephrine reuptake inhibitor) medications.

This essential amino acid is a common building block for proteins. An ordinary food source of 5-HTP is Thanksgiving turkey dinner. Most people consume much more than 100 milligrams of this amino acid then (proving its safety and lack of harmful side effects). Not only does 5-HTP help to elevate mood, it aids weight balance, and helps supply a good night's sleep.

You can break the vicious cycle of bingeing on carbohydrates and sugars while addressing your serotonin needs by adding a high quality form of 5-HTP to your morning supplements.

Some high quality brands of 5-hydroxytryptophan are from Thorne Research and Ultra Pure by Life Link. These can be found either through a reputable health care practitioner or ordered from your local health food store or Walmart has the best price. Further vital information is in

Chapter 9 on your Adrenal Glands and Chronic Stress, plus Chapter 14 contains insights on Addictions.

Pause and re-read the story of Tina. Use the resources of *Edge Effect, The Metabolic Typing Diet, Flatter Your Figure, Fitting Finesse,* and *The Mood Cure* to better understand where you're at and start feeling better about where you're going. Review the exercise that Carol used to find the answers she needed with her questions. See if you can think of some questions and begin opening yourself up to discovering the answers as they appear in your life this week. This is fun and surprising.

The next chapter covers more on how to connect your intuitive side with your feelings through inner exercises. When you safely explore the rich fertile ground of dealing with your feelings, you're on the way to having your life blossom in ways you've always wanted.

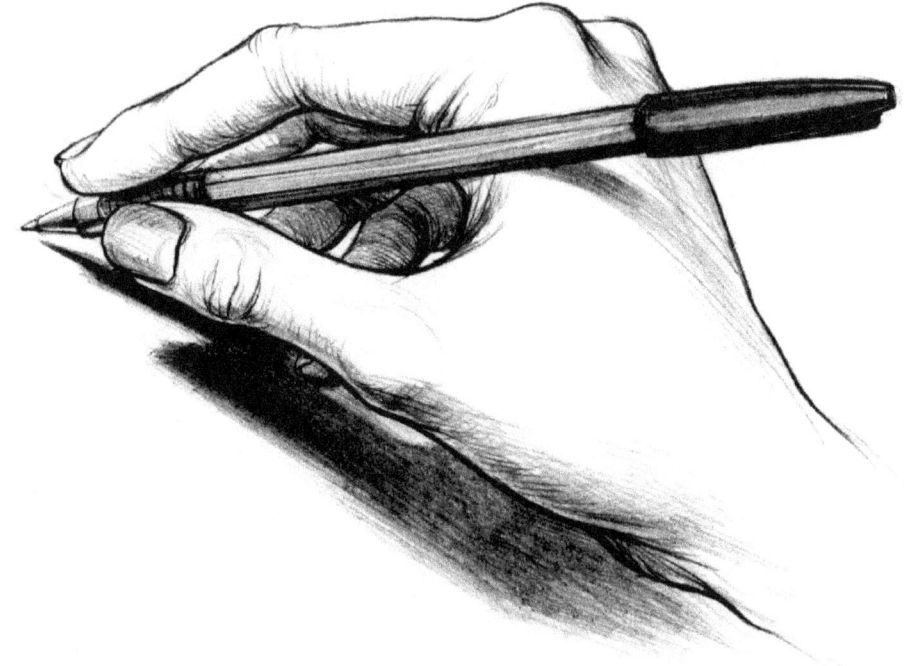

Journaling Can Open Your Awareness

Chapter 20

Honoring and Easy Clearing of Your Feelings While Connecting to Your Intuitive Side

Identifying Hidden Feelings So You Can Take Positive Action

> *Remember your feelings are a golden key in your quest for weight balance freedom.*

By now you've been checking your feelings every evening. If you've neglected to do this, use this as a gentle reminder to begin checking in with your feelings daily. When you feel guilt, strive to find the truth underneath that guilt. If you find anger comes up and you've never dealt with it before except by bingeing, find the deeper truth your intuitive self is trying to tell you.

The technique of getting in touch with your emotions is similar to healing an infection. An adhesive covering an infection just won't heal it. The infection needs to come to the surface and be addressed, so that the wound can heal from the inside out.

To cover it over is similar to stuffing feelings. Ignored and stuffed feelings create an infection in your subconscious. Eventually those stuffed feelings have to surface and be healed in appropriate ways. If not, they build up as ever-present subconscious stresses that cause major imbalances in your health, which eventually manifest as heart disease, cancer, and other serious diseases.

The following chart is *The Graduate Level Feeling Chart*. You can make copies of it to use for several weeks. Put a check mark by each feeling that you experience during the day. No second guessing or changing your first impression; the first hint or nudge is the honest truth for you. If you haven't made a habit of knowing your feelings, then you need to go back and do the exercise in Chapter 17 until you can recognize your true feelings.

Remember feelings aren't good or bad; they are just feelings. Do this exercise because you choose to show yourself love and take the best care of yourself that you can for now. You will benefit from this for the rest of your life.

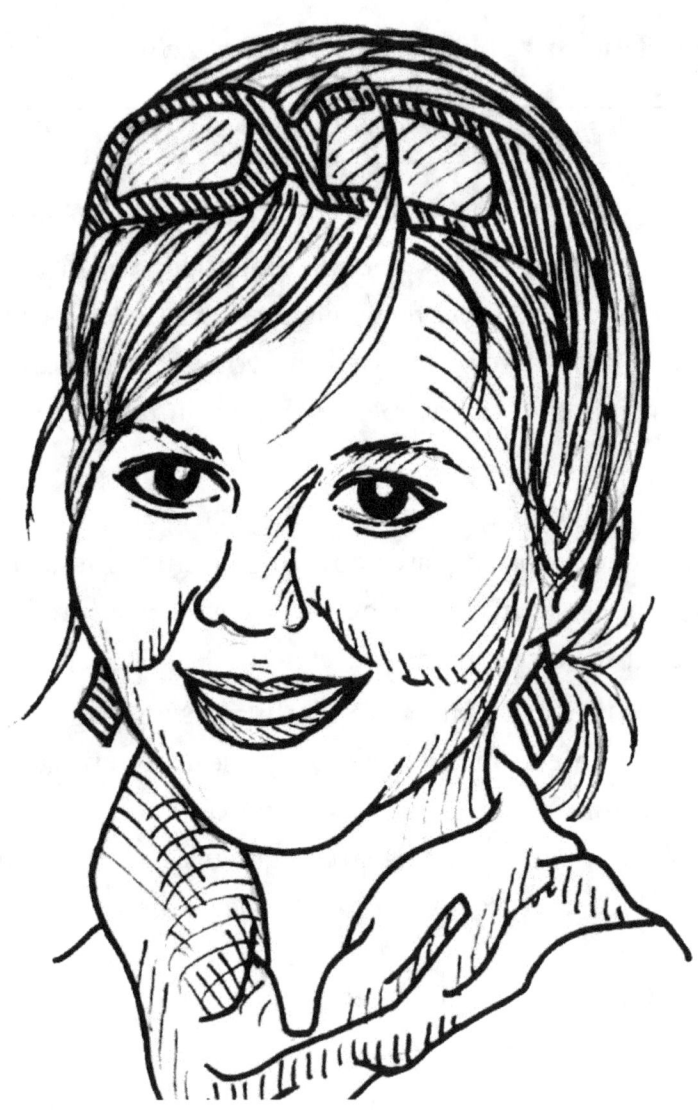

Connect With Your Intuitive Side

Graduate Level Feeling Chart

	Mon.	Tues.	Wed.	Thurs.	Fri.	Sat.	Sun.
Annoyed							
Fiery							
Fuming							
Rejected							
Embarrassed							
Confused							
Frustrated							
Sarcastic							
Disappointed							
Used/Abused							
Burdened							
Discouraged							
Self-punishing							
Bitter							
Hurt							
Attacked							
Adaptable							
Open							
Caring							
Amused							
Attractive							
Numb							
Involved							
Questioned							
Safe							
At peace							
Opposing							
Bothered							
Indignant							
Choosy							
Optimistic							

Graduate Level Feeling Chart (*continued*)

	Mon.	Tues.	Wed.	Thurs.	Fri.	Sat.	Sun.
Deserving							
Approachable							
Acceptable							
Hateful							
Overwrought							
Seething							
Belligerent							
Furious							
Hysterical							
Prepared							
Encouraging							
Invigorated							
Adequate							
Answerable							
Refreshed							
Aware							
Wounded							
Unappreciated							
Dumb							
Offended							
Fascinated							
Needed							
Understanding							
Essential							
Tuned-in							
Welcome							
Appreciated							
Trapped							
Put upon							
Deprived							
Vindictive							
Picked upon							
Excited							

Graduate Level Feeling Chart (continued)

	Mon.	Tues.	Wed.	Thurs.	Fri.	Sat.	Sun.
Trusting							
Let down							
Threatened							
Frightened							
Ignored							
Overlooked							
Unwelcome							
Brave							
Affectionate							
Daring							
Bold							
Considered							
Proud							
Betrayed							
Defeated							
Unacceptable							
Despondent							
Ruined							
Lucky							
Reliable							
Sincere							
Purposeful							
Concerned							
Productive							
Pessimistic							
Rigid							
Stagnant							
Destructive							
Immobilized							
Unfeeling							
Disconnected							
Attuned with							
In balance							

Graduate Level Feeling Chart (*continued*)

	Mon.	Tues.	Wed.	Thurs.	Fri.	Sat.	Sun.
Tender							
Congruent							
Creative							
Appreciative							
Gentle							
Neglected							
Unimportant							
Morbid							
Unloved							
Melancholy							
Deserted							
Quiet							
Unified							
Fulfilled							
Completed							
Connected							
At one							
Perceptive							

A Word about Perceiving and Judging Your Feelings

How you were taught to perceive and judge your feelings when you were growing up is what stops you from feeling and acknowledging the truth beneath those feelings right now. It is normal and human to experience many feelings throughout the day. What you want to learn from the practice of charting your feelings are ways to clear or process all feelings, so that you don't continued to carry them around in the background any more.

For example, if you don't seem to experience anger ever, this is a red flag warning you that you're in deep denial about your anger. Getting to the truth at the root of your anger is a key to being free of it.

The best time to chart your emotions is at the end of the day. If you continually find you're stuck in the same emotional bandwidth, ask yourself the following questions and write the answers to them in your journal. These questions will help you get clear about the facts regarding your emotions and feelings. The answers to these questions will help you reach freedom and balance eventually.

Journal Questions to Ask When You're Stuck in Your Emotions

Remember when you do this questioning part of the exercise, you need to make the effort and be persistent. Results will follow.

Question 1: What are my thoughts in connection to this feeling?

Question 2: What did I think next? How did I feel about it?

Keep asking the above questions and write down as many answers as you get, boiling it down for as long as it takes, until you get to the bottom where there are no more thoughts and no more feelings.

Drawing Can Uncover What's Hidden for You

Next draw a stick figure or something else that represents where you are after the last question. Put a dialogue balloon over its head and let the drawing speak to you. What would it say if you drew anything else?

Write three sentences that begin with, "I am _____" underneath the picture and finish the sentence with a different characteristic of what you felt when you drew the picture.

Remember to do the best you can. There is no right or wrong way to do this drawing. The important thing is to take action and do it. When you draw, use symbols and images—the easiest language for the subconscious to understand. This exercise is valuable in beginning to clear out feelings that are blocking you.

After you do this exercise, wait a few minutes and see if you start feeling better. Then check again later in the day to see if the feelings have decreased in intensity. Learn to look for shifts and little steps that will lead you to feeling better. You'll find as you check in with your feelings, you'll learn which ones lead to overeating, binging, starving or other compulsive eating behaviors. Acknowledging unconscious habits and fear of feelings, rather than denying them, puts you on your way to balancing them and finding out what will truly make you happy. Feelings are the key to your truth.

What to Expect When You First Begin to Chart Your Feelings

In the beginning, recognize that it is okay to feel unsafe about acknowledging your feelings. It is equally okay to feel disheartened when you first start to practice checking your feelings daily. These feelings need to come up in your awareness because they have been hiding too long in your subconscious where they have been causing trouble. Any discomfort you experience will pass as you continue to do the freeing techniques in book.

Freeing Hidden Emotions So You Can Take Positive Action

As you begin to ask for answers in your life, you'll encounter truth when you are ready. Working with hidden emotions can be difficult only because they haven't been dealt with before. The frustrations, anxiety, fearful and out-of-control feelings seem over-whelming, but the more you deal with them, the less difficult they will become until they loosen their hold on you. So how do you muster up the initial courage and approach this process with an adventurous spirit?

Connecting with Your Adventurous Spirit

The way to connect to an adventurous spirit is to first define what this state of mind or consciousness is for you. In other words, where is your attention? How do you feel in your attitude toward your quest? Remember the three keys of attitude, attention, and mechanics when tapping into your adventurous spirit.

A woman named Annie illustrated how she used these three keys to unlock her adventurous spirit. First she practiced an imaginative technique. Then she used her attention and imagination to complete the exercise, and finally she used an observer attitude in viewing herself doing the technique. The observer attitude comes from Soul, your true Self. This attitude will feel neutral and balanced. You can enhance the observer attitude by invoking a sense of anticipation, as if toward an adventure that is about to begin, heightening the fun.

Here's what Annie did: she started by closing her eyes and gently focusing on the imaginary spot in the center of her forehead where insight occurs in the brain. Then silently she asked her Higher Power to connect her to her hidden feelings. Next, she imagined walking in a beautiful, shady garden bordered by low granite walls and lacy wrought-iron gates.

As Annie walked the stone path through the garden, she noticed a huge weed growing in the middle of the walkway. She bent down and began to pull it up. The first part of it, composed of many small roots, came up easily. But Annie was surprised to find that there was a single, long taproot holding it in. She pulled with all her strength, pulling and pulling until the root let go.

Then she asked her Higher Power if this huge weed-like plant was poisonous. When she found that it *was,* she asked if she could transplant it in her garden and watch it change positively.

Annie found just the right place for the weed. As she transplanted it, she began to notice that it changed into something beautiful. She watched closely as its breathtaking beauty blossomed before her eyes.

You can try this technique, too. It makes you aware of any weedlike feelings you might have in the garden of your consciousness. It sets up an adventure consciousness similar to that of going on a vacation when you are excited and looking at everything in a new way. Try this imaginative exercise every night before you go to sleep, or in the morning just before your day begins. Set one time a day to do this routine. You'll be surprised at the results.

When you assume a goal of finding hidden feelings that have blocked you from taking positive action in the past, you can be assured that you'll find symbols of those feelings in your visualizations. Acting as if you have the means to deal with these images in symbolic ways paves the way for you to achieve this goal. In this case, setting up a regular time to practice the above technique works gradually on a subconscious level to free your life from the unconscious emotions that strive to stay hidden.

Taking the Technique One Step Further

Annie went further in the exercise by asking, "What does pulling up the taproot mean to my process?" Upon further reflection, Annie discovered the meaning of what pulling up the taproot meant for her: it was pulling out hidden, buried resentments toward the men in her life. These resentments had affected balance in her life with regard to eating.

In the past when she interacted with men, Annie felt over-whelmed. A few hours later, she would binge on muffins or jelly beans. Annie discovered that by doing this technique she was pulling up her resentments towards men and inviting them to transform. The more she practiced the visualization, the less overwhelmed she was around men. Annie became more aware of when she began to feel resentments in the moment and was able to calm herself by letting go of her guilt, taking charge of her response, and affecting the outcome of these interactions. Her muffin/jelly bean binges decreased with this change and she was on her way to being totally free of the binges.

Writing and Drawing Can Uncover What's Hidden from You

Put your attention on an area of your life and let the inner conflicts it elicits pop into your awareness. This could be anything about which you've had mixed feelings. Next, write the feelings down. Use "I feel statements" such as "I feel confused," "I feel guilty, anxious, afraid, sad, or out of control"; because these statements will help you take ownership and responsibility for your feelings. You can check your Graduate Level Feeling Chart to find out which emotions recur for you most often and use them. Chronicle them here or in your journal.

I feel ———————————————————————————————

———————————————————————————————————

———————————————————————————————————

———————————————————————————————————

———————————————————————————————————

Now draw a doodle picture of those feelings in your journal. You can pretend that you don't know how to draw even if you do. This attitude helps free your Spirit of Childhood to experiment and have fun. Then draw a funny stick doodle figure of your feelings. You can use a dialogue balloon above its head and write what the figure might want to say.

Next make a positive change in the picture or in what it wants to release. This technique works every time to uncover hidden feelings. It is enough to experience the feelings in this way for now. Feeling your emotions, recognizing them, then taking some action on those emotions will help you let them go.

Forming a Deeper Connection to Move through Your Emotions and Fears

In the next story, Annie used an exercise to help her form a deeper connection to her feelings in order to move through them and past her fears. She used it as a way to resolve a long-standing challenge that she'd never been able to face, let alone begin to address.

Annie had been working on several aspects of her process. However, one challenge remained for her—the challenge of encountering the void.

Annie described the void as complete vulnerability, which left her so helpless and without hope that she felt terror and thoughts of death. Annie would be stuck in panic while in this emotional state.

As a child, Annie had continual nightmares and she would hide under the covers. At this point, Annie recognized that this void was part of her fear of abandonment. A completely helpless feeling that no one was there for her would overcome her. Although she had asked her Higher Power many times to clear this black void and the intense irritation that she experienced when she got close to someone she cared about, Annie had no idea how to approach the process of resolving it. This was because on the other side of her defenses was an inner wall.

Then one night her Higher Power gave Annie a dream. She wrote the dream down as soon as she awoke. Then she went back into the dream and used imagination and visualization to address and resolve her fear of the void (abandonment). This is what she wrote:

"I went back into the dream in my imagination and just watched. Soon I remembered that I was standing behind a chain link fence. I moved towards the house and opened the gate in the fence. As I looked at the house, I knew I was walking to the house of my Higher Power-God's house. The door was wide open with warm light streaming out. I began clearing my emotions.

Mostly what I felt was overwhelming fear. I could hear myself saying, 'You can do it. You are always safe.' I used every effort of inner strength to step up on the first step of the stairway that led to the open door.

Next I felt like I had to move through an iron wall, just to step into the doorway. I entered and was catapulted into the void, into blackness, helplessness, terror, and complete vulnerability.

Then I sensed the soft whispers, the Voice of my Higher Power telling me what to do. I listened. I sensed my inner ears hearing these words, 'Trust that you are loved as you allow the blackness to engulf you. Just be, and know that in being, you are love.' This experience of being aware that I was love eliminated the illusion of blackness and the void."

Annie wrote how powerfully loving this experience was and how she felt uplifted for weeks later. That experience is part of her consciousness forever.

Try this exercise of going back into a dream with the help of your Higher Power. If experiences don't happen for you right away, try again. You may have to spend time playing at it. Sometimes you will meet your Higher Power in disguise on a street in your dreams. You will know this by a feeling of upliftment or love that accompanies the experience. You'll either feel lightness or joy when you are with your Higher Power, or when the experience is over. The upliftment and joy is a blessing given to you in divine love.

The Hidden Answers within Three Steps

1. Keep writing in your journal, asking questions to your Higher Power like, "What is my next step?" Chronicle the answers you receive.

2. Contemplate and pray as you connect to your Higher Power.

3. Taking courageous new actions out of compassion and true inner self-love once the foundation is set.

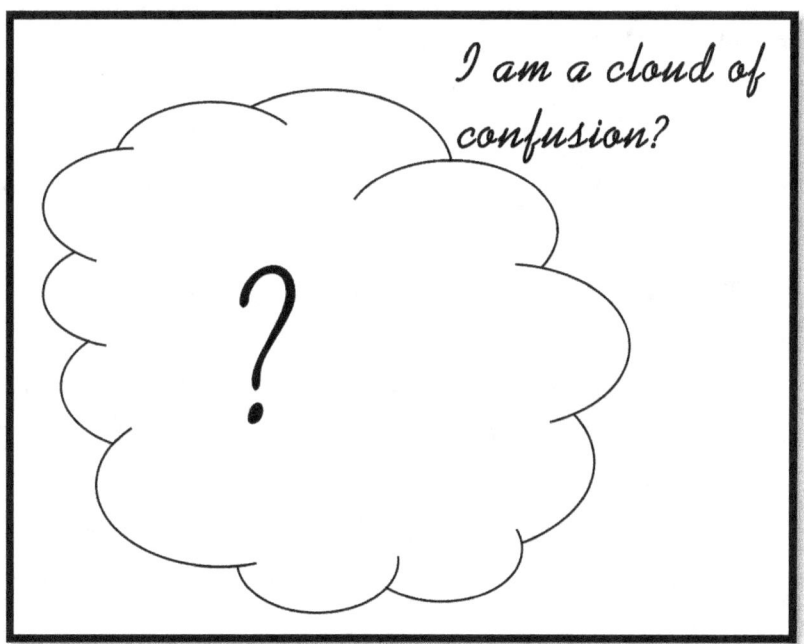

A Technique for Finding Answers in Your Dreams

1. *Before you go to sleep, write down in your journal a question for which you would like an answer. Ask to receive a dream with the answer in it, in a way you cannot possibly misunderstand. Keep your journal and a pen beside your bed.*

2. *Before you go to sleep, read your question over ten times with a strong feeling of love.*

3. *Be ready to write down your dream and the answers within it immediately upon awakening.*

To review:

1. Commit to singing your love song to yourself each day at the same time daily.

2. Get a physical examination and complete blood work if you think it's necessary and check out *The Metabolic Typing Diet* by William L. Wolcott with Trish Fahey, *The Mood Cure* by Julia Ross, and the first section of *Cut the Guilt*–Using Biology to Change Your Eating and Weight.

3. Ask and write down questions that arise naturally from your goal statement and go on an adventure to find the answers. Check out the wisdom contained in your local library, on the Internet, local bookstores, health food stores, and health centers and other businesses found in the Yellow Pages.

4. Use *The Graduate Level Feeling Chart* daily and journal the answers to the following questions when you become stuck in emotions:

Question 1: What are my thoughts in connection to this feeling?

Question 2: What did I think next? How did I feel about it?

5. Use the drawing exercise to uncover and release blockages from hidden emotions.

6. Remember to use the three keys of attitude, attention, and mechanics when connecting with your Higher Power during visualizations and dreams.

7. Practice the *Hidden Answers within Three Steps* exercise and *The Technique for Finding Answers in Dreams*. Write the results in your journal.

In Chapter 21, we'll explore successful techniques for getting unstuck emotionally and verbally, and discover more on how to process anger and other strong emotions.

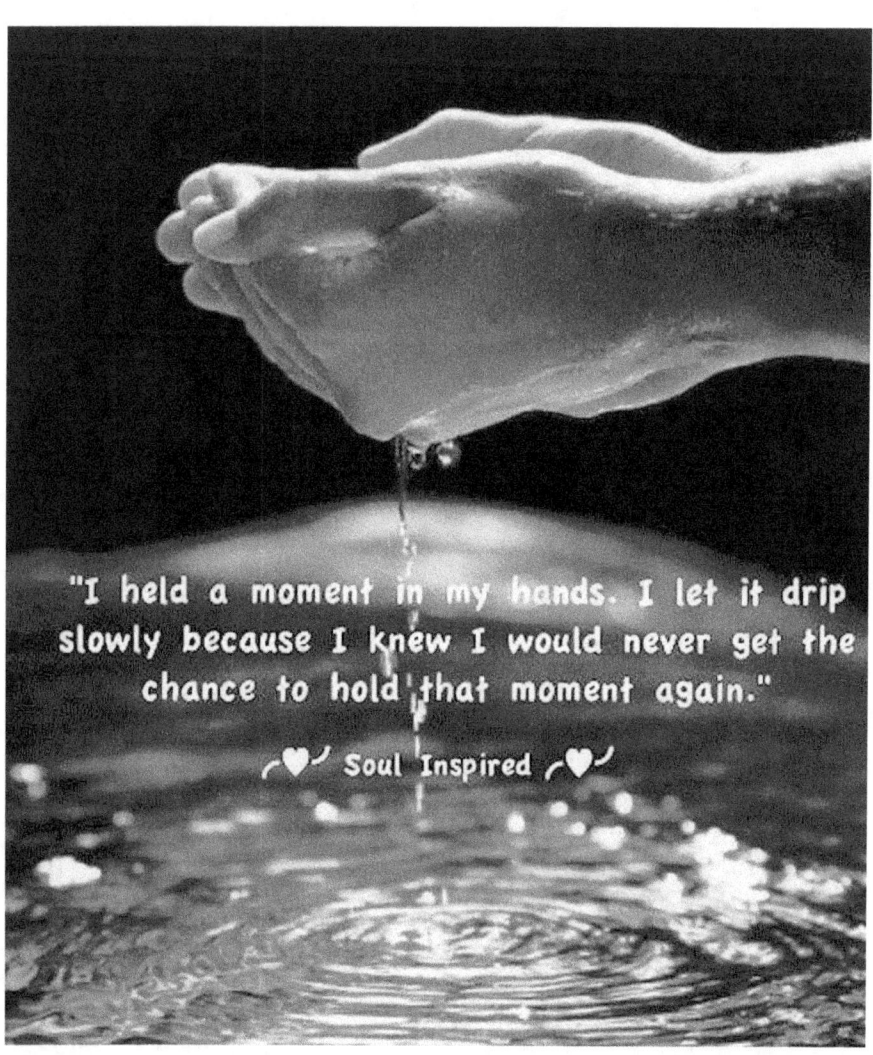

"I held a moment in my hands. I let it drip slowly because I knew I would never get the chance to hold that moment again."

♥ Soul Inspired ♥

Chapter 21

Getting Unstuck and Learning When to Say "No" (without guilt)

Tips for Getting Unstuck and Moving Beyond Discouragement

Annie has made excellent progress so far. After several sessions, she's recognized that she subconsciously relies upon the myths of "Dieting Will Make Others Proud of Me" and "Dieting Will Make My World All Right."

> *She has also uncovered her deeper truth behind this myth,*
> *which is the human need for love.*

Annie made her positive purpose statement *(I am on my way to being successful through learning the secrets to weight balance success)* and chose a personal symbol that represents her success (a star), which she uses in visualizations every day. Annie also incorporated the Five-plus Passkeys to Success (setting up her environment for success, committing herself to new behaviors and self-monitoring them).

In her session last week, Annie asked, "What changes can I make to jumpstart my weight balance success and resolve my fears?" She's begun applying principles from *The Metabolic Typing Diet* and started changing her eating habits and patterns. She also utilized some of the techniques, exercises, and visualizations offered in Chapter 19.

When Annie enters the room this week, I notice she's feeling defeated. Her body language loudly broadcasts discouragement as she slumps into a chair. As we talk, Annie's hands twist nervously and she looks down at the floor. She expresses disappointment about not losing as much weight as fast as she wanted.

"I just can't seem to lose any weight," she says. "I'm doing all the right things, such as balancing my carbohydrates, proteins and fats according to the *Metabolic Typing Diet.* I'm eating the right *kinds* of carbohydrates and three balanced meals a day without bingeing." She sighs as I listen.

"You didn't lose a *single* pound this week?" I ask for clarification.

Annie paused to reflect. "Well, I did lose a couple, but my secretary lost six pounds the first week she started her diet. This week I only lost two!"

"I understand," I said. "You sound discouraged. But a better indicator would be to evaluate your energy level and note how well your clothes are fitting."

"My energy level *is* good," Annie admitted, "and my clothes *are* much more comfortable."

"It sounds like you might be leaning toward buying into the myth of eating less to lose weight, but I think you already know where that will lead. If you stay on track and continue with your metabolic plan, I think you'll soon begin to see much more weight balance success. By the way, did you know the discouragement you're feeling right now is a positive sign?" I ask.

"It *is?*" Annie responds, incredulously.

"It's an indicator that we need to take different measures and be even more creative with techniques, exercises and visualizations to help you break through this bog of emotions. We need to do further fine-tuning to achieve your target. What would be more helpful for your attitude right now is to choose to trust in positive outcomes."

Annie sighs and slumps a little more as she looks at the floor. I can tell she's gotten herself into an emotional quagmire that's hard to shake.

"How are you feeling emotionally right now?" I ask.

"I feel like a failure," Annie says. "I'm scared, pessimistic, unacceptable, and frustrated. And I feel awful that I didn't do as well as my secretary."

I suggest to Annie that she visualize what feelings of discouragement look like. Notice I said to focus on *feelings* of discouragement, not the *thought* that she's a failure.

"What would discouragement look like to you?" I ask Annie. "Imagine a picture of your PAST discouragement." Since the subconscious mind doesn't differentiate between past and present, I verbally emphasize the word *past*. In this way, I'm encouraging Annie to move through this stage as quickly as possible and put it *in the past*.

I ask, "Does your past discouragement look like a sunny field of wild flowers?"

"No! It looks more like a dark warehouse. Everything is empty blackness." Annie is in deep distress, her hands and fingers are wringing with the intensity of her emotions.

"Take a few deep breaths, Annie, and let it go," I suggest gently. "That's right."

Then I begin to lead Annie out of the swamp of her emotions. Since the language of the subconscious is composed of pictures and images, I tap into a visualization technique that will help clear blocked energy and her feelings of failure.

"Annie, close your eyes and look up at the center of your forehead where insight occurs in your brain and connect with your Higher Power. Silently remember your purpose statement and your symbol as you look upward. Ask your Higher Power to help you by inviting this past discouragement that looks like a dark warehouse to change positively. Watch or sense it as it's changing," I say.

Annie was able to visualize the warehouse, but she was unable to allow it to change positively. Her hands and fingers told the story of how difficult this was for her to do.

"Take a few deep breaths, Annie, and it will relax you." "It's so empty and dark, and I'm scared."

"Stay connected to your Higher Power, Annie. Stay with it. Keep taking deep breaths . . . you're doing all right."

Not only did Annie have a hard time getting the empty warehouse to transform, she had even more difficulty verbalizing this, so we used another imaging tool.

I asked Annie to draw.

At first she did not want to because she felt she couldn't draw. I reassured her that it was not about drawing in an artistic sense. It was about putting down a symbol or stick drawing of whatever you experienced inside of you. Putting emotions down on paper in any visual way helps transform the feelings and get them out.

Annie did this willingly even though her hands still showed how nervous, anxious, and scared she was. By drawing, Annie broke through old mental traps that led her to believe and feel she was a failure. The first step of allowing the empty warehouse to transform in her imagination was to pour her feelings of emptiness onto the page.

Annie showed me her "empty feelings drawing" and explained what she had drawn. It was an empty toothpaste tube, shown from three different angles and an empty glass. This was powerful work for Annie. She cried for several minutes.

"It's OK to let that past go. It's safe to let it go. It's safe to grow and change," I said. Through this emotional flood, I saw Annie had released the negative block of emotions that commanded her to see herself as a failure in this situation.

To further help Annie transform the image of the dark, empty warehouse, I offered her *The Schoolteacher Technique.*

I asked her to write the following sentence 15 times every day in her journal for the next three weeks: *I am sincere and I choose to trust in positive outcomes.* These words concisely convey to Annie's subconscious her purity of purpose. Writing this continuously for three weeks is the first step to forming a positive habit that will endure. I urged her to practice this for as long as it took to integrate this truth into her cells, eventually causing a complete change in body, mind, and spirit.

At the close of this emotionally moving, clearing session, I told Annie we would work further on transforming the empty warehouse in future sessions. In conclusion, I encouraged Annie's progress and gave her a little more understanding about the process in which she was involved.

"Annie, you did some wonderful work today. I know you've been feeling anxious and discouraged about your perceived progress and you want to go faster, accomplishing your goals according to your expectations and timetable."

"However, please remember that it's important to hold realistic expectations. A part of the process is the rhythm of 'two steps forward, one back.' It's integral to attaining solid equilibrium on each new level you reach."

"It's also natural to feel discouraged at times, especially when you perceive you might be slipping backward. Any time you make any kind of change, the subconscious and the body knows there's safety of familiarity in the status quo. We often want to stay with old behaviors only because they're familiar—even though those behaviors may be hurtful or self-defeating to us in the long run. This is a part of the paradox of life. Please know that you're doing well and moving forward toward weight balance success," I concluded.

In a matter of six months, Annie balanced to her perfect weight.

Use the **Schoolteacher Technique** to Transform Yourself.

The Schoolteacher Technique

Write, I choose to trust in positive outcomes in your journal 15 times each day, at the same time every day, consistently for at least three weeks. Be aware during this period of time how your mind free-associates and connects this phrase with your purpose statement during the day. Look for changes in your life, attitudes, and outlook that reflect results with this exercise.

You can also add a purpose symbol to this statement, or draw a fun doodle image to go with the above statement. Make it silly and light; there's no right or wrong way to do this. Since the language of the subconscious is composed of symbol and image, this technique allows you to talk Soul to Soul (your true divine Self) with instant understanding.

> *The old habits of the mind are stubborn in their resistance to change. However, committing to practice these techniques and doing them—no matter what—ultimately brings lasting change. In this way, you say "No" to mental programming and old emotions that have held you back in the past. This is the way you choose to be free.*

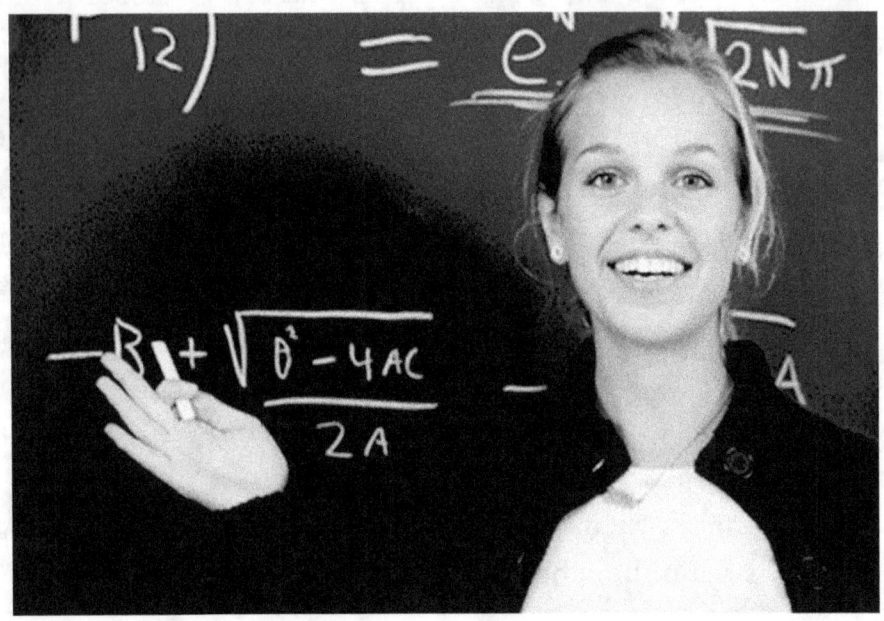

Taking Stock of Your Progress So Far

It's time to review what you've accomplished so far and take stock of your emotional state. Maybe you've been feeling discouraged like Annie. Maybe your discouragement even verges upon defeat, as hers did. At this point in the journey, it's a common pitfall for many people to minimize the positive steps they've already made. You're not alone if you're feeling this way.

> *So often the mind will skim over the small steps and minimize your progress as a way of denying the truth. The good news is you can choose to view this is a positive road sign.*

You can chose to release the denial and allow yourself the opportunity to be involved, motivated, and bold about your progress.

The affirmative statement that works in this case is the same one I gave Annie in *The Schoolteacher Technique*: "I choose to trust in positive outcomes." It also helps to say, "I am trust" 10, 100, or 1000 times a day. The operative principle here is to say it until it comes true.

This is part of your responsibility and your mission in attaining weight balance success—to deprogram the mind from myths as well as minimizing. You can use both of these affirmation statements with breathing exercises to release deep stress and nurture relaxation as you begin to trust yourself, trust the process, and trust in positive outcomes.

Review List Exercise

(1) Close your eyes, connect to your Higher Power, and ask, what steps have I taken so far?

(2) List all the small steps you have taken, such as buying, reading, and practicing the principles outlined in this book. Be sure to count making your purpose statement and every technique, exercise, activity, and visualization you have done in the course of reading this book

(3) Read your list aloud to yourself and really understand deep in your heart all you have done in the quest for your goal.

(4) Again, close your eyes and ask your Higher Power if you missed any steps. Then add any missed steps to your list.

(5) Ask your Higher Power, "How can I better accept my progress and stay reliable to myself?" Write down the wisdom you receive.

(6) Ask your Higher Power, "What is my next step?" jot down what you receive.

Take a deep breath and open your eyes when you're ready.

I like to tell the following metaphorical story about the journey to weight balance. In order to traverse the half-mile bridge across my street, I have to take one small step right now to get out the door and start moving toward it. My steps are small. Some people have a larger stride while others have a smaller, slower stride than mine. Yet the way to walk this bridge for everyone is simply by taking one step after another. Maybe it's necessary to take time to rest midway through, and then take more steps. I may stop at the crest of the bridge and want to turn around because I become discouraged. Yet resting refreshes me. Since the remainder of the journey is downhill, it's easier from now on.

You are on a similar journey of weight balance. The Review List Exercise is one rest stop. You can choose to stay on course after this rest stop by choosing to be reliable to yourself and your greater purpose.

How to Eliminate Being Stuck

When I think about ways to eliminate being stuck, a thousand possibilities flood my mind. What I've learned from experience is to keep it simple. The following techniques are simple and yet powerful in their ability to free you from being stuck. Choose one or more you'd like to use and practice them.

Brainstorm for Activities

When you're feeling stuck, you can use a brainstorming technique to gather as many ideas and techniques for getting unstuck as you can imagine. The most important thing to do with this technique is to "turn off the censor." *Any* idea has the potential to lead you to the one thing it will take to get unstuck.

To brainstorm, take a large sheet of paper and write "How to Become Unstuck" in the center of the page. Draw a circle around the topic. Next, put any ideas that pop into your mind around it, drawing circles around each idea with a line connecting it to the concept that led to, generated, or helped inspire it in the first place.

When I did this exercise, one of the first ideas I got was to call a supportive person. Reach for the phone and call. Keep your mind free of doubts or thoughts of fear that might have stopped you in the past.

Another idea is to imagine a nearby beautiful place. Get ready and go for a walk where there is beauty. Enjoy the surroundings as best you can. See if anything unusual happens that might relate to your being stuck. Maybe you'll see an animal that's stuck. Maybe you'll decide to help it get unstuck. You could have a number of adventures as you open your eyes and see in a whole new way (maybe the world around you has a symbolic, image-rich message for you about how to get unstuck).

Another idea is to scout around and find a support group. Ask the members if there are other groups they know of and when do they meet? Or turn to the members in your discussion group on this book. Keep pursuing your quest for support.

Another thing to do is draw a stick figure that is stuck using colored markers. Put the title *Being Stuck* into the picture. Ask the figure in the drawing for some insight into the deeper reasons why it is stuck or how to get unstuck. Write down what you receive. Then journal your explanation of your drawing as if you were sharing it with a close, trusted friend or a therapist. Be sure to date your work. Reflect on it for the next week as you look for greater insight and understanding.

As soon as possible, take out your journal and write about being stuck. Write a prayer question, pray for help from your Higher Power, or contemplate on the answer. You can use any of these techniques to help move beyond any feeling of being stuck that you might have.

Before Dealing with Rage and Pain

Gabrielle Roth explores dancing as a release and prayer of emotion in her latest book, *Maps to Ecstasy*. She also has videotapes (*The Wave: Ecstatic Dance for Body and Soul*), and compact discs (CDs) (*The Endless Wave*) that explore using movement as a spiritual practice. She describes releasing feelings in an ancient, profound way through moving meditatively and creatively to music. Free yourself from stuck feelings using her music or select your favorite musical songs to create your own ecstatic dance. The only requirement is being willing to move and let the music direct you.

Dealing with Rage, Anger, and Pain

I once worked with a successful business man (who was consistently stuck in anger and rage) as I did with Annie in the opening example of this chapter. I asked him to get a visual picture of his anger and rage, leaving himself out of the picture. He saw these emotions embodied in the image of an exploding volcano.

I suggested he continue with the example of the exploding volcano, close his eyes, look upward to the center of his forehead (where insight occurs in the brain), and connect with his Higher Power as he knew it.

Then I said, "Silently ask your Higher Power to help you invite this picture of your past anger and rage to change positively. Watch it change to more closely reflect your purpose statement. Let go of forcing it to change, invite it to change positively, and watch what happens."

He took his time (it works even better when you take more time), and watched. To his amazement, the volcano started to erupt even more.

I asked him to just keep watching the volcano release all of the anger and rage, and tell me what he was experiencing with each change. This is what he described: "At first the volcano exploded more, then it finally stopped, cooled, and began to change geologically into two rolling hills. Then green grass started growing. Finally the sun came out."

"Does that feel complete for you?"

"Yes," he said.

This technique is especially helpful for releasing and moving beyond strong emotions that have set up chronic patterns throughout your lifetime.

Punch a Hologram

The next technique is great for releasing individual episodes of past angers or frustrations. You'll be surprised at the positive results you will have breaking free once you use this technique. One woman remarked she was able to sleep better than she had in years. Another said she was calmer throughout the week and no longer turned her past anger upon herself in self-punishing behavior. By feeling calmer, she felt motivated to eventually take her next step toward a healthier, balanced diet.

First find a comfortable, safe place where you will be undisturbed for at least 20 minutes. Close your eyes and look upward to the center of your forehead where insight occurs in your brain. Ask your subconscious mind to scan back through the many past angers or frustrations you've experienced in your life. Let the subconscious pick one for you to release now.

Keeping your eyes closed, allow both of your hands to form fists. Make them tight, as if you are clenching the past anger or frustration you want released. Consciously be aware of how tight and tense your fists are. Feel this tightness in your belly and your legs.

In front of you is a hologram. It may be a person you are still angry with, or it may be a symbol of a situation that angers you. Step closer to it. Feel your fists hitting the hologram in your imagination. Hear the slap, smack, or pop sounds. Each time you hit this hologram, release more of your past angers or frustrations. Keep on doing this until you feel you've released all of it. You may yell silently in your imagination to release even more past anger. It is important to take all the time you need. The more time you take to do this, the better.

When you feel the exercise is complete, take a deep cleansing breath. Relax your hands and body. The image of the hologram will disappear and once again, you are in your safe, quiet place.

Say aloud, "I choose to trust in positive outcomes." Connect again with your Higher Power and ask for help in reflecting on what you have learned. After you do this, write the answers to the following questions in your journal:

(1) What did I learn?

(2) What is different now from my releasing all this anger and frustration?

Feel, Question, Change Technique

For this exercise, let's explore a specific emotion, such as guilt. Suppose you feel guilty. Ask yourself, what does guilt look like? Let the first picture of what guilt looks like pop into your mind. Guilt probably wouldn't look like a dozen red roses. Maybe it looks more like rust eating a fairly new car.

Close your eyes and look upward to the insight area between your eyes. Ask your Higher Power to help you to allow this past guilty feeling to change in an uplifting way. Maybe you start to become part of changing the situation by sanding away the rust and preparing the car for a new paint job in your imagination. After you finish sanding, maybe you spray on a few coats of paint in your favorite color, until the car looks brand—new. Take your time; keep asking for more change, keep watching and imagining. You'll know when it's complete. When it is finished, thank your Higher Power for helping you be free of this past guilt.

Now picture or sense a door in front of you. Notice the color and any other details, like the knob, how it is made, or its finish. As you open the door and walk through it, know that you are stepping into a new level of awareness and freedom, furthering you on your journey to weight balance success.

The Five Senses Technique

What the *Five Senses Technique* does is elevate the thought of being stuck to a higher level of the brain in order to clear it. To do this, you'll be using all five senses as passkeys to create an image or symbol that speaks to the subconscious while sweeping it clean.

Let's say you are feeling stuck with the negative thought *Nothing is ever going to change*. Close you eyes and look upward to connect to your Higher Power. Ask yourself, what color is this feeling of being stuck, as you allow the first thing you think of to pop into your mind. Now think to yourself, where do I keep this feeling in my body?

Next, let an image connected to this feeling just pop into your mind (even if it doesn't make sense). Now this stuck feeling that's a certain color which you keep in a certain place in your body that's connected to an image, how big does it feel? Does it feel as big as this room? Define how big this feeling is in relation to you.

Now let a sound pop into your mind. Then think of a smell and or a taste. Express this feeling of being stuck with a hand movement of some kind. If you believe "I don't know how," just imagine you *do* know how and let your hands express the movement. Do it now.

Finally, ask your Higher Power to give you a tool to get rid of this feeling of being stuck and all the negative thoughts and images that tag along with it. Conceive of using the tool to get rid of every single piece of this feeling, the negative thoughts, and the images, down to the essence of your cells.

If you need to use your imagination or your creativity to make yourself huge or your tool gigantic, then do so—whatever works. Take your time and make sure every atom of the feeling is gone.

Take a deep cleansing breath. See yourself and know you are accomplishing your purpose. Think about your purpose symbol and see yourself taking one more step toward your goal.

In summary, any one of these techniques will help free you from being stuck in any negative emotion. Each technique is simple but powerful in its results. You'll alter the dynamic and change the cycle after you do one of these techniques. Saying aloud "I choose to trust in positive outcomes" afterward will help bring a wind of change into your life.

Now remember a time in your life when you felt free. Tap into that feeling and try one of the techniques mentioned previously right now. Try it and feel free.

If You're Doubtful at Times, Here's What to Do

This doubt-busting technique is relatively simple. Just choose one inwardly to be open to a new spiritual awareness or answer. It's often in the humblest of places that we find answers. It's just a matter of having the humility to bend down and look for them.

This story about a phone man illustrates this "do it with love" attitude. It occurred about two weeks after I began using a new phrase (*I am love*) with "The Schoolteacher Technique." I was thinking of this phrase as I directed the phone repair man to check out the phone jack in the bedroom.

Although he was relatively young (in his mid-thirties, dressed in a T-shirt and jeans), he had already developed a large potbelly. When he saw the stairs, he said, "I wouldn't want to climb these very often."

The phone man resented the stairs and the concept of any extra physical effort. His resentments stopped him from getting into better physical shape and moving forward in consciousness. Resentments, like doubts, can hold us back. To me, the stairs represented an opportunity to give myself more health through physical effort.

I said, "I love them. They help me keep in shape. I like to run up and down them. My heart loves the aerobic action, too."

Putting love into all you do will help you progress physically, emotionally, mentally, and spiritually. Even stairs can be seen as a blessing of health when accepted with eyes of loving awareness.

You Always Have a Choice in How You Respond

When you're feeling hopelessness, helpless, powerless, and don't know consciously how to access your power and leave these feelings behind, it's often easy to act in controlling ways toward yourself and toward others. In the following example, Jenny discovers that she has a choice in how she responds.

Once during a business meeting, a co-worker asked Jenny to pick up a client at the airport. Inwardly Jenny felt this was a hassle, beneath her job description, and she just didn't want to do it. Jenny was furious at her friend for asking but found she couldn't say no, so she agreed to meet the plane. Then Jenny felt hurt, trapped, and hostile. She began to pout by looking down at her notebook and stopped interacting at the meeting.

Situations such as this had happened many times in the past. Usually Jenny would go home and eat, stuffing her anger. However this time, Jenny's boss confronted her.

"You're controlling everyone in this room," she said. "You haven't said a word, but you've had everyone's attention for the last fifteen minutes. You know it too-you're smiling."

Shocked and ashamed, Jenny knew it was true, for she felt like laughing even as she was being confronted about her angry, controlling behavior.

Her boss continued, "If you make the choice to use that energy in a positive, purposeful way, you'd be a powerful being who could accomplish anything."

Jenny was hit with the truth. Powerful? Angry and controlling? Accomplish anything? She knew she felt like an ashamed little girl and began to wonder about the dynamics of the dichotomy that triggered her urge to laugh.

This was turning point for Jenny. She gradually became more aware of her behavior and its effect on others, even when she felt helpless and didn't fully know what she was doing. Deep inside, Jenny knew she was a powerful spiritual being. But she also knew she had bought too heavily into the societal belief that it was more acceptable to be helpless.

That day Jenny learned what it feels like to be on the dark side of control, allowing herself to be controlled and the flip side of manipulating and controlling others. When Jenny negated her feelings by agreeing to do what she did not want to do, she denied her own truth and undermined her true self.

Jenny might have handled the situation differently. She could have asked for support and help from others at the meeting—but she didn't. It was easier for Jenny to act out of past habits and patterns. Well after the event, Jenny realized she had a choice in how she could respond. The simple truth is this: Jenny could have responded by just saying, "No."

Learning to Say No and Feel Good about It

The following story is about using creativity to learn ways to say "No" to what you don't want in your life so that there's more room for you to say "Yes" to what you do want.

A woman named Kathryn wrote in her new journal, "I'd like to dedicate this journal to creating spiritual writing exercises to bring more freedom into my life."

Inwardly Kathryn knew what was keeping her from experiencing the level of freedom she wanted, since she had struggled with guilt most of her life. This guilt connected to many weed-like beliefs and behaviors, such as (1) Kathryn believed she wasn't good enough; (2) she thought everything that went wrong was her fault; (3) she felt compelled to please others; (4) she felt responsible for fixing everyone's problems; and (5) she couldn't say no to other people's requests for her time and energy. Underlying these beliefs, Kathryn discovered she held unrealistic expectations of herself, namely that she needed to be perfect and liked by everyone. Both of these expectations stemmed from a false sense of vanity rooted in low self-esteem.

Kathryn's first step to healing her faulty belief system was learning to say no to the many demands on her resources. She began this process by writing NO in eight-inch high, black letters across her front door to remind her to say it whenever she could. Whenever Kathryn *did* say no however, she noticed a high degree of anxiety and guilt would result.

Kathryn realized her underlying guilt was blocking her progress toward developing the ability to say no. She knew the only way she could feel good about herself was to go deeper in her quest, simultaneously confronting and dealing with both major issues (learning to say no *and* absolving her guilt). Here's how she did it.

Kathryn wrote the words "LET IT GO" on several yellow index cards and placed them at strategic points around house. Whenever she saw these cards, it reminded her subconscious to let go of guilty feelings. Also, whenever she started to feel guilty, she would command herself in loud, forcible words to "LET IT GO!" She practiced saying this throughout the day.

She not only found that the command words helped her release feelings of guilt and perfectionism, today she only has to hear these words and she instantly relaxes. These command words will work for you in a similar manner once you've mastered this technique.

Kathryn also practiced many different ways of saying "No" using the *Assertiveness Scripts* that follow (see sidebar on page 352) until it became comfortable for her to segue them into casual conversation. All of this happened gradually in a natural cycle of change. Kathryn took the process of change little by little, step-by-step, all the while receiving just what she could handle, at the pace she could handle.

Kathryn found when she mastered the ability to say no, she was finally free of the guilt that had once plagued her. And when most of her energy wasn't tied up emotionally with faulty beliefs, her eating habits began to improve too.

Kathryn used the following journal technique to stay on target in mastering ways to say "No" in disagreements and discussions.

Targeting the Bull's-Eye Technique

First she drew a picture of a bull's-eye target in her journal. She wrote the word NO in bold letters directly in the center. Then she drew long arrows, reaching from the edge of the page to the center of the target. Then Kathryn drifted into a light contemplation and thought about the last opportunity she'd had to say no and failed(a weekly phone call from her mother complaining about other members of the family). In her mind, she replayed the conversation from start to finish.

Instead of clenching her jaw and allowing the situation to frustrate her, Kathryn focused on what she wanted to change about the conversation—namely her responses. Again, she used the *Assertiveness* Scripts to help prompt her. Each time Kathryn came up with a good counter-response to her mother's complaining, she wrote it down in her journal along the shaft of one of the arrows that pointed to the bull's-eye NO. She knew as she did this exercise, she was getting closer to her goal of being able to say "No" in actual conversation. Kathryn used this exercise, drawing a new bull's-eye target for each life situation she encountered where she wanted more clarity on how she could have handled it better by saying "No."

Assertiveness Scripts

(1) Disagree *with a straightforward statement ("I don't agree with your understanding of . . .")*

(2) Confront *by denying the statement is relevant to the conversation ("That's not the point.")*

(3) Reword *negative labels by framing it in positive words ("I am not being childish; I'm stating my view.")*

(4) Repeat *your main point until it is heard without anger*

(5) Ask Questions *if you're not comfortable with a point, or ask for clarification ("How do you see me as childish?")*

(6) State Feelings *by using "I" statements that reflect your opinion about the situation ("I really feel this is important!")*

(7) Be Short and Quick *by just saying "NO" directly*

You may look at these scripts and think to yourself, "That's all well and good, but it won't work in my situation because (fill in your specific reason why it won't work here)."

After mentally explaining your doubts to yourself, stop for a moment and ask, "Do I feel better or worse after explaining why it won't work for me?" In other words, do you feel more motivated toward your goal after explaining why it won't work, or do you feel let-down and a loss of energy? What did you discover? If you skimmed over these questions, didn't weigh the answers for yourself, or didn't do the targeting exercise, go back, read them again, and do the exercise with a willingness to measure your inner energetic results. You might learn something new about yourself.

Using an assertive script is the first step. You'll find when you learn to say "No" to the things you no longer want in your life, it makes much more room for you to say "Yes" to the things you do want.

A Simple Technique of Choice

(1) Upon rising go to the mirror, look into your eyes and say with determination, "I have a choice."

(2) Look into your right eye first and say, "I have a choice" three times.

(3) Next look into your left eye and say "I have a choice" three times.

(4) Then look at your whole face and say, "I have a choice" three times.

(5) Do this morning, noon, and before bedtime. Each time say it with passion Act "as-if" your attitude toward being open, prepared, and purposeful in your quest toward weight balance success is manifesting more every minute. You will get what you expect.

(6) Stay open during the day and be aware of how your attitude changes. Be willing to honor yourself, your style, and your intuition. Be ready to be flexible to unforeseen circumstances as reality shifts in unexpected ways to ultimately accommodate your goals.

Being Willing to Do Whatever Is Needed

What comes next is learning to say "No" to negative feelings and behaviors *while feeling good within yourself and about yourself.* Ask yourself, "Am I willing? Am I willing to do whatever is needed to reach my goal, staying firm and on purpose?" With as much emotion as you can imagine or conceive of, say or silently think this affirmation: "I am willing to do whatever is needed to reach my goal and support my purpose with my actions." Remember your subconscious is listening, so give it your sincere best.

How to "Feel Good"

If you've never felt really positive about who you are during your whole life, it's a tall order to fill when you first start to want to feel good. Try right now to recall some memories of when you felt good. Maybe you remember feeling good when you ate ice cream with Dad. Or maybe you felt good from a lover's touch or from a hot bath. Maybe you felt good after reaching a goal that's taken months or years to accomplish. Maybe engaging in your favorite hobby or competing in a sport makes you feel good.

Ask yourself the following questions: "What feels good to me? What qualities would be part of an experience of feeling good?" One woman started this exercise by listing the things she knew did *not* make her feel good-things she no longer wanted in her life. Her list looked like the following:

"What I Do *Not* Want" List

(1) No morbid thoughts about my body

(2) No more exhaustion

(3) No more stuffing myself until I sleep

(4) No more thoughts of hating myself or my mate

(5) No more abusing my body with purging or restricting

(6) No more stuffing my anger and not talking about it

(7) No more second-guessing or doubting myself in my thoughts or feelings

(8) No more isolating myself due to fear or grief

(9) No more reacting to guilt arising from habit, based on faulty beliefs—not true reality

These points of what she did not want in her life anymore were prompted by the *43 Symptoms to Heed* in Chapter 17. By practicing the following exercise, you can turn your "don't wants" into affirmative keys that unlock knowing what you do want in your life.

"What I *Do* Want" List

(1) "No more morbid thoughts about my body" transforms into "I choose to accept my body. I choose to feel complete and at peace inside my body."

(2) "No more exhaustion" transforms into "I choose to feel relaxed in my body. I choose to feel balanced in all my activities."

(3) "No more stuffing myself until I sleep" transforms into "I choose actions to make me feel better about myself."

(4) "No more thoughts of hating myself or my mate" transforms into "I choose to be gentle and loving with myself and others."

(5) "No more abusing my body with purging or restricting" transforms into "I choose to be kinder to myself. I can discover ways to be my own best friend more every day."

(6) "No more stuffing my anger and not talking about it" transforms into "I choose to be willing to learn the steps to safely change and grow in understanding my anger."

(7) "No more doubting (second-guessing) my thoughts or feelings" transforms into "I am on my way to letting go of doubting myself."

(8) "No more isolating myself due to fear or grief" transforms into "I choose to be willing to create a ladder that begins to put me into healthy activities and around supportive people who nurture the new me."

(9) "No more reacting to guilt arising from habit, based on faulty beliefs—not true reality" transforms into "I choose to catch my reactions to my doubts and my guilt before I act upon them. I choose to actively seek new, life-enhancing behaviors."

These affirmations change what you don't want into what you do want. Take a deep breath. As you let your breath out, silently tell yourself to relax. Take another deep breath and slowly breath the air out, all the while saying to yourself, "Relax" Really *mean it* as you tell your shoulders to relax.

Then tell your jaw to relax and feel it. Say, "I give myself permission to relax. It is safe to relax and grow."

Any one of these transformed statements can be made into a reality and brought more quickly into your life by using it in *The Schoolteacher Technique*. This is one way to say *yes* to bring good things into your life.

Resisting the Urge to Quit

A woman named Joyce tried the previous exercise. However, after doing the "don't want list," she became overwhelmed, over-wrought, and felt just plain inadequate.

In the past, whenever Joyce felt overwhelmed, overwrought, or inadequate, she would drop whatever was overwhelming her, go fix herself a big plate of pasta, pizza, or bagels, (and a chocolate bar or two), and eat it. After she'd finished eating, the feeling of being overwhelmed would completely disappear. Joyce didn't realize this escape mechanism of "turning on" to food was her way to magically make the negative feelings go away.

Joyce never took the time to transform the statements into positive affirmations by completing the "do want list" part of the exercise. Her reaction at this point was to just quit: quit doing the affirmation exercises and quit striving for weight balance.

When old feelings of being overwhelmed, overwrought, inadequate, and guilt kick in, old behavioral coping mechanisms and habits automatically take over, unless you choose to act in a take-charge kind of way to change that right now.

Start your own list. Change all the reasons why you can't do it and want to quit into transformational statements of affirmation, such as, "I am choosing to be open, prepared, and purposeful in my quest for weight balance success." Choose to be open and on target with your actions-keep reading! You can do it by first taking a series of deep belly breaths. Belly breaths help center and relax you.

Like a book, when we stay open, we have the opportunity to gain more tools, knowledge, and wisdom. If we're closed, there is no way to gain these gifts of greater understanding from the universe or our Higher Power. This is a most important key. Stay open, keep this book open, and keep reading!

Practical Tools to Find More Answers

Recently, Annie often felt stuck and frustrated. She was trying hard to choose different actions so that she didn't return to escaping her emotions by eating, or distracting herself in endless pursuits of pleasure as she had done in the past.

I found the biggest clue as to why Annie was stuck and frustrated is in her word "trying." Trying is not doing; it is simply attempting, yet failing once again. When someone is trying, they're really not ready to take action toward change. There's a subtle shift between trying and doing, but it makes all the difference in the world between staying stuck and attaining your dreams.

This is what it takes to be free of the old mental patterns that enslave us without our conscious awareness. It is mysterious because it remains unknown, hidden in the subconscious of the person experiencing enslaving thought patterns. So Annie was caught once again in the self-defeating, negative inner self-talk of her unconscious.

In the following story, Annie manifests a breakthrough contemplation experience, reflecting her willingness to change. It also shows the ever-present support and assistance of her Higher Power, which is just waiting for a sign from Annie that she's ready and willing to move into a state of transformation.

Annie wrote to me about some experiential work she was doing. One morning she had a vision during contemplation. She wrote, "I was in a chrysalis and a couple of helpers in my life were there to support me. I was aware of them energetically around the chrysalis, cheering me on. However, even though I pushed my head backward against the encasing energy, the chrysalis was too solid for me to break through."

Because Annie journals, practices the techniques in this book, and relies on her Higher Power for daily guidance, she spontaneously knew she could ask for help and get it at this critical time. "Please, I need help," she wrote in her journal. Because she surrendered enough to ask for help, the message broke through to her subconscious, illuminating the deeper meaning of the vision in her mind.

What Annie didn't realize at the time was she was observing the situation as she was taking action. It was only when she reviewed her journal account of the experience later that she stumbled on the insight that the helpers surrounding her were connected to her Higher Power.

The symbol of the chrysalis showed not only how trapped she was in hostility, but that the process of transformation was imminent. I explained how she could work with the chrysalis image in her imagination to stop "trying" to free herself from the old mental thought patterns and start actually doing it. Here's the next step of this creative process that you can do, too.

The Butterfly Technique: An Imaginative Exercise for Empowering the Next Step

1. *Before going to sleep, record in your journal that you want to invite the state of being in a chrysalis to change positively.*
2. *Imagine putting this request into the hands of your Higher Power.*
3. *Now close your eyes and imagine yourself in a warm, relaxed, comfortable state encased inside a chrysalis.*
4. *Visualize your Higher Power and Its helpers surrounding the chrysalis. Each of them has a tube of chrysalis-dissolving fluid.*
5. *Observe carefully how each helper squeezes some fluid on the tip of the chrysalis and rubs it in. See the chrysalis-dissolving fluid begin to dissolve the material encasing you in everyday problems and stuck behavioral responses this lifetime. Your Higher Power and Its helpers are gently and thoroughly rubbing the dissolving fluid on the surface of the chrysalis. Remember, you are the spiritual butterfly within the chrysalis.*

Now shift attention from watching what is happening outside the chrysalis to being inside the chrysalis. Feel the dissolving fluid rubbed into the area surrounding your head. Feel the encasement of a lifetime begin to dissolve. Soon your head is free. Your Higher Power and Its helpers cheer you, "Hey, you in there, come on out."

They watch as you break free of the human emotions and behaviors that have trapped you in the past. When this happens, the sun seems to come from behind a cloud and shines brilliantly upon you melting the remainder of the chrysalis. You hear the sounds of nature (use your imagination to manifest this). Do this exercise each night for about a month. You'll experience progress and more freedom in your life.

Allow Change

Practice *The Butterfly Technique* to help free yourself from hardened attitudes and old states of consciousness connected to diet myths, as well as empower your next step toward a new consciousness—one which embraces weight balance success. Be patient with yourself and keep in mind that the process of transformation is often a gradual one (like the butterfly breaking free of the chrysalis).

To expedite change, say the following words five times a day: "I allow these changes into my life." Saying these words is a way to allow yourself to experience and learn new things. It is a way you can be supportive of yourself as you take the time to become skilled at something new.

To review:

1. Commit to singing your love song to yourself each day at the same time daily.

2. Practice *The Schoolteacher Technique* by writing "I choose to trust in positive outcomes" or another affirmative statement that furthers you toward your goal, contributes to clearing blocks, or frees you from feeling stuck. Write the positive affirmation at least 15 times daily.

3. List all the positive, small steps you have taken toward your goal. Write down everything you can remember. Ask your Higher Power, "How can I better accept my progress and stay reliable to myself?" Write down what you receive. Ask your Higher Power, "What is my next step?" Jot down what you receive.

4. Brainstorm possible ways to move beyond being stuck. Experiment with one or more of the imaginative techniques and visualizations given in the brainstorming section of this chapter.

5. Do one practical, down-to-earth thing each day with love, while asking inwardly to be open to a new spiritual awareness or answer.

6. Journal about the situations or events in your life which you have a choice about how you respond. If appropriate, practice *The Bull's-Eye*

Target Technique with the *Assertiveness Scripts* to foster the ability to say no to those things you no longer want in your life. Briefly record your experiences with this in your journal.

7. Practice *The Butterfly Technique* to get unstuck and empower your next step. While keeping in mind that transformation is a gradual process (like the butterfly), say the following words five times a day: "I allow these changes in my life." Practice patience with yourself on your journey to weight balance success.

Chapter 22 explores a dozen ways to interpret your dreams and rediscover your true self. It also offers techniques for combining creativity and imagination to make your dreams come true, as well as sharing ways to receive the love you need while maintaining your success.

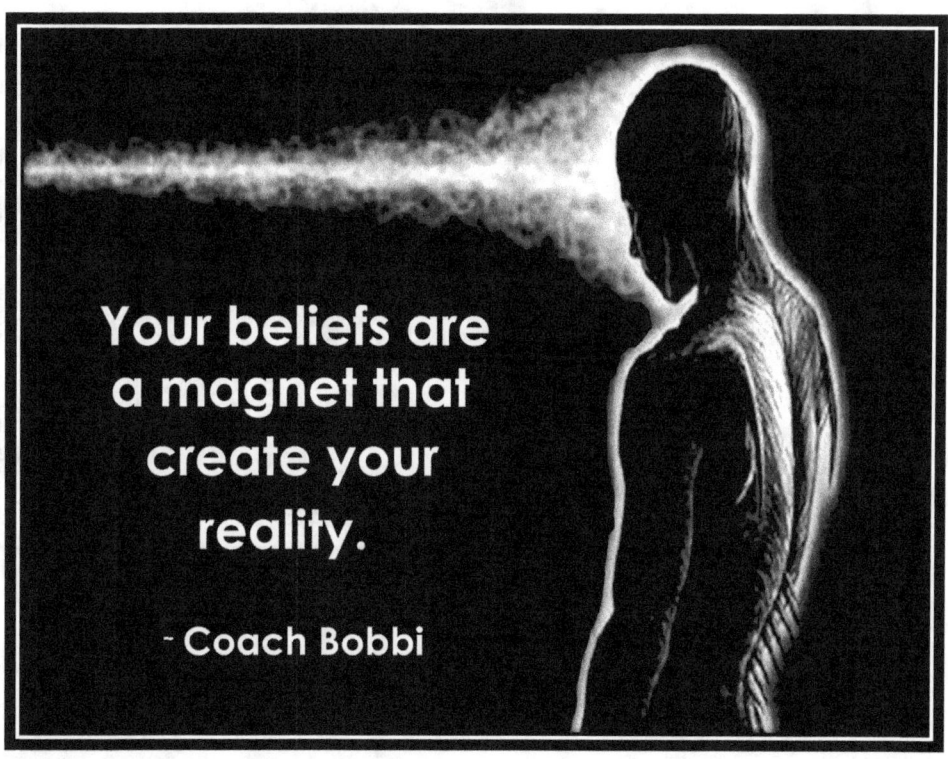

Your beliefs are a magnet that create your reality.

- Coach Bobbi

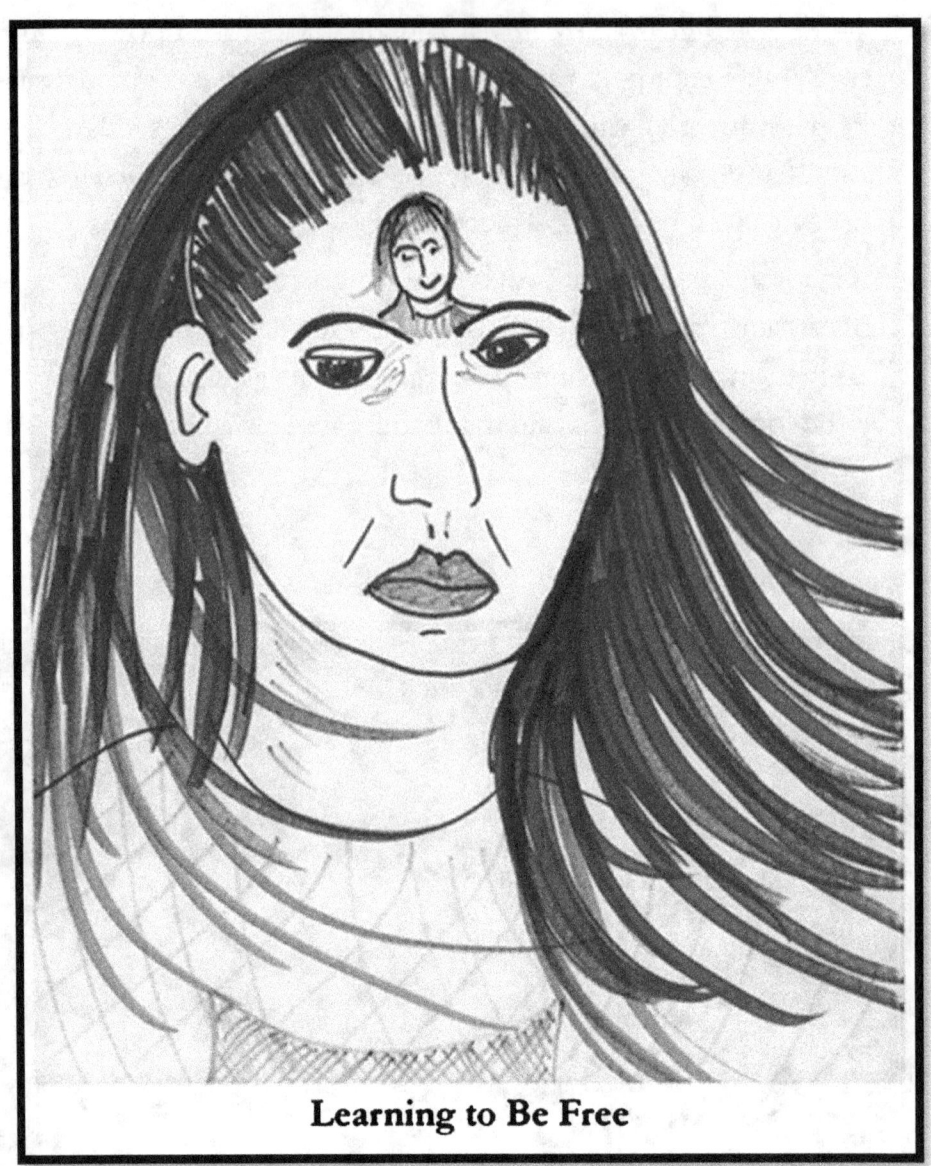

Learning to Be Free

Part 2

Learning To Be Free

Chapter 22

Three Powerful Tools: Secret Dream Technnques, Creativity Enhancement, and Learning to Use Your Imagination In Secret Ways

Getting Clear on How You Want To Be

Where do you start? Just the thought of dreaming how you want to be can conjure up images of living your wildest dreams, So let the wildest dreams come out! A woman named Katie said, "I'd like to be slim and healthy, have clear skin, a boyfriend, and tons of fun experiences," Try the following fun, imaginative, writing exercise and see how far it takes you in establishing a vision of your future—the first step to making your dreams come true.

My Wildest Dreams Come True Writing Exercise

1. My wildest dream is to be _____.
2. My wildest dream is to be _____.
3. My wildest dream is to be _____.
4. In my wildest dream, I have _____.
5. In my wildest dream, I have _____.
6. In my wildest dream, I have _____.
7. In my wildest dream, I look like _____.
8. In my wildest dream, I feel like _____.
9. In my wildest dream, I think _____.
10. In my wildest dream, I know _____.

You can make this a continuing writing exercise by adding to it in your journal for as long as you like. In fact, this is an excellent tool for uplifting your thoughts and focusing your attitudes and actions toward shaping your future in an ongoing daily vision quest, regular attention on dreaming, believing, and infusing the future of your life with love will help bring a new tomorrow into reality sooner.

The following story illustrates how faith and imagination combined with creativity and action helped Katie bring her dreams of the future one step closer as she changed her life.

Katie came from a home where her mother constantly criticized her. Katie's mom would say, "You aren't like me. You eat too much and you're stupid. Why can't you do things right? You're no better than white trash people; you don't belong here with me." Katie's mom pushed her away and threw Katie into her room. She yelled at her and beat her, telling her she was a bad girl. Katie tried to be good and do all her chores, but she was always hungry because her mother gave her so little to eat.

One day Katie went into the woods, sat down, and began to cry. She cried so hard it seemed that she would never stop. The more she cried, the more hopeless and distressed she felt.

This cycle continued all through her adolescent years until her mother became ill and needed Katie to take care of her. Katie did the best she could. She washed the clothes, the dishes, and cleaned the house. She even tried to prepare the food. However, she didn't know how to since her mother had fed her so poorly and she never learned.

One night Katie had a dream. In the dream she was outside sitting in the woods, crying because she felt so miserable about her life. She looked up once and found a woman standing beside her who asked, "Why are you crying?"

Katie answered, "Nothing I do seems good enough. My mother is sick and I can't even take care of her properly. All I want to do is stuff myself with any food I can find and when I can't stop, I feel awful. I hate that I'm so fat. If only I could do something right, be thin, have beautiful skin and a boyfriend like the other girls at school."

The woman said, "Katie, dry your eyes and I will tell you how to reverse your feelings of deprivation. Say to your Higher Power, 'I am choosing to be fulfilled. I am choosing to be complete within myself.' Write these statements fifteen times a day for three weeks. Watch your life for changes and be grateful as the changes come, knowing they'll bring the highest good into your life."

The woman assured Katie that her life would change for the better if she did this. She also encouraged Katie to check out some books from the library on improving her food choices and her health. Then the woman vanished.

Katie thought, "I must try this at once. I'm so tired of being sad." She looked up through the trees to the blue sky and with all her heart she called out, "Higher Power I choose to be fulfilled; I choose to be complete within myself." Scarcely had she uttered the words when a purring cat appeared beside her, rubbing up against her leg. Katie picked up the cat. So much love flowed from this cat to Katie in her dream that Katie started feeling wonderful. She sat and petted the cat for a long time, feeling more love and contentment as she did.

The dream affected Katie profoundly. From this dream, she knew she could always connect with the love inside her, as symbolized in her dream by the cat. When she woke up the next morning however, her mother was still sick in bed.

Katie did the housework and began to change how she ate. She started to write the statement the wise woman had given her in the dream in her journal fifteen times every day before she went to bed. In time, Katie's weight balanced and her skin cleared up-mainly because she chose to align her actions with a changed attitude by including more wholesome foods in her life.

One night Katie dreamed she and the cat were walking through the woods when a handsome young man drove up in his Jeep. The man stopped and asked Katie to show him the way to the north road. "Sure," Katie said, agreeing to ride along with him. As they drove along Katie smiled and chatted comfortably with him. She was having a great time. She sensed he really liked her. The dream was so vivid and real. When Katie awoke, she said, "Wow, what an experience." She knew she had been dreaming one of her possible futures, a future filled with love.

What you hold in your consciousness, even on the subtlest, subscious level of your dreams, gives you the ability to write your own future. Understanding this to the finite cells of your being enables you to make your dreams come true. All it requires is the skill to focus and take one purposeful step after another in the direction you want to go. Everything you need to make your wildest dreams come true is *already inside you.*

Dream Time

Do you remember your dreams? Do you believe dreams hold powerful messages? Have your dreams come true? Have you dreamed of the past or the future? How can dreams help you shape your body/your life? What techniques can you use to better remember your dreams?

Dreaming is not just rest-and-unwind downtime.

> *Dreams can access higher levels of wisdom that directly benefit all aspects of your daily life. These higher levels also allow you to explore the world from a much wider perspective.*

This chapter highlights techniques you can use to expand your dream time for greater experiences, and gives tools you can use to better interpret and understand those experiences, among other things.

What follows is only a small part of the totality of dream knowledge. If you practice the simple techniques described here, you will learn ways to use them for your growth and purpose. Have fun using these techniques and greater peace of mind will follow.

Higher Power Technique

1. *Say to your Higher Power, "I am choosing to be fulfilled. I am choosing to be complete within myself."*
2. *Write this same statement fifteen times a day for three weeks.*
3. *Be willing to receive the changes in whatever form they come. Record the changes in your journal.*
4. *After three months, review what you have recorded by looking at it from a spiritual perspective.*

Accessing Higher Insight and Understanding the Messages of Dreams

At a spiritual level, we can access answers to anything we want to know. Here is a technique you can use before you go to sleep to help you access higher insight through your dreams.

Before going to bed, relax and decide upon awakening that you will know the answer to whatever you specifically want to know. Put this in the form of a request addressed to your Higher Power, such as "Higher Power, if it's for the greater good, please show me the reason why (fill in your specific request here)."

Maybe you'll ask your Higher Power for the next step on your journey. Maybe you'll ask your Higher Power to show you insights about what you're doing. Maybe you'll ask to understand the reason why you resent the choices you've made in your life. Or you might ask to be shown how to let go of self-hatred, which is the truth hiding beneath the attitudes of regret, annoyance, frustration, or guilt.

These clever disguises for self-hatred are dangerous in that they subliminally undermine your efforts to birth the life you need. They often lead you to act out or escape into old destructive patterns, such as eating, spending, drinking, or looking for love through sex.

By asking for answers in your dreams and expecting to know the answers when you awaken, you can create your new self and birth the life you need with the love that's already inside of you. The following story shows how I came face-to-face with my self-hate and found the means to defeat it by using this simple technique.

Feeling of hate and self-destruction accompanied me for some time, sapping my energy and leaving me with a lingering depression. One day I wrote in my journal, "All I see around me is useless structures everywhere, ways I minimize my years of hard work. I am obsessed with asking myself, 'Is it worth it?' and it takes all my energy to muster up the strength to yell, 'Yes, it is!' I have to break free of this morass and reverse the negative mind set."

That night I wrote, "What I have built is good overall, only it needs to be polished and restructured. I clear these past negative thoughts and surrender them to my Higher Power."

Then I invited myself to be peaceful and take a moment to appreciate myself and all that I had accomplished. Before I went to sleep, I relaxed and decided that when I woke up I would have the answer to peace and self-appreciation. I went to sleep with my dream journal near my bed, knowing that at the moment of my awakening direct truth would be in my conscious awareness.

When I awoke, the dream I'd been dreaming was in the forefront of my mind. A feeling of peace and acceptance pervaded my being and I knew the dream I'd been having held the answer to the question I'd brought up the previous night. Immediately I began to take notes on my dream in my journal.

I dreamed I was descending an escalator with a friend whom I love and admire with all my heart. Carol was behind me, criticizing the one man in the world whom I most admire and love more than anything or anyone else. Surprisingly, I wanted to know more about my friend's negative insights about this much admired man's ego defects as she saw them.

Inwardly I was shocked. It disturbed me deeply to feel that a part of me expressed these negative attitudes in the dream. I realized from this dream experience what vanity feels like. I recognized gossip and criticism as the most blatant forms of vanity. I also realized that they always reflect back destructively upon the sender.

Then I got another shock and tears began to pour down my face. *This is what I am doing to myself.* The man I love and admire most in the dream symbolized what I love and admire most in myself (my spiritual side). I realized I destroy myself daily through self-hate and by demeaning what I have accomplished in life. And every time I criticize someone I love, I do the same to myself spiritually. I really got the truth of the situation in that moment. I decided then and there to take action and let go of criticizing myself, as well as others. I knew I needed to forgive myself for what I had unconsciously done. I did so in writing at the end of chronicling the dream. Then I thanked my Higher Power in writing for giving me the truth through this dream experience.

In the past I had read about this idea of loving yourself more, *but I needed to have the experience* to know the truth about really loving myself. The dream state can be an invaluable tool for giving us the experiences we need to move on and feel good about ourselves, if only we have the ears to listen. We each have our own dream symbols with special meanings for us. The following example illustrates this.

Releasing Destructive Patterns by Diagramming Dreams

The following night I relaxed and decided I'd have the answer to resolving the depression that had arisen from feeding these useless, unproductive attitudes when I awoke.

The next morning I wrote about a series of dreams I had. First I wrote them out longhand, synopsis-style. Then I set up a four-column chart to analyze them.

Here's what I wrote:

I dreamed I was a young mother at a dark party. I felt trapped in a hot tub with a gang of teenage boys. One killed me by slicing a knife across my throat. I flew out of my body and over their heads, circling them as I scared them back.

In the next dream scene I was looking through my mother's jewelry box. I was searching for a specific pearl bracelet I wanted my daughter to wear in her wedding. I found many pearls, but persisted until I found the right pearl bracelet.

In the third scene of the dream, I pulled up a plant to bring home. Some women at my house discounted my treasured plant. I took it into another room and saw its stem turn bright purple like pokeweed. The young leaves resembled baby spinach leaves. I knew the pokeweed plant is poisonous; only the new leaves or root tubers can be eaten safely.

After I wrote down the dreams, I divided the next page into four columns. I designated the first column for dream symbols, the second column for free-associating the meaning of the symbols, the third column for questions that arose from the perceived meanings, and the fourth column for answers to the questions. During the process of filling in the diagram, I found the answer to understanding and resolving my depression.

First, I listed each dream symbol in the left column, allowing plenty of room between them. In the second column, I wrote the very first thing I associated with each symbol—even if it didn't make sense. Next, I let a question evolve from the free-associated meanings. Lastly, I turned to my Higher Power in contemplation for answers to the questions. The combined answers to the questions gave me a few sentences that succinctly answered my original question of how to resolve the depression I had fostered from feeding useless attitudes. My example follows. You can try this technique at home with your dreams, too.

Dreaming Can Give You Answers

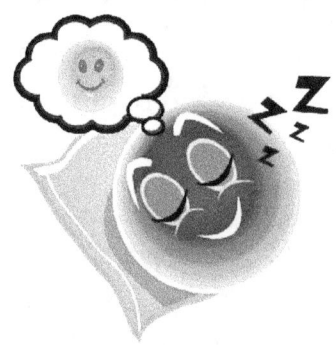

Dream Symbol	Meaning	Question	Answer
MOTHER	Mothering Overprotective	What part of me mothers? What do I care for most in myself?	My discipline My spiritual journey
HOT TUB	Contained heat	What hot feelings do I safely contain?	Self-hate
KNIFE KILLED	Stabbing, cutting in a violent ending	What do I want to eliminate or cut out of my life? Will I do anything to end?	My hate
THROAT	Trust	How is trust killed?	Hate kills trust I put in my creative spirit
FLEW	To freely rise above	What do I rise above and become free of?	I want to rise above and let go of self-hate
BRACELET	Commitment	What commitment do I make?	To continue with my spiritual growth
PEARL	Irritant transformed in radial beauty	What irritation can be transformed into beauty?	Resentments
DAUGHTER	Feminine youth	What part of me is youthful and feminine?	My renewed joy of life
WEDDING	To publically commit to wed or united	What do I want to be drawn more closely to through a public commitment?	My spiritual growth
TREASURED PLANT	Valued growth	What values grow naturally within?	Understanding and spiritual expansion
POKEWEED	Poisonous with age	What grows more poisonous and destructive with maturity?	Unresolved resentment

Here's the message I received from the analysis: I must use self-discipline to protect my growth and progress on my spiritual journey. Self-hatred or any kind of hate I allow myself to feel kills trust and my creative spirit. I can rise above and let go of hate and resentment in order to continue to grow on my spiritual journey. Resentment can be transformed into a renewed joy of life with understanding. Long-standing resentments can be recognized, resolved, and risen above with spiritual expansion as another step in my spiritual growth.

Journal Pages to Prompt Dream Wisdom and Help You Find Change

Date: Question:

Purpose:

Dream(s) or Waking Dreams Synopsis:

Diagram (on the back of the page)

Insight:

Action taken:

The analogy of the pearl bracelet is also my commitment to purity in my spiritual goals. I try to continually turn life's irritations into pearls of wisdom, love and mercy towards all life-like oysters turn specks of sand into beauty. By resolving resentments with truth and kindness when it's necessary, I can be like that pure pearl, too.

I've given my daughter the symbolism of pearls so that she will understand the process of turning life's troubles and sorrows into precious gems of strength. The process of writing down, analyzing, and interpreting your dreams is one way to develop this strength.

Persistence in Journaling

When you start journaling your dreams, you may find that your writing voice is undeveloped, even awkward, like a small child's—mine was too when I began journaling dreams in the 1980s. Your first dream writings may make little sense to you at first. I admit this was true for me, too.

However when you persevere in recording and analyzing your dreams, they will tell you exactly what you need to know to live a freer, happier, more fulfilled life. Persist in writing and analyzing your dream wisdom so blessings may continue to come into your life, turning your dreams of the future into realities.

The Power of Taking Just One More Step

Sometimes the art of taking just one more step can radically change the course of your life for the better forever. It can be as simple as getting a good night's rest so you can begin with a new outlook the next day or as dramatic and life-changing as the following dream and its accompanying life story illustrates.

About sixteen years ago, I dreamed I survived an enormous hurricane and found myself struggling with the aftermath. Rubble surrounded me and a strange smell hung in the air. I climbed over beams and under roofs. I fell and scratched my knees and legs, and even twisted an ankle. Yet I knew I needed and wanted to keep moving forward. I knew I wanted to survive.

The path soon became steep. I leaned forward and willed my legs to keep walking. Yet I wondered about the prospect of going back. "Why am I doing this?" I asked myself. "This is crazy. I could go back." Yet I felt compelled to keep moving forward, taking just one more step, and then another, through the rubble.

I felt frustrated and hopeless. I was so tired I could barely see where I was going. I almost turned back. Finally the path opened into a valley nestled between two foothills. I realized I had entered a bowl shaped crater carved out by the forceful hurricane winds.

The devastation from the hurricane lay strewn around me. I started looking for things I could use to survive. I found a leather tool belt—the kind carpenters wear—and buckled it around my hips. I scanned the surrounding countryside and saw scattered tools and supplies: an ax, a hammer, a pocket utility knife, a plastic jug of water, and some rope.

I gathered the tools and hung them in the leather holders and pockets of the tool belt. Each time I put one into my belt, I felt the power of its possibilities. The events made sense on a profound level. I stood tall with the leather belt supported on my hips, feeling completely safe. I knew I was entering another stage of my journey and felt excited about getting started.

I opened up to the highest possibilities in a spiritual sense. I knew whatever I undertook, I would be successful at it with the help and guidance of my Higher Power. I woke up from the dream feeling excited and filled with trust for what life had to offer.

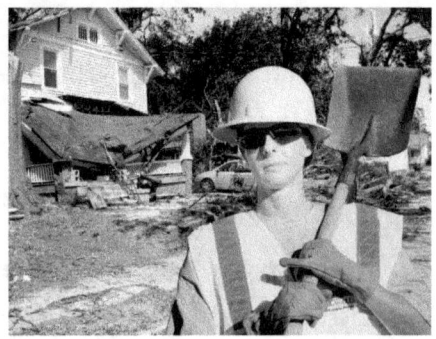

> ## A Notable Dream Key
>
> *Notice how you feel when you awaken from a dream. Write in your dream journal not only the elements and analysis of your dreams, but also your mood or emotional state immediately upon awakening. This is often a clue or a key to the hidden wisdom of your dream.*

Analyze Dreams in Concert with Your Current Life Events

This dream occurred during a time of dramatic life change for me. When I dreamed of walking the steep path after the hurricane, I had just left my marriage—an investment of more than two decades in an abusive relationship.

The journey I embarked upon ultimately turned out to be starting my own counseling practice. From this, I would build skills with the tools I'd gathered, eventually sharing the results of my harvest with others. With the ax I'd be able to powerfully sever ties of the past as a victim. The hammer would help me construct and rebuild my life after the divorce. The knife represented cutting away past anger and resentments. The portable water jug was a cleansing symbol of spiritual renewal and survival. The rope symbolized learning to connect to my Higher Power while reining in the character flaws of my smaller self. The tool belt balances and centers my life from a position of strength.

I have grown in success and skills, taking the experience of cleaning up the aftermath of the dream hurricane and transforming it into tools to help others on their journey of self-discovery as they birth lives of more health, balance, and love.

Dreams of the Future and a New Way of Life

The following example illustrates a symbolic dream of the future and reassurance for adopting a new way of life. Three weeks after I left my marriage, I dreamed I was giving birth in a hospital. A doctor checked my progress, but I knew I was not yet ready to give birth. I left the hospital and returned home for a more natural birth. At home, an Indian woman put down two grass mats—one for my head and one for my body—in a shaded outdoor setting that reflected openness and freedom.

In the next year, this dream came to fruition as a major turning point. I birthed a new life when I graduated with a double master's degree in the sciences of Human Services and Mental Health Counseling. Instead of choosing a traditional hospital setting for my career, I decided to try pursuing alternative healing paths.

The dream I had about giving birth was a dream of healing for what I had experienced in my marriage. The Indian woman in the dream was a mentor or midwife, guiding my physical body back toward healing. If I hadn't had this kind of help inwardly, I believe I would have died from the sheer physical, mental and emotional traumas I had experienced.

Waking Dreams and Divine Protection

Often the most poignant dreams are the ones we receive when we're awake. Waking dreams involve unusual occurrences that seem to further highlight an incident in our lives. The elements of waking dreams are interpreted symbolically like the elements of a sleeping dream, to bring greater insight into what's happening in your life. Waking dreams messages can also provide divine protection, as shown in the following example.

Just after I left my marriage, I stayed at a friend's house until I could decide what to do. Her boyfriend, who had been practicing psychotherapy in another state, soon arrived. I didn't know it, but he wasn't licensed or qualified to practice psychotherapy anywhere at that time. He had created an experimental approach to therapy that wasn't based on any traditional therapeutic modalities. From the get-go, I was leery of him. He started asking me questions and even offered me his unsolicited opinion.

"You could go home," he suggested.

My eyes widened as my throat choked, and my lower jaw dropped slightly. I was confused and instantly felt a concrete wall erect itself in my gut against this unwanted advice. It was as if he had flippantly said, "Here's a quick fix for you today."

At that moment a loud thunder bolt broke the silence. We heard a crashing, splintering sound in an adjacent room and ran to see what happened.

A tree branch that overhung the roof had broken off and shattered the skylight. As I looked up at the remains of broken glass, I noticed the outline left by the break formed the shape of an angel with a broken wing. The boyfriend was distracted by the incident and went outside to assess the damage. Mercifully I was spared any more of his overt pressure.

"God damn it!" he yelped, and I saw him grabbed his finger in pain as he inadvertently cut himself on the glass.

The waking dream message here was clear and I soon moved to another friend's house. A therapist who is full of anger and advises returning to an abusive situation is derelict in responsible professional behavior. Later I realized any anger I had about leaving my husband would break me in a similar way that the branch broke the window.

The way I chose to use my awareness in this situation (by interpreting it as a waking dream) gave me the wisdom to leave a crisis behind instead of getting more deeply mired within it or return to a bad situation. I chose to use this moment as an opportunity to learn more and grow more loving. This I know: life encounters strive to teach us more about loving—always.

There is an answer for every situation or question in the journey of your life. The only thing that holds us back from realizing these answers is our attitudes. Learn the value of recording your dreams. Make a short note about every dream you recall, whether it's a waking dream or a sleeping one.

Asking for and Receiving Golden Messages

An extension of the waking dream is the golden message. Answers to your problems or questions may come from other people in your waking hours during the day. Be on the lookout for these golden messages; your Higher Power can be subtly working through them, too.

Sometimes golden messages come from an article you're reading or a sentence or two from a radio announcer. You may meet someone at the store who says something that stands out in your mind. All these instances and the following story are examples of golden messages.

A Golden Message from God

A woman was stressed out due to her weight and out-of-control eating. The stress of these health concerns was just too much for her and she felt overwhelmed. Often she wrestled with where she was with her life during counseling sessions, feeling the pressure to change.

She thought a move might help. "Maybe a change in location could help me find my purpose in life and get me away from this bad situation." But every time she asked for a message from God, the only thing she received was, "Stay where you are."

One night, she awoke from a fitful sleep of tossing and turning. She decided to connect with her Higher Power for counsel. She practiced a visualization and contemplated, asking her Higher Power, "Every time I have asked, you tell me to stay where I am. If I am to stay, I need another message from you. I need even more encouragement because I feel so hopeless."

She wondered how to get back to sleep again without visiting the refrigerator. She glanced at the radio/CD player next to the bed and decided to listen to relaxation CDs for a while. She hoped the CDs would put her to sleep.

When she turned on the player, she inadvertently turned on the radio. The first words she heard were, "Are you waiting for a message from God? Stay tuned."

This caught her attention. The announcer gave an advertisement for a local church, then came back to the initial question as promised.

"Are you looking for a change? Here's a message from God to you: Bloom where you're planted. God wants you to stay right where you are. God has a plan for you right where you are."

What an incredible golden message!

Be Aware and Listen for the Next Step

One morning I wrote the following passage to my Higher Power in my journal: "Please show me what I am to do next. I feel too eager. How can I slow down and enjoy the present?"

That day's mail contained an organization newsletter with world-wide distribution. I took time to read it during lunch. During the course of reading it, several thoughts bubbled to the forefront of my consciousness about the requests I had posed in my journal that morning. The following golden messages occurred to me:

(1) You'll know the answer when the right spiritual experience is you.

(2) Everything comes in its natural course in due time.

(3) Relax and stop worrying about the next step for now.

I was surprised to find that connecting with these insights cleared the confusion from my mind. I began to perceive life more calmly from a much fresher perspective from then on.

Soul Knows Everything in Dream Time

At the highest levels of unity, Soul knows everything. If you want to bring this inner wisdom to your consciousness, try the following technique tonight.

Before going to sleep, take time to check in with your breathing, counting down from five to one. Tell yourself to let go or relax, and decide upon awakening you'll have an answer to what you want to know.

Then check in with your purpose symbol. Think of someone or something you love. Lightly hold that feeling of love in your heart. Now remember your favorite music or sound. Next conceive a favorite smell, and finally a favorite healthy taste. Finish by asking your Higher Power to help you find the answers during your dream time, and slip off to sleep, knowing in the morning you'll awaken refreshed. When you awaken, the answers will be in the forefront of your thoughts.

At the moment of slipping to or from sleep, your psyche is open to truth and in direct contact with it. It is at this point that you are most able to perceive answers. Immediately note them in your dream journal. Record any insights or changes that happen in the weeks to come.

The Power of Awareness and Control

Two keys that help you consistently reap quality wisdom from your dreams are your level of awareness and control of your attention. This means developing a focus for dreaming in your life.

The difference between scattered attention and concentrated attention can be compared to the power of a 40-watt light bulb and the precision of a medical-quality laser instrument. Some people have scattered attention when they seek counseling. They jump randomly from one subject to another.

Other people come for a little polishing on a specific problem. Their attention is laser-like in its approach. It is so powerful that they accomplish their goals quickly. Which kind of attention would you prefer to use for your purpose?

Ways to Develop More Focus

Practicing the exercises and techniques outlined in this book is one way to develop more focused attention. Most request that you look upward, to the center of your forehead, when you close your eyes before you begin the exercise. This helps concentrate your highest attention on the part of the brain where insight occurs—a good focal point for sharpening your attention to laser strength. Doing this while connecting to your Higher Power as you know it exponentially increases your focus and intent.

One further way you can implement the exercises in this book is to record them and then play them back softly as you fall asleep. That way they can leave gentle impressions, further preparing you for dreaming by focusing your mind before you sleep. Remember you are *not* your mind. Your mind is the tool you choose to sharpen to achieve more of what you want in your life.

Making Room for More in Your Life

The following exercise helps you explore a larger awareness of yourself as you make room for more possibilities in your life.

Have someone you trust read the following exercise/visualization to you or digitally record it in advance for your bedtime listening. As you listen to the exercise, let yourself go in creating a safe space to experience this larger awareness.

An Exercise to Experience a Larger Awareness

Close your eyes and gently look upward to the point where insight occurs in your brain. Gently notice your breathing. Let your breath relax you. Now conceive of a safe place for you. This can be anywhere on earth. Your safe place could be outdoors or indoors. Maybe it is near the ocean or in the mountains. Or maybe it is your bedroom. Invite the child you were long ago to join you. Ask your shoulders to let go and relax. Ask your jaw to let go and relax.

Again notice your breathing. Feel it as it comes in through your nose and down into your lungs. Gently send your breath into your belly. Notice how your belly expands.

Now check your feelings. Silently ask yourself, "What am I feeling now?" Ask yourself, "What was I feeling earlier today?" Ask yourself, "Do I have feelings about my future?"

Ask yourself, "Am I only my feelings?" Then ask yourself, "If I can know my feelings, then what else am I?"

Begin to ask for the cause of your feelings. Let the first thing pop into your mind. What happened before the feelings began? What happened after your feelings? Let this awareness be a part of your consciousness. Then let it go.

Ask yourself, "How is it I can be aware of the cause of my feelings?"

Begin to check in with your thoughts. Observe your thoughts as they go across the screen of your mind. Let this checking in with your thoughts be part of your consciousness. Ask yourself, "Am I more than my thoughts?"

Begin to notice sounds in the room where you are. Are the sounds outside? Now expand your awareness beyond the building you are in. Go outside with only your consciousness. Is it night or day? If it's daytime, make it night. Look around you. What do you see or sense? Maybe there are houses, buildings, parks, highways, rivers or the countryside. Now conceive of looking or sensing the whole area from a bird's eye view. See or sense the whole state. Now view the whole country. Ask yourself, "Am I viewing the whole?" See your family, friends or relatives in their everyday lives. Expand your consciousness to view the whole earth. Enjoy the experience.

See the whole solar system. See the earth revolving around the sun. See other planets revolving around the sun. Everything is in balance. Conceive of yourself existing in that balance.

Again notice your breathing. Feel it as it comes in your nose and down into your lungs. Expanding and contracting your lungs as you breathe. Ask yourself, "How do I know myself as consciousness? Am I more than my thoughts, feelings and body?"

Conceive of expanding yourself to two times your size, now three times your size. Ask yourself, "How do I feel and what do I think as I expand and become larger?" (Give yourself a moment to reflect on this.) Now be your current size again.

Ask yourself, "How do I feel now after being so large? How does this awareness affect my attitude about my present size?" Now conceive of yourself at your *perfect, balanced, realistic* weight.

What does your body feel like at this size? Hold that image of yourself lightly in your mind while remembering your purpose image or picture. Do this at least three times daily for three weeks and journal the results of your experience.

What moved you the most with this experience? Apply what moved you the most to your purpose. How can holding a larger awareness help you maintain a more balanced life?

Each time you do an exercise such as this, it builds creative muscles. Those creative muscles are keys to reaching a balanced diet and maintaining a balanced body through an expanded awareness.

Creativity and Imagination: Your Keys to Manifesting Change

Consider for a moment how creativity could be your weight balance secret for success. Is creativity a mysterious quality only artists, writers, and performers have? Do you even need artistic talent to be creative?

Creativity is a God-given right of everyone. By accessing your creativy, you can do almost anything. To create i s simply to bring something new into existence. Individuals use creativity to manifest change all the time.

Deep inside you have a natural urge to create and change, as all things in the world do. That urge is a natural talent of Soul. Reading this book is a catalyst for creativity and making change happen.

So how do you become more creative? How can you apply creativity to your goal of deepening and sustaining your results?

The Creative Principle

Let's talk about the three aspects of the creative principle: *knowingness, intention, and imagination.* When you allow these three aspects to shape your thoughts, you choose creativity.

Knowingness is knowing something with all your heart. "I just know I'm ready to do this." If you *hope* or *wish* or *try* to do a thing, then you will fail. Thoughts of hoping and wishing are creating a lack of something and trying isn't really doing it. In other words, what you hope or wish for, your subconscious is hearing you don't have. What you try isn't done. Your attention is focused on lack.

Whatever you put your attention upon, you will get. So it is better to simply know it is yours or know you can do it. For example, instead of saying, "I wish I had better eating habits," (thinking from a lack of things) say, "I know I'm developing good eating habits." Then strive to align your actions with your words and make it true! See the difference?

Knowingness is not easy. In reality, knowingness has many saboteurs. The worst enemy of knowingness is opinion based on past fact. For example, an opinion based on past fact may say you have no creativity or will power. If your current beliefs are based on this, you'll sabotage yourself from the start. These assumptions are really only *past opinions*.

Change happens simply by starting with a different knowingness and then following through with it. Go ahead and do an exercise from this book to prove it to yourself.

A Simple Story about the Power of Intentional Dreaming

In 1986 I dreamed of living and working in a historic home on the St. Lucie River. It didn't make sense to me at that time because I was still married to my husband, but I wrote it down anyway and even made a sketch of the dream house.

Later I could not afford to buy a home like this because of past complications from the divorce. At first, I believed such a millionaire's home was beyond my means. Yet I simply chose to trust my prayers and asked for the best location for my business and home while surrendering the outcome to God.

Ten years later, I found a historic home up for lease overlooking the expansive St. Lucie River. I looked at this opportunity as an earned blessing on many levels for many reasons.

Although leasing the mansion was still beyond my means, I brain-stormed, negotiated, and generally impressed the landlady with what I had to offer the home and what a great tenant I would be. As the manager of her family trust, she could tell how much I loved this historic home and she knew that I would take the best of care with it. The details of how I came to lease this house are too numerous to list, but it was truly an amazing experience and an example of the power of creativity and intentional dreaming. It's a joy for me to share this haven for healing with others on the St. Lucie River.

Intention Is Simply Your Purpose

The aspect that helps you create is *intention*. Intention is simply your purpose which can be identified as "inner action." Remember when you use images, you're speaking the language of the subconscious mind and talking to the subconscious is dealing directly with 97% of your total mind.

The Shaping Force of Imagination

The third shaping aspect of creativity is *imagination*. When you know what you want, and you know it is possible and your intention is clear, *then you can imagine yourself doing it*. This is the reason why I ask you to specifically see yourself doing certain activities when you practice the exercises, techniques, and visualizations in this book.

For example, if you want to eat healthy foods to sustain your balanced weight (a logical conclusion), use your imagination to see, feel, and experience yourself eating healthy foods, maintaining your best balanced weight. This way, your inner pictures and feelings send clear messages to your mind that match your intention and purpose.

Matching the inner pictures with outer goals is crucial. The way to reach your goal, whether it is balancing your weight, your life, or feeling good about yourself, is by matching the force of your imagination with your intentions and purpose.

Using Imagination to Prepare a Contingency Plan

Another way to use the imagination for your success is to look ahead and take steps to correct any problems the future might bring to derail you. One example of this is to imagine arriving home from work. You're tired. This is a dangerous time because you can see yourself grabbing some fast foods. What can you do to prepare for this likelihood?

Imagine preparing food in advance. Then take time twice a week to prepare the nourishing whole foods you imagine in a way that they can be served quickly after a long workday. Use this imaginative technique to head off potential stumbling blocks in anything you do. This basic technique for empowerment is one way to be dynamically creativite in all aspects of your life.

Using Purpose, Intention, and Imagination for Exercising Made Easy

Find an outdoor passion you love. For example, I love to walk at night through the historic city with a friend and my dog. First is my purpose: walking for easy exercise. Second is my intention: "I know I'll do it." Third, I imagine and see myself walking where, when and what time of day. Then I simply make myself do it until it becomes a habit (do it routinely for at least 21 consecutive days and it becomes easier to do it than *not* to do it).

I chose to know I could do it. Once the pattern is set, it becomes customary and easy for the body to do. Joy comes from following the pattern and looking forward to each walk as an adventure.

Strengthening Your Muscles for Active Creativity

Please note that if you have been passive for some time, passive activities easily become the most uncontrolled habits. The result is you become the effect of them. The most common passive habits are overeating, spending money and shopping, too much radio, television or movies.

In a balance these activities are okay, but too much results in your creative abilities becoming weak. Like physical muscles (which are dormant when healing a broken bone), your creative abilities have a tendency to atrophy, too. So start slowly with creative exercises and let them gradually build up your "creative muscles."

Making Things Happen with a Plan of Action

To maintain good results, form a plan of action. The first step is to *access the resources you have now*. For example, to slim down your thighs you might want to find someone who could give you instruction in the proper exercises.

Next, *imagine yourself having fun while exercising*. Imagine how you will look in a realistic way. Then, *imagine how you can maintain exercise as a part of your daily routine*, similar to brushing your teeth. Finally, *implement it*. This is the way to be a catalyst for creativity in loving yourself and changing your life.

Live Happily Forever After

> *The elements of dreams, creativity and imagination are spiritual first steps to birthing the life you need.*

Feel free to draw upon the techniques and exercises in this chapter whenever you need the upliftment and joy they can bring. It's important to play with these light, fun activities; they help show you the ebbs and flows that are a natural balance on any journey of life.

Low points do exist in the best of success stories. The greatest heroes inevitably reach complicated times of being stuck in negative feelings and pessimistic thought patterns. At times they deny themselves excitement and joy, or may feel unappreciated, threatened, or disconnected from life, without quite knowing why.

At these times, it's important to be gentle with yourself. In Chapter 23, you'll find ways to confront dark times and the shadows of life while rediscovering your hidden talents and strengths. Chapter 23 also reveals more than a dozen exercises to help you develop attitudes and acquire skills that keep you in balance as you further deepen and sustain your success.

Keypoint to contemplate—"Imagination is stronger than willpower! Most people don't know that our imagination is much stronger than willpower." (Chapter 2)

Chapter 23

How to Clear Your Shadow Side's Hidden Angers, Denial and Resentments

The last chapter revealed deeper ways to manifest the life we dream through waking dreams, sleeping dreams, and dreams of the future. We explored ways to harness our energies and talents by using creativity and imagination. Now let's dispel the hidden reasons

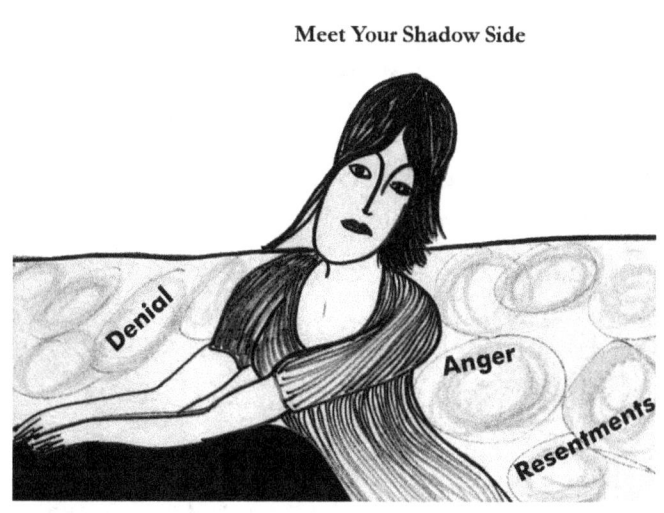

Meet Your Shadow Side

why some mental and emotional responses, such as frustration or fear, may continue to persist. This chapter covers ways to keep the shadow of their influence from further holding you back from your best future.

The Tinsmith' s Escape

The Spiritual Dimension of the Enneagram: Nine Faces of the Soul by Sandra Maitri opens with a parable from the recently deceased Sufi teacher Indries Shah. It's about an unjustly imprisoned tinsmith who miraculously escapes from prison. The following synopsis tells the methods he used for escaping when asked about it years later.

> When the tinsmith was asked how he escaped, he replied that his wife (a weaver) had woven the design of the lock to his prison cell into the prayer rug upon which he prayed five times a day. He realized that the rug contained the lock design, so he struck a deal with his jailers to get tools to make small artifacts, which the jailers then

sold for a profit. He surreptitiously used the tools to fashion a key, by which he eventually made his escape.

The moral of the story? Understanding the design of the lock that keeps us imprisoned can help us create the key that opens it.

Moving Past Blockages and Denial

Basically because the mind functions like a machine, experiences, facts, feelings, or beliefs that are unacceptable to it are routinely blocked out or denied. This happens in even the best of minds because the whole purpose of denial is to keep experiences, facts, feelings, or beliefs which which would *most likely overwhelm or disrupt you* out of your everyday consciousness.

The Emotional Fallout That Precedes Destructive Patterns

People become overwhelmed most often when the worst of circumstances come into their lives. Upon reaching a state of overwhelm, they will tend to drop into hopeless or helpless states more easily. It's dangerous to remain in either of these states for any period of time because they often induce the destructive life patterns which were addressed in Chapter 22 (i.e. overeating, overspending, too much radio, television or movies).

Elizabeth Kubler-Ross' pioneering books on death and dying helped establish the modern hospice movement and brought to mass awareness the five stages that precede and give closure to the act of dying (1) denial and isolation, (2) anger, (3) bargaining, (4) depression, and (5) acceptance.

Take note of these five stages. When people let go of preciously held beliefs, many times they will pass through these same stages before reaching and accepting a new awareness. Often each loss, whether the death of a loved one, dropping an old belief, or releasing a limiting behavior pattern, needs to be grieved and honored in the natural process of the five stages before the individual can move to a higher level.

Sometimes dreams help facilitate the transition that begins with these five stages. At other times the exercises in this book can help. In certain cases a support system of friends who understand the process can offer assistance to you, as you would for them.

The ideal way to shift to new states of consciousness is to move alternately between the five stages in a random pattern that's comfortable for you, until you reach a state of acceptance gradually. It's imperative to avoid getting stuck in any one state for too long (which can bring on feelings of confusion or hopeless before you default to a destructive life pattern).

When you do feel confused, helpless, or hopeless, reach out to friends, a support group, or turn to the exercises and techniques in this book for help. Often it's just a matter of trying different tools, techniques, and support systems until you find a combination that works for you.

Stopping the Cycle of Destructive Patterns

A woman named Debbie wants to feel satisfied with eating more fresh vegetables and fruits in a balanced diet. Yet she is pulled back to old mental patterns and body habits, thinking she needs only meat and potatoes for satisfaction. In other words, she reacts as a victim of her thought patterns for meat and potatoes. At the time she thought this, she was overtired and her energy was down. When her energy gets low, she typically reacts from discouragement.

Given this situation, anyone would slip backward. When you're weak, it's relatively easy for an avalanche to occur. However, Debbie decided to be aware of her mental state and take responsibility to stop the slip. She connected with this book and friends again, both of whom successfully helped her to keep the slip from turning into an avalanche.

Freeing Yourself from the Bedrock of Destructive Patterns

When fears come up and bring with them your deepest worries and doubts, how do you usually react? Do you tend to isolate yourself and nurse your emotional state in a feedback loop of depression or guilt? Do you react with anger by lashing out at everyone closest to you—your family, friends, and co-workers? Or do you deny you're depressed, frustrated, or angry and eventually draw up a deal with the devil, bargaining away all your hard-earned weight balance success in exchange for eating habits designed to rocket your serotonin levels? Delving into the foundation reasons why these emotional states persist is the first step to permanently clearing them.

Beating Mind Games

The mind can take a warm memory and in the short space of a minute, trick you into turning it into one that produces guilt or resentment. This is because memories and emotions are intricately linked in the mind.

One way to free yourself from their influence and move beyond them is to heal resentments of the past by exposing their shadow sides, then find one way to take the next small step. Using the techniques outlined in this chapter, my patients learn to let go of their resentments gradually, one by one.

I was amazed to find that even within myself many resentments grew, numerous as weeds in a driveway. A man rode by on his bicycle yesterday morning as I was weeding and called, "It's a never-ending job!" I agreed as he passed and continued weeding. But after he passed I found I no longer resented the job. Instead I chose to change my perspective and weed out of love for my home. What a different attitude to take! A changed outlook made the job a joy for me!

A Flash of Insight from the Past about Resentment and Guilt

I searched for more truth on the origin of my guilt feelings three years ago. Because I had spent several years exploring this in my quest for understanding, I got a flash of insight as I was reading an article on the many lifetimes that the priests of the day used guilt to imprint control over the masses. As I read this, I felt an intense, fiery pain, as if I was awash in waves of agony.

These waves were past rips and scars of how I bought into the guilt that was handed down from three or four generations of ministers in my maternal family history. Due to the strong influence guilt has had upon members of my family, I always bought into the feeling that I was never good enough. I also knew from this insight that if something in the past was implied or judged as wrong, I'd feel guilty about it.

After this insight, I built even stronger boundaries to protect my understanding of my true Self. As I felt stronger and stronger, I noticed that food began to taste better than ever and my eating habits improved. I started to deeply savor the flavors of foods in a similar way that a gourmand would. I was no longer driven by an unseen force to eat my way out of the "Land of Guilt." Gradually the guilt in my gut disappeared.

You can take the approach of savoring your meals like a gourmet too, simply by slowing down to completely enjoy every flavor and every moment of the experience. This will help you feel fuller sooner, discouraging you from eating until you're stuffed.

Sometimes it seems we must move mountains of resentments that have been handed down through the generations. Emotions of resentment, anger, guilt, doubt, or fear which are passed on to you second hand from relatives are as destructive as a knife to the throat or poisonous acid eating away your peace of mind.

Understanding How We Adopt Family Shadows

Rejuvenation is defined as "to make young again." You can rejuvenate yourself and your current relationships when you strive to live more consciously with a balanced awareness of the legacy of your past generations.

Depending on personal family history, the cycles and dynamics within families bear fruit every fourth through sixth generation. When a family unit is tight, strong, and loving, the members of that family enjoy the strength of cohesiveness and support from familial love, which helps them ride through the hard times of the currents of life better.

However when a family unit is not close (antagonistic), or displays emotional fusion (lack of boundaries, poorly differentiated relationships), or is dysfunctional, then the family dynamic becomes more of a liability than an asset to its members. The more closed the family system is, the more rigid and automatic the family responses and patterns become. Family members who identify strongly with or idolize other members may be prone to continue destructive behavior patterns throughout generations.

How does this happen? Family behavior patterns can be passed along in stories, as well as through attitudes, liaisons and affinities between family members for generations. The intensity of these patterns often unconsciously pulls at our attention and influences our lives on a subconscious level. Sometimes they interfere with the ability to make wise, conscious, decisions and undermine the ability to live fully and function truthfully in the present modern world. One way to discern and understand your family dynamic is through a charting method known as the *genogram*.

The Genogram

A genogram is similar to a family tree in that it describes family relationships between its members. Primarily used by mental health experts, physicians, and clergy, a genogram maps biological processes (such as birth order, marriages, pregnancies, deaths, households, and other historical and medical events).

A genogram can also map the emotional dynamics in relationships between family members, such as whose relationship was conflict ridden, which relationships were close, the incidence of physical abuse or incest, as well as other patterns of dysfunction within the family history for generations. When used effectively, this tool gives a "snapshot" of the historical and dynamic influences at work in a family. You can benefit from this information. Simply draw your own family genogram and use it to become more conscious of the hidden influences within your family.

The Genogram Survey

Draw up a history of your family in your journal, using circles to signify females and squares to delineate males. Record at least four generations of your family, beginning with your grandparents. Add each generation (your parents, their brothers and sisters, you and your brothers and sisters, your children and their cousins) and their spouses or significant others. Do your best to fill in the relationship dynamic by answering the following questions in the genogram survey.

(1) Label addictions such as alcoholism or drug abuse (recreational or over-the-counter).

(2) Note any medical information you can. Look for chronic illness, eating disorders, depression, or other mental health problems. Some health concerns you might be aware of are the following: allergies, arteriosclerosis, arthritis, asthma, cancer (what kind), cataracts, cystic fibrosis, diabetes, Down's syndrome, dwarfism, emphysema, epilepsy, heart disease or heart attack, hemophilia (or other blood disorders), hypertension, hepatitis (or other liver ailments), multiple sclerosis, muscular dystrophy, sickle-cell anemia, Tay-Sachs, and tuberculosis. Add any others that apply to your family that are not listed.

(3) Label any emotions that might define certain members or that they might be stuck in. For instance did you parents argue? Did you mother remain bitter? Did either of your parents experience loss and grief? If so, how did they teach you to handle it by their example? Did either parent have difficulty overcoming fears?

(4) Using straight lines, connect the relationships in your family which were loving and close. Which relatives do you identify with or idolize?

(5) Connect all the conflict ridden relationships with jagged or wavy lines. How much of what you do today is directly or indirectly influenced by unresolved issues in these relationships?

(6) If possible, ask the family for more history. What were their lives like? How did their lives turn out? Successful or tragic? In what ways? As sensitively as possible, ask for specific details. What "family secrets" do members choose *not* to talk about? Fill out your chart accordingly.

Emotional History

In addition, answer the following questions to determine the past messages your family sent you. Understanding these things consciously takes them from being stumbling blocks and turns them into personal stepping stones out of unconscious behaviors.

(1) Ask yourself, what message or belief did my mother pass on to me?

(2) Ask yourself, what message or belief did my father pass on to me?

(3) Ask this same question for each grandparent, both maternal and paternal.

(4) Write each in a boxed area that relates to the relative on your genogram.

(5) Then reflect on background factors in your family that are always at work.

The emotional beliefs passed on to you by previous generations are powerful coercive forces that affect you and your choices in life. Knowing your family background can help you understand where some of your feelings and actions originate and allow you to make more conscious, satisfying, rewarding choices in the way you react or behave, tremendously effecting the course of the rest of your life.

Standard Symbols for Genograms

Male:

Female:

Identified Patient:

Divorce Date:

Living Together or an Affair:

Children: Place in birth order with the oldest to the right:

Twins:

Stillbirth:

Miscarriage:

Abortion:

Foster Child:

Adopted Child:

Symbols Denoting Interactional Patterns between People:

Close Relationship:

Very Close/Fused Relationship:

Distant Relationship:

Conflictual Relationship:

Fused & Conflicted:

Estranged/Cut off:

Sexual Abuse:

Addictions:

List Family Losses:

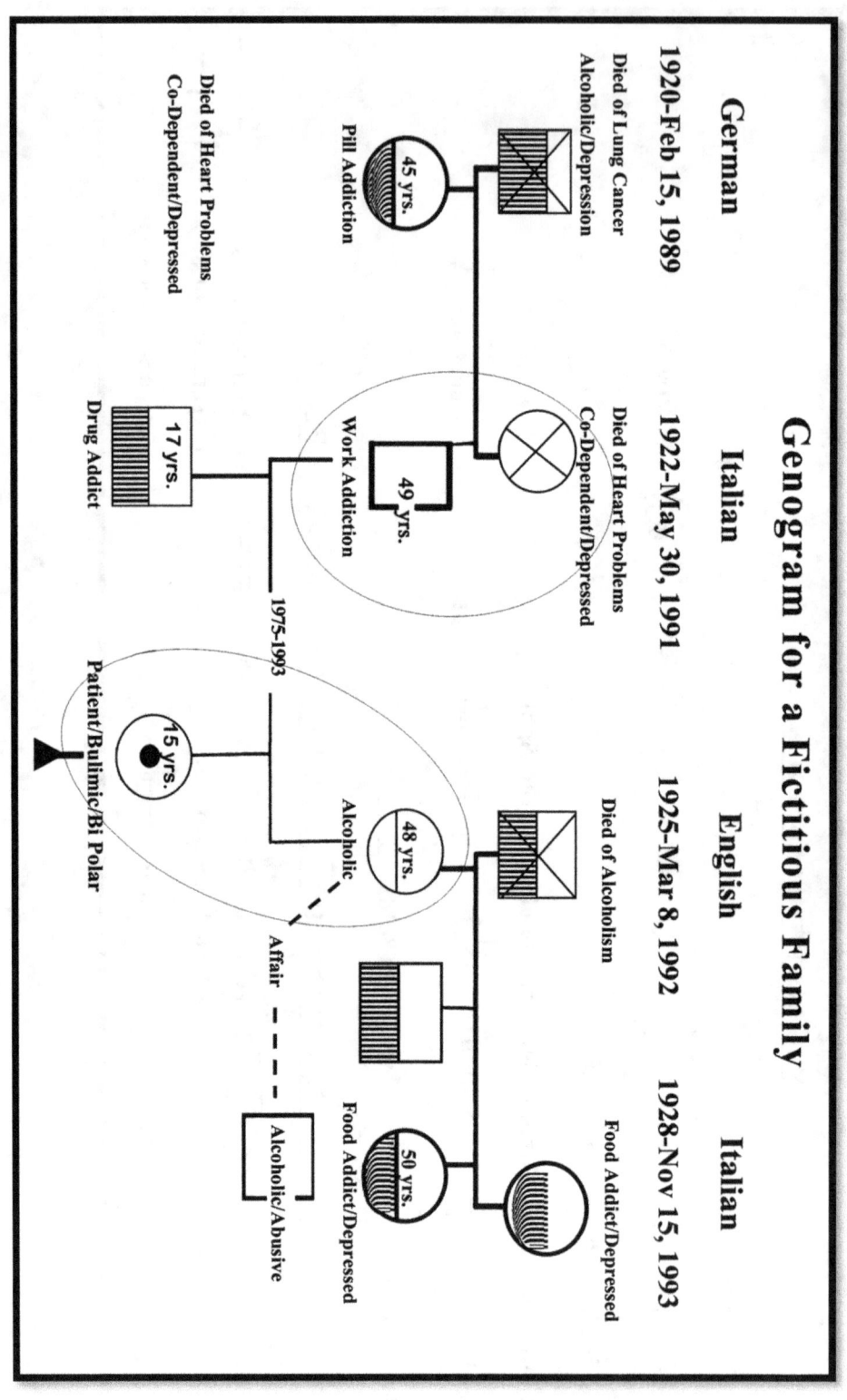

Genogram for a Fictitious Family

Genogram Analysis

- Self-harm or non-suicidal self-injury (SI) are common among adolescents, particularly among adolescents with eating disorders. Previous studies have shown that self-injury seems to be associated with sexual trauma, mood disorders, and substance abuse.

- Patient started bulimic behaviors when she was 12 years old. At that time her parents were arguing and a year later divorced.

- Patient defiant and became pregnant when she was 14 and had an abortion.

- Her mood disorder is generational, starting with her grandparents.

- Her maternal grandmother was a food addict.

- Father is demanding and distant.

- Her mother is an alcoholic, needy, overprotective, controlling and cannot be truly empathic.

- Emotionally, what did her father teach her about life?

- Emotionally, what did her mother teach her about life?

Your Family History

This is your family history in a nutshell. It tells a lot about the tides of power and the relationship dynamics within your family, as well as your family resilience to dealing with stress and the cycles of life. It also shows behavior patterns and emotional choices that often repeat themselves, passed on from family members across generations. (Editor's note: For examples of famous family genograms, please refer to Monica McGoldrick's book *Genograms: Assessment and Intervention*. See Genogram drawing and legend on pages 399 and 401.)

A Story of Accepting My Own Personal Shadows

Earlier in this chapter, you read about how my maternal grandfather and the men in the ministry in my family lineage spread guilt and fostered resentment through being overly judgmental. On the flip side is the story about the women on my paternal side of the family and the legacy they passed down to me. Both sides are pertinent to who I am today and reflect the double whammy that guilt and resentment has played in my life.

It's often easy to blame our mothers, believing they have slighted us in so many ways. After all, isn't it the mother who stereotypically provides unconditional, nurturing love? This nurturing is the wellspring that supplies both a basis for self-worth and acceptance of others. Mothers who use their feminine creative energy for birthing, sustaining, and nurturing their offspring epitomize this ideal.

I was totally astonished to discover that my paternal grandmother and great-grandmother had much more influence on my self-worth and acceptance of others in this regard.

In the beginning of the 1890s, my paternal grandmother and her younger brother were abandoned by their mother on the steps of an orphanage. Her mother told the nuns that she would return for her children.

In the late 1950s, my grandmother discovered her mother had said this and that she eventually *did* return to claim her children, but by the time she did, it was too late. My grandmother and her brother had been separated and adopted with no traceable records long before that.

I can only imagine the trauma my grandmother must have felt from first being separated from her mother and then her younger brother. I feel empathy for what she must have gone through at the age of five in coming to terms with this tremendous loss and its associated grief.

Later on my grandmother married and gave birth to a child—my father. Although she became pregnant a second time, the family secret is that she used a coat hanger to induce premature labor and consequently aborted that child.

My father married my mother and she gave birth to my older brother. Three years later my mother became pregnant with me. At that time my grandmother's beliefs strongly influenced my father's insistence that I too, should be aborted. Living in close proximity to my father's parents, my mother succumbed to their influence and set up an appointment for the abortion.

My mother has told me this story several times, so much so that it is engraved upon my heart. She was on the table about to undergo the procedure when the doctor arrived wearing a bloody apron. Terrified that he was going to butcher her, my mother jumped up and ran out of the room in tears.

The source of the guilt and abandonment I felt for most of my life sprang from my mother and the emotions I experienced through her as a fetus. I had a direct link to the emotions she struggled with during her pregnancy with me. For most of my life I deeply resented and hated my mother for the legacy of this emotional backlash.

I didn't realize until much later that the self-hate and rejection I felt originally stemmed from my paternal great-grandmother's action of abandoning her children. Everything started with that single, long ago abandonment. Beliefs and attitudes are primarily based on feelings and the illogic children sometimes use to rationalize things to themselves (such as feeling worthless, thinking that boys have more value than girls) or to blame themselves, as if they somehow could have done something different to change the outcome.

I have vivid memories of visiting my grandparents as a child. After returning home, I'd ask my mother, "Why doesn't Grandma ever talk to me? She just tells me to go lie down and take a nap."

I always felt she loved my older brother so much and that I was unimportant and unacceptable to her. I always tried so hard to please everyone, yet I felt such unresolved guilt.

What had I done? It must have been something terrible. I concluded, "It's all my fault," as any child would. Only compulsive eating patterns gave a clue to the unbalanced state and constantly striving for control that I felt (which existed within me constantly from as early as six years old).

Throughout my life I experienced repeated losses, as if I were caught in a never-ending grieving process, in much the same manner as the Sisyphus myth (of rolling the stone up the hill, only to have it roll back down, endlessly repeating this cycle, again and again). Perhaps you have experienced similar endless cycles.

I know I enacted cycles of loss and abandonment within myself continuously, buying into the myth of *Dieting Will Give Me Self Esteem and Acceptance,* until I learned the lessons contained in this book. Isn't it better to make these cycles conscious, in order to face and overcome them than to allow them to stay subconscious while you endlessly repeat the cycles? I overcame my belief in these myths. You can do it, too.

Discovering Your Shadow Side

Like Alice in Wonderland, you might be ready to go down the rabbit hole and explore more about the shadow side of your feelings and the memories connected with them. Uncovering the deeper personal reasons why these cycles continue to persist in your life may be the first step to change.

The White Rabbit Technique

Here's an exercise to try. Imagine that, like Alice, you have dived into the darkness of the rabbit hole. At the bottom you'll find your favorite fears and worries, those you continually pull out from time to time. What do you think, feel, or say to yourself *from the shadow side?* Write about what your fears and worries have to say to you in your journal. Strive to know them objectively. Ask, "Why are you in my life?" and "What wisdom do you have to share with me?" Write down their answers in your journal.

What I've found is that each problem or worry in life actually has a gift for you, once you learn to perceive it. Ask each fear or worry, "What gift or personal strength are you trying to bring to my attention? What do I need to develop more of in order to balance and bring this fear or worry to normal size?"

Make an effort to mock up feeling the personal strength which will balance your problem or weakness. For instance, if you feel threatened or fearful, ask your Higher Power, "How can I feel more brave?" Then choose to feel brave. See what happens. Choose to use the imaginative capacity you have and, like Alice in Wonderland, feel big, strong, and brave.

Living in a Sea of Experience with the Influence of Your Higher Power

This sea of substance is forever alive and active. It is sensitive beyond our mind's wildest dreams or imaginings. The thought pictures of the mind can mold this substance into expression.

Ask yourself, "How can I choose to see things in a more amusing way? How can I be more trusting of my process? How can I choose to be excited about new changes?"

Then take the words and say "I am choosing to be amused. I'm choosing to be excited more and more. I am choosing to trust in positive outcomes."

What you give out is what you get back. It's time to let go of the past. What could stop you now? Only the hostility you harbor inside your own heart.

Turning Anger or Primal Rage into Energy that Works for You

Does your anger strike you as being like a burning coal? Or do you just end up confused and hurt without understanding? What can you do about this? By knowing the heart of your anger better, you can become free.

The Heart of Resentment and Rage

The illusion at the heart of rage, denial, and resentment is that you can exert control over people, places, and events in your world when in reality you have no control over anything outside of yourself.

This faulty impression about power and control comes from the small self, the ego. Believing in this only keeps you confused, frustrated, and disappointed. Confusion is another word for resenting yourself, resenting the flow of life, and resenting the choices you've made in the past, which were dictated by past shadows.

Confusion and resentment lead to frustration, hostility, and stress—attitudes that release bodily manufactured chemicals (such as the steroid hormones of adrenaline and cortisol) and propagate them through the body, creating emotional level addictions within your body to those chemical reactions. (The stress hormone cortisol has also been known to lead to carbohydrate cravings and overeating, as well as abdominal fat).

Your mind and emotions may dislike what's going on, but your body is driven to seek out life situations and replay personal interactions with people, places, and things that stimulate the release of the body chemicals to which it is physically addicted. This theory forms the basis of Stress Pattern Processing.

Indulging emotional level addictions over time speeds biological aging, debilitates your immune system, and leads to disordered eating habits. It's fairly well accepted that long held stress from destructive attitudes (resentment, guilt, and anger) are actually precursors for cancerous conditions that develop later in life.

Be aware! Take charge of those things which you *do* control! Time to change old thinking and feeling patterns-time to reveal another layer of your true self hidden in the shadows of your dark side.

Hidden Rage

Hidden rage frequently elevates itself in order to be noticed, often expanding to many times its actual size. Many shadow traits you may have ignored, disavowed, or disowned over the years will do this in order to get your attention. The traits that you may considered your worst often have a "positive side" that's just begging for acknowledgment. When you embrace your rage and realize all the good qualities it has to offer you on the flip side, it reduces in size and nature, allowing you to manifest it in appropriate amounts in suitable situations. In many cases, rage becomes normal anger and no longer controls you—you manage it.

Rage can be hidden so consider this: did you have temper tantrums when you were young? Ask, "In what ways did I get angry when I was a toddler?" Rage is so undercover for most people that they can't acknowledge how much of a hold it has over their lives.

Remember repressed anger turns into guilt, self-loathing and self-hate. It may take months, years, or a lifetime but eventually repressed emotions will turn self-destructive. Some people spend a lifetime coming to this conclusion, but you can choose to understand it right now. You are worth whatever it takes to get it.

Feel good about yourself right now. Feel good that you've come this far. Ask yourself, "Do I want to move forward and be free?" If so, say aloud, "I choose to be willing to do whatever it takes to be free."

Embracing the Heart of Rage

Take the same exercise as before and go down the rabbit hole to meet your rage. Ask, "What wisdom do you have to share with me?" Write down the answer in your journal.

Ask your rage, "What gift or strength are you trying to bring to my attention? What do I need to acknowledge or what positive aspects come with the gifts that rage brings me?" Write down what you receive. Acknowledge, honor and embrace the positive gifts you find in the shadow of your rage.

Write a Poem About Anger

Another simple tool to use to expel repressed anger or resentment is to write an anger poem. The following poem is an example of anger being expressed instead of repressed. When you read the poem, listen to the compassion and courage Sally used in confessing her heartfelt anger. When you are finished, write a poem about a strong emotion that you experienced this week. Here's one example.

The Great Debate

by Sally G.

I am so irate because I hate to work late and since I don't rate,

It is my fate and my joy to be and love a reprobate.

When I ate and ate nothing would sate my appetite, so my weight

Kept growing, turning away my bedmate, which would exacerbate /exaggerate,

The situation so I needed to placate my anxiety and quiet the great debate

In my mind and allocate my energy if I quit lying prostrate

And not gestate or stagnate and endlessly berate.

Myself as I have in the past so I must not hesitate

To right away activate an exercise plan with my housemate

And not complicate it by issuing a mandate

Too immense and great that I would immediately deviate

From any plan to help me recreate

My mind and body because I want to medicate myself and not tolerate

Life on life's terms, and obliterate the world around me, hoping to terminate

All thoughts and actions to rehabilitate me. So I don't want to participate

In anything, but just vegetate and hibernate.

Take a Divine Shower—A Simple Technique for Disengaging from Anger

For many years Lorraine loved her husband and family life. She was proud of the fact that she wed such a successful man. After many years of marriage, Lorraine developed an intense dislike for her husband as he did for her. Lorraine began to eat to stuff her anger. She gained over eighty pounds.

As time went by, these feelings grew into a rage, the likes of which she had never before experienced. She couldn't understand why she felt so enraged whenever her husband said or did anything. Although her husband had addictive problems and she had eating problems, they still remained married.

Through spiritual study, Lorraine learned about the Law of Cause and Effect (karma). In her dreams, Lorraine became aware that she had been instrumental in destroying her husband's character and marriage in a past life. As a result, both of them had created a spiritual debt for this lifetime. She saw this situation as an opportunity to pay off that debt. However, even though she was aware of this, she was too emotional to sustain this higher awareness. She tried to let it go, to give it to God. She would say, "I turn this over to you, God." Yet she always took it back the next time she thought of her husband.

Lorraine decided to attend a spiritual seminar. Knowing that she always felt divine love at these seminars, she was eager to go. She asked her Higher Power to show her a technique to use to let go of the anger she felt toward her husband.

At the seminar she learned about a Divine Shower Technique. She practiced it each morning before the day began. While she showered, she sang the word HU, which is an ancient prayer song to God. Then she imagined the Holy Spirit pouring thousands of shimmering stars over her, showering her from head to toe with the divine love of God.

Lorraine explained to me that the water became for her the love of the Holy Spirit. The most peaceful feeling overtook her in these moments, cleansing her of inner and outer anger and frustration. She sensed anger flowing out of her body, out each fingertip, spiraling down the drain. She continued with her daily life, beaming with joy and love for all of life. She let go of her animosity and stopped reacting to her husband.

However, I continued to do this technique every day. Little by little, I gained more control of my emotions," Lorraine said.

Lorraine also realized that as she surrendered this anger more and more to her Higher Power, an inner healing was taking place, so gradually that she barely noticed. Her attitude was changing, and so was her husband's.

Eventually she was able to give her husband unconditional love, even laugh at his jokes, and once again he could smile at her. To her surprise, the extra weight she had gained started to drop off naturally and gradually.

Soon they were both on friendly terms. During this time, they both realized it was best to move on with their lives without each other. Lorraine knew in her heart that the karmic debt (of destroying his character and marriage in a past life) had been balanced, repaid, and eventually put to rest, totally resolved. She was grateful for the experience and at peace with the outcome.

Seeds of Doubt

The seeds of doubt are all around us continually. Do you want to see the vision of yourself that disparages you or do you choose to see a person who acknowledges and boosts your self-esteem?

Linda had deep seated doubts about her worthiness. She used a visual technique to help clear the self-doubt that plagued her for this lifetime. It took a long time for Linda to isolate self-doubt as a major contributor to her need for therapy over the years, but this discovery gave Linda the opportunity to use the following technique to finally clear it.

Visual Picturing Technique

(1) Linda asked herself, "What does this self-doubt and self-punishment look like?" She pictured a pioneer wagon stuck in two deep ruts. Then she focused on the symbol for her purpose image.

(2) Next she closed her eyes and looked up at the center of her forehead where insight occurs within the brain. She asked her Higher Power to help her with her tendency to get caught in attitudes of self-doubt and self-blame. She asked for this symbol (that resembled a wagon stuck in two ruts) to change positively. She watched it change. She took her time with this technique and kept asking it to change positively.

When Linda tried this exercise, she saw a figure get out of the wagon and ask for more help. Three more people arrived and helped lift the back of the wagon. Then they lifted the front of the wagon so it could turn in a new direction.

Linda went about her life, but afterward she was transformed by this inner experience. She had turned a corner. The experience was so deep that Linda continued to have fresh insights about it for the next six months.

Are you plagued by doubts? Imagine an image that symbolizes your doubt. Then kick that symbol (in the metaphorical butt) and laugh.

Freedom is being able to be you and to love yourself as you are now. The rest of your dreams will come true as you start loving yourself more.

Confronting the Shadow Cynic

What could stop you now? Only *not recognizing* the Shadow Cynic within yourself. A cynic is someone who denies the sincerity of other's motives and actions. A cynic sneers or is sarcastic about people and life in general.

What is behind sarcasm? Do you know of anyone who automatically comes to mind (by their actions and attitudes) when you think of what it is to be sarcastic? Stand back and get a better look at this person. If you know their background, you may see that they survived a tough trauma while growing up. Trauma continues to exist within a person's subconscious mind in the way he or she views the world. Their perception of reality as seen through the lens of trauma is, most simply, a hostile one.

In fact, all information coming into a traumatized person's mind goes first through the mental filter of the mind's programmed hostility response. Then they judge the world as being insincere through their mental lens of hostility. Nothing can get past this filter until they first consciously choose to willingly surrender their old beliefs, attitudes, and actions.

So often we equate surrender with defeat. It's a common human response, a battle that has been fought all our lives where we're always trying to win something that was lost long ago (when the trauma was first initiated). However, you can choose to look at surrender not as defeat, but as *doing things differently*.

If you've been doing things one way all your life and you're still unhappy, why not try something different? The imagination is wonderful in that it can free us from our limitations and inhibitions, and lead to more freedom with body images.

Four Techniques to Stay Clear on Your Inner Body Image

The following techniques work easily and with efficiency. Suspend your disbelief and trust the process. Just follow the directions and try each exercise in the order given. Each one builds on the results of the one before, working in concert to help you attain your purpose.

Loading Your Ship Technique

Imagine giving up everything that's holding you back in your world. Give up old patterns of self-pity, anger at yourself or the world, or thinking you have to do everything for everyone. Make a fantasy of constructing a ship. After it is built, the captain directs you to load it up with all your old baggage, the stuff that weighs you down in the past or present. Thank the crew and captain for their help. Then wave goodbye to it from the dock and see it sail away.

You may do this as often as necessary to keep releasing feelings that drive you to hopelessness. Trust and keep doing it. You are worth the effort to get free.

Where Am I Right Now Technique

Take out a drawing marker or pen. In a drawing, answer the question, "Where am I right now?" This is not about art. Draw whatever first comes to mind, even if it is just stick figures. Then, give the drawing a voice by writing the following sentences and completing them.

The three sentences begin the same. "I am . . . I am . . . I am . . ."

Now, journal as if you are talking to your best friend, explaining how you felt when you were drawing. Open your awareness like a wide river to the sea, and stay with the experience without having to have all the answers right now.

Bottoming Out Technique

In a second drawing, answer the question, "What is blocking me?" Use symbols, colors, shapes, textures, and lines in whatever way you like. Give yourself permission to dare to draw any way and anything you want. Give the drawing a voice and complete the following sentences, "I am . . . I am . . . I am . . . ."

Free Your Attitude Technique

Here's how you determine if an attitude you have grown up with works for you. Ask yourself the following questions. No second guessing. Again let the first answer pop into your mind and write it down.

(1) Write your intent or purpose.

(2) Write your limiting beliefs. For example, "I have to think before take action and get active for my health." (This thinking will talk you out of taking action.) Or "I have to feel anxious to get motivated." Or another belief is, "I need to know 'why' before I can let it go!" Or "It's no good, I'll never be able to do it." Write down all your strong attitudes and limiting beliefs.

(3) Ask yourself to be willing to suspend your disbelief for now while you use this technique. (If you don't have the willingness or intent, the exercise is assured to fail.) Get honest and find your willingness.

(4) Imagine you have written this statement in the hardest material or substance known to man. What is it? A brick wall, a granite cliff, or a huge boulder. Whatever it is, see it.

(5) Sense the attitude or belief carved in the substance. How is it carved? How big are the letters? Do the letters have a color? In what font or typeface are the letters written?

Now answer either Yes or No to the following four questions.

(1) Does this attitude or belief produce *positive, joyful feelings or actions* for you on your way to your purpose?

(2) Does this attitude or belief take you *towards your purpose?*

(3) Does this attitude or belief have value in leading you *to your purpose?*

(4) Is this attitude or belief pertinent to *where you want to go* in your purpose statement?

I'll bet all the answers are no. If these beliefs were working, you wouldn't be reading this book. If you have trouble getting clear with this technique, share it with a trusted friend. Do this again and again for all your limiting beliefs.

Next, ask your Higher Power to help you see the carved belief change positively. Watch it change with your eyes closed as you focus on the center point just above your eyes where insight occurs in the brain. Sense it and allow it to change while giving yourself some time to do this. You can work with a partner or do this as a silent contemplation for healing.

Watch it change for several minutes, keeping your eyes closed. Keep asking it to change positively as you just watch. Any slight change is good. It may need to get worse before you understand that it is changing for the better. Do this several times during the week. Change either the stone or the message, whichever works for you.

"I've Got You, Babe" Surrender Technique

Cut out magazine pictures of images or symbols that have hypnotized or bound you in the past. Be aware of how these pictures have shaped your desires to look or be like a favorite actress or model. Make a collage of all the pictures you can find.

Now stand back and see what has "got you, babe" from the past. Finally take this collage outside and set it on fire. Let it go. All the while, ask your Higher Power to help you be free of those hypnotizing body images. Let it go!

Release Fear on the Way to Healing

This exercise is for healing tension and extreme stress for the mind, body, and will. For a reference point, the color red is used to strengthen the life force of the body and to give self-confidence to the mind and will.

Close your eyes. Say, "I love my Higher Power. I love Spirit. I love God." Imagine seeing all your past worst stresses rolled into the image of a huge gray cloud. The cloud is filled with all your fears, terrors, and worries. The cloud follows you as you hurry away. You enter a forest. All the while you know that God is near you always.

Now imagine you hear a soft inner sound. Surrender and trust that you can creatively follow that inner sound as it threads through the forest. Soon you come to a huge cement building. It's got an open entranceway with two twin pillars on each side. You walk in, still following the inner sound.

Next you enter a bathing area. Proceed to wash yourself under a gently falling waterfall. In this refreshing shower, you release all stress and fear. Imagine the stress pouring away from you.

As you step out of this cleansing area, someone safe drapes a Red Cloak of Consciousness around you. This renews your will, life force, and your mental strength. This image of this cloak can be used as a tool for further healing you as Soul.

The Mystery of Dying to the Old

The mystery of dying to the old begins with exposing the dark energy of your anger, your fears, your resentments, and surrendering all these aspects of yourself. This emptying time gives you the opportunity to strengthen your inner balance. Letting go of the old makes room for the new.

Let go of being seduced by the ways of old habits and allow the new energy of upliftment to shine like the morning sunrise after a dark, stormy night. Trust that the new energy will be available. The sun always rises and so do you.

Vision Quest

Nicki, a dark haired, fragile looking woman, has a history of repressed anger and aggression. Her years of bingeing, over-exercising, and starvation diets lead her to look for ways to break free. A therapist recommended that she sign up for a week long workshop retreat in the Black Mountains of North Carolina.

One outstanding part of this workshop was the use of a vision quest as a way to break free of old habits. The initial assignment was to collect things that represent everything in your life that was shamed, rejected, or used to blame or betray you. Nicki put these symbolic shadow items in a black bag to show how she kept these parts of herself hidden from herself, where she thought no one else could see them.

Nicki found a variety of items and a symbolic meaning she attribute to each one. In her journal Nicki wrote the following passage with her list, which follows: "In all respect and humble reverence for the reality of life and ego, I choose to purify my memories and free myself from any attachments in my mind, emotions, and body. I release what is no longer a way of life for me. I gladly give up tokens of the old as I make room for new awareness as the Soul that I am."

(1) Death Symbol—a fallen leaf, crumbling after finishing its creative cycle, will transform into fertile soil, nourishing new growth over time

(2) "Why" symbol—a dried-up branch shaped like a 'Y' that represents forever asking "Why?" I never got an answer to this constant question, only more confusion

(3) Illumination Symbol—a stone with a face on it that looked like its crown chakra was opened represented 'weird-crazy' label. The gift of being 'weird' is really visionary

(4) Surrender Symbols—twelve seed pods represent the secret ways to surrender on the way to freedom

(5) Dream—Not—Planted Symbol—an acorn. Aspects of life put on hold

(6) Symbol of Openness—an exquisite fluttering butterfly came to rest and spread its wings in all its beauty, sharing beauty without an ounce of shame

(7) Symbol of Illusions—a pink mushroom hidden under a leaf spoke to me through my intuition, as I remembered a line from Alice in Wonderland

(8) Symbol of the Fall—a yellow leaf reminds me of the contemplating Soul and wanting to travel to the stars and breathe in the beauty of God

(9) Symbol of the Void—a totally black, shiny pod from the stream that reminded me that I am always drawn to understand the void

(10) Symbol of Rejection—a discarded bubble gum wrapper

The Surrender Ritual

The next part of the ritual involved letting go. At the evening bonfire, a white-haired, spry old man began to play a trance like rhythm on the drums. Nicki's turn came. As she slowly stood before the group of twenty, she felt powerful. She addressed the fire: "I give up my attachments, one by one, to be purified and dispersed to the winds of change." The fire sparked and smoke curled up into space and time.

"I give up my anger at myself for being judgmental when I am a beautiful Soul."

"I freely give up anger and sadness at my life choices, for they are meant to be."

"I give up my anger and release its habit of catching my attention, telling me what's not fair and what's wrong, rather than what is good."

The drum thundered its response.

"I give up my anger to rest in the arms of the essence of life as it is."

"I give up my anger at wanting to understand the lessons I have learned." Nicki threw this symbol as hard as she could into the leaping flames.

"I give up wanting to understand with my mind. I choose to trust it to be." "In all of this I respect with humble reverence the process of purifying my memories and freeing myself."

"This copy of my marriage certificate symbolizes love/hate and pain/pleasure and something that is no longer. I close the debt as I burn this copy in neutral divine action."

Nicki originally gathered the symbols for the bonfire to facilitate sharing her shadow story with the group at the communal gathering. She compiled a medicine bag that contained these symbols so she could carry the power of the wisdom that she had gained with her. Some of the older, out-dated symbols that she wanted to divest herself of were burned in the fire. These were things she no longer needed in her life.

You can choose to experience the freedom of this exercise for yourself. Gather your shadow symbols for a vision quest. Create it with several others or by yourself, the way you want it to be.

Prepare for Opportunity Disguised As Loss

The process of surrender is not a lesson in loss as much as it's an opportunity in disguise. Here are four "how-to" clues on navigating the process of surrender.

(1) Ask for an experience to learn surrender

(2) Be open to opportunity

(3) Be willing to surrender all that is holding you back

(4) Have patience and the conviction in your beliefs, knowing this will transpire with time.

Looking at Loss as an Opportunity to Make Room for the New

When you get caught in a series of losses you may tend to start to look at life as a victim. You might become machine like in your automatic thoughts and habitual actions. This is slavery to the negativity of the mind. Continue to take positive actions and be sure to ask for help, if you need it.

When I faced my deepest shadows, I found losses accompanied my deepest fears. Those losses read like a dirty laundry list of life messes. The losses included my marriage, my oldest daughter, my ten acre dressage center, three show horses, my dog and four cats, and my financial base. A few years later, I faced the loss of my sense of safety due to a stalker, loss of face when I had to file a restraining order and appear in the state attorney general's office. Four court appearances later resulted in a prison term for the offender, finally re-establishing my safety.

Yet these losses were hidden opportunities.

Higher Power knew I needed to face my gravest fears in order to put them to rest forever.

What I received in the way of gifts by going through those devastating losses were the deepest strength and freedom I have ever known. These spiritual qualities of strength and wisdom abide in me today and I share it with whomever I contact. The culmination of these experiences opened my heart in a way that wasn't possible previously. I couldn't have gained these riches of spirit in any other way than to go through the experiences I did. It was well worth it!

Chapter 24 explores the companion to the shadow side, a way to true balance. By learning more about how to embody the elusive qualities of forgiveness, gratitude, and grace, you'll take the next step toward embracing true freedom.

Chapter 24

Three Spiritual Truths to Open Your Heart: Forgiveness, Gratitude, and Grace

Accepting the Full Magnitude of Life

> *Understanding and accepting the full magnitude of life, both the shadow and its flip side, brings true balance.*

Chapter 23 revealed how shadows of anger, denial, and resentment limit life whenever they rule. It also highlighted how processing and releasing shadows makes room for new ways of being. The next step to living a life of more freedom is fully understanding and adopting spiritual qualities of forgiveness, gratitude, and grace.

Forgiveness—The Most Misunderstood Quality

Often people believe forgiveness implies full *exoneration* meaning "to relieve of responsibility," suggesting that alleged offenders are fully vindicated and not accountable. Nothing could be further from the truth. [Editor's note: Definition from *Webster's Ninth Collegiate Dictionary*, Private Library edition.]

In the world in which we live where the laws of physics rule, *every action begets an equal and opposite reaction*. In other words, the Law of Karma governs. However, the ultimate time, place and price of karmic debt against others (in word, thought or deed) is a divine decision, one that's weighed in a court where the scales of justice are exquisitely balanced and completely free from the taint of error or perjury.

Forgiveness—The Gift You Give Yourself

Forgiveness doesn't need two or more participants. Forgiveness doesn't need witnesses. It doesn't need to make an outward appearance.

Forgiveness isn't interested in the outcome, retribution, recompense, or revenge. *True forgiveness* means "to cease to feel resentment against (an offender)."

All forgiveness takes is *you*—and a changed attitude.

Forgiveness primarily revolves around a changed consciousness, a changed heart. Fully and unconditionally forgiving others can make all the difference in the world to your life.

As difficult as it may seem, the skill to *truly forgive* everyone who has done wrong against you is a valuable one to develop. By fully releasing everyone involved in situations from blame, you'll have the key to keeping resentment out of your heart. This is the greatest gift you can ever give yourself, a life free from the emotional fallout of your own aggression.

A Story of Forgiveness

As I floated in a Florida pool one heavenly winter day, I found myself thinking in an expansive way. I reached inside my consciousness, wanting to find the cause of some chronic shoulder pain. What I found was leftover resentments in my consciousness towards a surgeon for mistakes that I thought he'd made during an operation. (He was supposed to do it perfectly and I always suspected that he didn't.)

I decided to try this forgiveness technique, so I focused on letting go of feelings of resentment and forgiving him fully. As I did, my shoulder freed. Then I began forgiving each person involved in the operation. Not that I haven't forgiven them for this situation a hundred times before. But the mind has a curious way of taking resentment back.

This time, as I forgave each person with all the love in my heart, my shoulder began to release even more. I floated more buoyantly in the water as I did this. I was in ecstasy.

Then I forgave myself for any role I might have played in the situation. I accepted the current state of things today as the way they are meant to be.

I accepted myself in my current condition and realized that whatever had happened, the experience was what I needed to become the person I am today, the person who will be able to complete my life's work on earth. I know that what is *now* is what is divinely meant to be.

During the next few months, I watched for ways this change of consciousness affected my life. I found that the more I accepted myself this way, the more my body began to change in appearance. At times I truly felt like a goddess. All previous self-images which were tied into societal beliefs about what is popular today were gone. Forgiveness is a powerfull tool for shaping the body from the inside out.

Floating in a Pool of Forgiveness Technique

Try this forgiveness technique out for yourself the next time you have an opportunity to float in water or *now*. Lay on your bed and imagine you're floating in the most warm wonderful ocean of forgiveness, an ocean of love and mercy. Recall situations you would like to forgive. Fully forgive everyone involved and forgive yourself for your part in it. Finally, accept the current way things are today as the way they are meant to be, part of the Divine Plan. Practice this technique until it becomes a part of you.

Are You Ready to Forgive?

So often the forgiveness technique is put aside because people are just not ready to forgive. However, forgiveness is integral to healing, becoming whole, and taking back all your energy that is tied up in the emotions that go with *not forgiving*.

If you are not ready, know that when you reach a point of being tired of all the sadness in your life, or the addiction to food, relationships, shopping, or media consumption, then you will be ready to accept the gift of forgiveness.

Be watchful for the quick fix. Be careful of anyone who says, "I can make that better for you in one or two sessions," or any other quick fix scenario. Fast ways are not always permanent ways. Wouldn't you rather address things permanently with a mended heart? Quick fixes seldom give you feelings of empowerment, such as, "I did this myself. I did the work and now the solution is permanently imprinted in my heart for all time."

Forgiveness Like a Mantra

I took another step and practiced a forgiveness technique with a friend I have known for 19 years. I shared a variation of the forgiveness technique with her over some herb tea. First I said, "I accept you for who you are."

Then I stated, "I forgive you for whatever you have thought, said, or done in this lifetime and all past lifetimes." Third I added, "I forgive myself for all I've thought, said, or done in this lifetime and all past lifetimes." Finally I said, "I send you spiritual love and I accept spiritual love."

I told her that I had been saying these forgiveness statements every day, even several times a day. I really wanted to let it all go. Yet, I added with a frown, "It seems like I'll be saying these statements like a mantra for the rest of my life!"

"I know," she said. We had a good laugh over that.

What I found is that doing the forgiveness technique like a mantra helped me open my heart in gentle waves of bliss and purity until I *got it* in a way that can't ever be taken away from me. This is the most precious gift.

Visualization and Progressive Relaxation to Shape the Body

Make a recording of the following script in a slow, relaxed voice. Then play the recording for yourself each night as you go to sleep. If you feel you can never relax, tell yourself, "Please do not relax. Simply enjoy listening to my voice" at the beginning of the recording. Start your recording with the following paragraph.

State your purpose with your symbol. Take three deep belly breaths and tell yourself, it is safe to relax. Close your eyes and conceive of a safe place. This safe place can be real or imaginary.

Look around your safe place and notice details. What sounds do you hear? What can you reach out and touch? Feel the texture of whatever you are touching. This is your safe place where you can go to lower your fears or anxieties.

Accept in your mind this visualization is not about trying to relax, just allow it to happen. Know you are safe. You can hold on as much as you like or you can let go and relax—deeply relax. That's right.

Let your hands rest easily in your lap, at your sides, or on the arms of your chair. Close your eyes, and think of your whole body growing limp and relaxed.

Accept in your mind that the muscles in the scalp and forehead are growing comfortable and relaxed. You may find that as you think of these muscles relaxing, they will.

As the muscles of the forehead relax you may notice a slight increase in tension around the eyebrows. Concentrate on the eyebrows and all around the eye and this tension will fade away. Accept in your mind the tiny muscles of the eyelids relax. Let the relaxation move deep inside the eyes and deep in back of the eyes.

Let all the facial muscles relax; over the cheekbones and the cheeks, the jaw and chin, the lips and mouth—all relax. The relaxation moves deep inside the mouth. As the muscles of the mouth relax, you may find that your mouth automatically becomes not too moist and not too dry, but just moist enough to keep you perfectly comfortable. The relaxation spreads deep in back of the throat, deep in back of the head and neck, deep into the neck and shoulders.

Let the arms relax. Relax the upper arms. Focus on the forearms and feel them relax. All the muscles between the elbows and wrists relax. The relaxation spreading across the tops of the hands and deep into the hands, deeply through the hands to the palms. Now the fingers relax all the way to the fingertips. As the fingers relax you may or may not experience a slight tingling in the fingers. If you do, you may find it to be a pleasing feeling.

Bring your attention back again to the relaxed muscles of the neck and shoulders. The relaxation flows into the chest and lungs. Your breathing is easy and gentle. You feel yourself relaxing more and more with each gentle breath.

You may relax more and more with each sound of my voice. All outside sounds are unimportant. Only the sound of my voice is important now.

Let the relaxation spread into the back. Feel it move gently down the back to the small of the back. Let all the muscles of the body go to sleep in a sense while you remain aware and focused. Feel the relaxation spreading around and deep into the sides of your torso. The muscles of the abdomen are relaxing deep into the abdomen.

As the muscles of the abdomen and hips relax, feel your subconscious open. This opening grows wider and wider. Accept my words into your mind. Gently conceive of the muscles in your belly and hips becoming firmer and firmer with a younger, leaner form and feel happy.

Now let the legs relax. The relaxation spreading into the thighs and knees. The calves of the legs relax, all the way to the ankles. In this relaxed state open your mind to conceive of how firm your legs are becoming.

Now let the feet relax, the heels of the feet, the soles of the feet, deep through the feet to the tops, and finally even the toes relax. It feels so good to relax and release all tension and care.

Enjoy a few moments of relaxation now as I slowly count from ten down to one. As I count, let your body relax more and more with each count. At the count of five, you may be more deeply relaxed than ever before. Then you may go even deeper as each number becomes smaller. Counting now: ten ... nine ... eight ... seven ... six ... five ... four ... three ... two ... one ... Rest.

Allow a wonderful peacefulness to surround your body as it becomes leaner and stronger. Feel good about this. Remember a favorite feeling and memory as your body effortlessly does the work.

As you drift and relax with your favorite feeling, your body can start becoming leaner, healthier, and stronger. Even as you soundly sleep, your body and mind are working on becoming leaner, healthier, and stronger. You will awaken in the morning feeling refreshed and ready for your day.

Play this audio nightly for three to eight weeks and then weekly for three months. Finally, play it once every three months for a year. Compare how far you progress from when you start to when you finish.

Gratitude—The Gift that Keeps on Giving

If you want to have more joy in your life, then look for joy in all things. If you want more grace in your life, surrender woe and be willing to look for grace. Granted, it's not always easy to do this. However, you can find the courage by rising to the challenge.

In the beginning it may be difficult to surrender an attitude of 'woe is me.' The key is to look for what's working in your life. This key is as simple as being thankful for even the smallest things every day.

Start small. Be grateful that you have a toothbrush and toothpaste. Make a list of everything for which you are grateful. Add to your list in incremental degrees every day.

Gratitude Technique

Write a letter to your Higher Power requesting, "Show me gratitude." Then go about your day, expecting insights about gratitude and being ready for them to surprise you. At the end of the day, write down in your journal what insights and experiences you received.

Gratitude Is Here and Now

Express gratitude for everything that is in your life today. On the most basic level, gratitude is simply accepting what is.

A woman named Janet wrote in her journal about all she had learned during the past month. She wrote of gratitude for her deepening ability to listen with her heart as she prayed to God. Once, as she was driving along Interstate Highway 95 on her way to work, she was reflecting on how thankful she was for her life. She noticed how her eating habits had been much more balanced recently. It seemed effortless because she was willing for it to be so. Her heart opened with joy and bliss.

She enjoyed this feeling of bliss for the rest of the half hour drive. She said, "Even now I can feel the bliss in my heart in remembrance."

This was significant for Janet because she had struggled with hardship in her life in the past. For many years she asked, "Why? Why me? Why do I have so much trouble opening my heart?"

When she finally began to practice gratitude and did an exercise that taught her how to perceive from Soul (her true observant Self), she could see much more clearly than before. She saw without judgment that she had chosen to strengthen her emotional body through the experiences of this lifetime. Furthermore, as she released grief, fear, and rage, they were replaced by a feeling of expansiveness. She felt focused and connected to an open heart.

"Thank you," she whispered, realizing her Higher Power had been and always would be there to help her. "I am blessed," she wrote. "God's grace is with me." This was the gift that came with acceptance and being grateful.

The Three Rings of Forgiveness, Gratitude, and Grace

This technique involves gathering three rings that are meaningful to you. One ring symbolizes forgiveness, one ring symbolizes gratitude, and the third ring symbolizes grace.

Each morning hold these three rings and think of someone or something you love. Let the feeling of love fill and pour from your heart, encompassing the rings. As you place the rings on your fingers, say the following affirmations.

(1) Gratitude: "I am thankful for all the gifts in my life."

(2) Forgiveness: "I forgive myself and I forgive all life, fully and unconditionally."

(3) Grace: "I welcome joy into my mind, heart and body and lovingly accept all life."

Picture accepting your natural, healthy body image as you say these affirmations and put the rings on every morning and take them off every night. Wearing the rings daily can act as a reminder for you to practice the qualities of forgiveness, gratitude, and grace every day. Perform this ritual with the accompanying affirmations for three weeks to foster attitudes of forgiveness, gratitude, and grace.

The Gift of Grace

According to *Webster's Ninth Collegiate Dictionary*, grace relates to gratitude and goodwill. It is also a virtue coming from God, unmerited divine assistance, and a blessing that is an act of divine favor or compassion. Grace is an act of kindness or the quality of being considerate or thoughtful.

Grace can be passively accepted, but let's also look at it from an alternative, more active viewpoint, taking it one step beyond a passive state of waiting for divine intervention. Let's view grace as a quality that can be courted by taking action, and not expecting God to do for you what you can do for yourself. Courting grace gives Divine Spirit an active vortex through which to work.

Let's think of grace as being in accord with the ways of Divine Spirit. By doing so, we'd know how and when to behave in a more graceful manner, and when to act with forgiveness and gratitude. We'd know where, when and how to be more loving with ourselves and with others. By taking a dynamic role, we could become conduits for grace throughout the world.

Exploring the Parameters of Grace

To find out more about grace, answer the following questions in your journal. You can ask a trusted friend to help by reading the questions aloud to you. This way you can write down the first thing that pops into your mind. No second guessing! The first thing that pops into your mind is your honest inclination.

(1) What does humility offer to help you understand grace?

(2) Who comes to mind when you think of the embodiment of humility and goodwill?

(3) How does this person show compassion for life?

(4) Does this person also illustrate self-realization and self-acceptance? How?

(5) How can you see yourself more honestly with compassion and love?

(6) How can you accept love for yourself as the initiation of receiving grace?

(7) How can you sustain the gift of grace on a daily basis? What can you do to further serve or realize this gift?

(8) What are you willing to do on a day-to-day basis to receive the grace that is always there for you because God loves you?

A Technique for Touching Grace

Stop and take several minutes to concentrate on grace. Close your eyes and imagine the feeling of grace. If it had a color, what would it be? What is the sound of grace? What is its scent? Does grace have a taste? How big is the grace that you are feeling? Can you compare it to something in the everyday world? Draw a picture that embodies the sight, sound, scent, taste, touch and feeling of grace.

Being More Open to Learning about Grace

How do you receive grace? In other words, the *process of receiving* is of foremost value and importance. How can you receive grace if you always give and never receive?

Let's imagine exploring a vast unknown vista with a flashlight, spotlighting one area at a time. Three elements I'd like to shine a light on will help you prepare to receive grace and understanding as love from your Higher Power.

The Flashlight Technique

(1) Ask to be open to receive an understanding about grace.

(2) Do your part by taking action. In other words, don't expect God to do for you what you won't do for yourself.

(3) Surrender the outcome to God, yet be ready to catch surprising insights moving into your life.

You can change the rate of your vibration using this flashlight technique. *Asking* opens you to the grace of Your Higher Power. *Doing* your part gives Spirit some action items with which to work. *Surrendering* the outcome is your way of allowing for God or Your Higher Power to work the outcome in the way, manner, order and time frame that's the best for all involved.

Many Sides of the Coin Called Grace

I need to practice all the subtleties of grace to really catch it. Part of the subtlety of grace is balance and acceptance.

Balance is integration of opposites or all things. The point of balance is at the center, where love is. When you catch true balance, your relationship with yourself changes. Your attitudes change as well as your beliefs about yourself and reality. You become equal to, instead of less than. The truth is that learning this state of balance deep in your heart is part of the price of earning freedom. To connect more deeply to the many-sided coin called grace, try incorporating the following three balances into your life starting today.

(1) Do something restful and calming that you enjoy every day.

(2) Do something kind for someone else each day, without letting anyone know about it.

(3) Say three times a day for the next four weeks, "I choose to be complete within myself and complete within my world."

Say this last affirmation until you believe it. Say it no matter what you may feel. Tape reminder cards on your bathroom mirror, computer, steering wheel, or whatever else is in your field of vision on a daily basis; anything to remind you to say it and believe it.

Control Panel Technique for Balance and Grace

Close your eyes. Look up at the imaginary spot in the center of your forehead where insight occurs in your brain. Conceive of yourself behind the wheel of the vehicle you most want in the world. A driving teacher sits next to you to help with the controls. You are now driving across a narrow floating bridge.

A half-circle gauge with the numbers one through twelve on its face dominates the control panel behind the wheel. See what number the red indicator arrow registers. Now ask the teacher to help you get the arrow to point to six in the center (your point of balance). Take your time doing this. When you feel completely balanced, thank the teacher for his or her help. Then open your eyes.

Take a drink of pure water to toast the health of your new body. Practice the control panel technique as often as you want so you can learn balance from the inside out. Balance is the key that opens the lock to the door of freedom.

When you accept and fully realize the attributes of forgiveness, gratitude and grace and make them your own, your heart will open wide like a river delta flowing to the sea. What an incredible feeling!

Attaining Freedom—The Next Step on Your Journey

I know part of the reason you are reading this book is because you want to feel better while you balance your life and weight. But you'll find at this point in the journey that the adventure is just beginning on a much different level. In Chapter 25, discover how accepting self-responsibility and fostering self-love can empower you to cross the threshold to freedom.

Chapter 25

Spiritual Laws of Consciousness, Self-Responsibility and Self-Love

Learning To Be Free—The Next Step on Your Journey

By this time, you have progressed far in your journey toward weight balance. The following testimonials paint a picture of the before-and-after change of consciousness that occurs when you actively apply the principles outlined in this book. See if you can find the steps of realization, adjustment, and subsequent change to a higher level of consciousness in these stories of personal success.

"When I was in college, I dealt with the pressure of papers and exams by getting a pizza, a pint of chocolate ice cream, and a bag of cookies, eating them all and then writing or studying like a maniac all night.

"As a result, my weight constantly fluctuated. I'd put on ten or more pounds from bingeing, then starve myself to take it off fast, then put it on again. Thank goodness this pattern slowed down and took a turn for the better when I realized that pigging out wouldn't ease my real world work stress. Once I admitted that binges didn't do much for me in my life now, they were easier to let go. I found other ways to relieve stress." - Jennifer, 30

"I used to have chocolate kisses on the counter, just to welcome customers. Candy wasn't my weakness, but pretty soon I became a social nibbler, grabbing a kiss with a customer every time we chatted about a printing job. "I stopped doing this one day when a friend who was having problems with her husband came by four or five times to vent. By the end of the day, we had emptied the entire bowl of kisses.

"I went home that evening with a gross, sugar and fat feeling in my mouth and stomach. That gross sugar feeling woke me up to how much

I ate while gabbing and made me think about all the food I unconsciously pop into my mouth at social gatherings (such as peanuts at bars and chips at parties). Through hypnosis I've made a point to be careful about what I pop into my mouth when I'm listening to others."- Heather, 26

"By the time I get home from work and all the stress there, it's 6:30 p.m. I'm exhausted and starving. I used to throw my stuff down and head to the kitchen, grabbing this and that—leftover noodles, cold cuts, bread— and eat as if I was inhaling them. But then one day, with a mouthful of granola, I thought, 'I don't want to eat this stuff. Why am I doing this?' I realized that frenzied snacking or shoveling it in was my way of releasing the stress of the day.
"Now I stay out of the kitchen until I calm down by using techniques that relieve my emotional stress. I take some time to figure out what I want to eat. That usually gets me eating healthier meals and has led to a better body weight." - Susan, 49

"My husband and I travel in our recreational vehicle while he writes books and consults with financial institutions. I don't particularly like accompanying him under these conditions. I realized that my resentments toward my husband were about giving up my previous way of life. lSacrificing everything to accommodate his second career caused me me to feel rejected, angry, and hurt. It was only when I began to appreciate myself and renew my past interests that I found the metabolic menus started working and my weight began to come off." -Fran, 60

"I learned to feel my anger by letting go of stubbornness. That was hard to do, but I did it. Before I'd just yell, hold on to the anger, and feel really guilty afterwards. Next I'd blame my parents or step-mom. Or I'd be sarcastic and make everything worse. When I stopped yelling and began talking about what was wrong, I found I felt better about me. That's when my eating balanced and I gave up purging." - Brittany, 16

"Every avenue I went down seemed blocked. All the people I knew were stuck in the past. I stayed home and ate out of loneliness. Then I learned to face my fear of people rejecting me. I practiced speaking up for my needs and wants. As I did this, I began to have more energy. I even tried new things, starting with having a cup of coffee at a Victorian tea room. Eventually, I began a yoga class and dance lessons. My weight gradually slimmed down. I feel like a new person." - Mary, 72

Julie learned to love herself by taking time to make different, healthy food choices. Heather made unconscious snacking habits conscious in order to stop them. Jennifer dealt with stress realistically and found it easier to quit engaging in cycles of bingeing and dieting.

Fran reconnected with her true inner self and gracefully gave up resentments toward her husband. When she did, her weight balanced naturally. Brittany found inner coping skills that helped her process intense emotions. As a result, she balanced her weight *and* stopped her purging behavior.

Mary committed to face her fear of rejection, which led to having more fun in life as she became a slimmer woman of balance. These stories share real life ways you too can overcome stumbling blocks that keep you from reaching your weight balance goals.

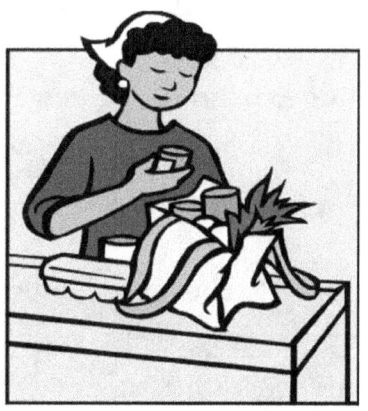

Choose to Eat Healthy

See How Far You've Come (What You've Achieved So Far)

I invite you to once again be aware of all the changes and the results, large and small, that you have attained so far. Feel good about your progress. By choosing to feel good about each change (and not wanting your whole body to transform magically in three weeks), you are on your way to a new body, a new state of consciousness, and loving it. I invite you to keep going for more. By reviewing your progress in this way, you'll be surprised to find your new body shifting each step along the way.

What the Techniques in This Chapter Will Do for You

The specific skill you'll glean from this chapter is a feeling of clarity in connection with your body image. The clearer you are, the more successful you'll become with manifesting your new body image. The insights you'll gain from this chapter will leave you feeling uplifted and calm. You'll be able to choose and manifest what you want in your life more each day.

Being in the Present Right Now

We all have ancestors. Last year's "you" could be your ancestor. However, because it is the past, it exists in memories. Only the present exists now. All else is irrational because the past does not exist for you now. Declare yourself alive and growing. Choose to be aware of endlessly giving birth to yourself in new and better ways.

An example of the need to continually expand into a newer state of being is illustrated in the following parable about seeing beyond your comfort zone. It is excerpted from Karen La Puma's book, *Awakening Female Power*.

Once upon a time, a frog lived in a deep well. She loved her home. It felt safe and secure and it was all she had ever known. She knew every corner, every crack, and every cranny of the well. One of her favorite things was to share what she knew about her well with others.

One day a sailor fetched water from the well. When he lowered the bucket, a curious thing jumped out and made a huge splash. With surprise, the well frog watched as the thing climbed onto the rock upon which she was sitting. It was another frog.

"Where did you come from?" asked the startled well frog.

"I came from a place far away, near a large body of water called the ocean."

"Oh! Is it this large?" the well frog asked, as she jumped to another rock across the well.

"No, it's really huge. Very big," answered the ocean frog.

The well frog thought *that* could not be true. That's wrong, she thought in total denial. She puffed herself up and used all her energy to jump from the rock all the way across to the wall of the well. With pride she announced, "Well, it can't be any bigger than this!"

The well frog limited her state of consciousness to what was known and familiar to her based on her past experience. She also got caught in the trap of vanity that her perspective about reality was *the* one and only right perspective.

Seeing from the Viewpoint of Soul

When we see with a more omniscient viewpoint (as the observer of life or Soul), then we see that the mind merely has likes and dislikes, without perceiving any "rights" or "wrongs" about a situation. A more Soul-oriented viewpoint can assist us in letting go of the past (even though it may be safe and familiar) to allow a larger and better view of what's possible to unfold before us.

Only by letting go of limiting past beliefs can we learn to discriminate and decide what is *best for the whole* in our purpose and goals. Holding the viewpoint of *what is best for the whole* helps us gain a larger awareness that *we* are part of a larger whole. Trusting this awareness allows us to begin to feel more complete within the entire universe and ourselves. Feeling complete also helps guide your actions effortlessly toward balancing your diet or eating style in a way that's naturally attuned to what's best for your whole body.

Learning Spiritual Intelligence

The key to weight balance depends on gaining a certain amount of spiritual intelligence that's based on how much control *you*, as Soul, have over your mind. When you learn and apply weight balance secrets for success, you're working with the Creative Force, which can be called your higher Power, God, or any term you might use for the Divine.

Like the well frog, first we are trapped into believing our will or mind knows the only truth. Though we're secure in this knowledge, a much larger truth awaits discovery. The many techniques offered in this book give you the choice of experiencing a larger awareness in your quest for weight balance success. This larger awareness is balance.

You can choose to progress in spiritual intelligence by making a choice statement, such as, "I choose to be creative in reaching my goals." Then follow it with an appropriate action so your mind knows that you are serious.

Telling the Story of Your Life

What universal truth about human nature is presented here? The truth is this: The conscious and unconscious choices, and the ultimate actions you take based on them, results in telling the story of your life.

As this book revealed in Chapter 23, everything that's happening to you at this present moment is a result of choices (conscious as well as unconscious) made in the past. Every choice that you make *now* generates your future. Why not write your life story in your journal and discover ways you can begin to make more self-empowered choices for your health and new body, for yourself now and for future generations?

Self-responsibility Is the First Step to Grasping Change

One of the most crucial universal truths contained in this book is accepting responsibility. I know you've heard this with your ears and mind previously. Can you now hear this universal truth with your heart?

When we accept responsibility for the circumstances we face in the events that occur in our lives, *without blaming others or ourselves,* we change the perception of illusion in our lives forever. Taking responsibilty is the first step to viewing all the "terrible situations" in life as opportunities to create something wonderful.

The More Self-Responsibility You Accept, the More Freedom You'll Have

Accepting self-responsibility is acknowledging and accepting truth for yourself. Acknowledging truth and freeing yourself from the quagmire of illusion is one way to show more love for yourself.

Do you remember how it felt to be caught in illusion? Remember believing that you had to be this size or that? Remember the limitations on your life when you perceived that doing something for yourself meant depriving or hurting someone else? Remember how self-defeating and constraining the illusion of "dieting will work this time" was? As you know, these illusions are hypnotic traps of preoccupation for the mind and ego. Choosing a persistent path *away* from illusion can lead you toward more success and more open doorways to weight balance.

Illusion-Busting Technique

(1) *Close your eyes and look upward at the insight area of your brain while connecting to your Higher Power. Imagine your Higher Power in front of you.*

(2) *Chant a word that means love while asking to perceive an insight that is true and helpful to your unfoldment as Soul right now. Do this for about five to ten minutes, then fall into silent contemplation.*

(3) *Listen for an answer from your Higher Power. When you are ready, open your eyes and write down what you perceived.*

A Tale of Self-responsibility in Action

A patient named Michelle felt stagnant in her life. She had trouble applying all she had learned about empowering herself toward improving her life. She was on the verge of making a major decision about marrying the man she had been dating for the past two years.

After seven weeks of gathering information and having experiences that showed her what she needed to know to make the decision, I asked, "What do you feel in your gut?"

"I'm not happy in this relationship," she said. "What do you want to do about it?" I asked.

"I want to avoid facing this and talking to him. Yet, I know talking to him is what I most need to do," she admitted.

"How is this the best course of action for you?"

"If I keep avoiding, it will eat at me. I'll end up compulsively eating just to numb out and make my mind be still," she explained.

"What could you do about that?"

"Face it and get it over with," she said firmly. "I will talk to him soon."

Michelle knew that it was time to move on from the relationship. She took responsibility for herself and her actions to get what she wanted from the relationship, not settling for less. She used patience up to this point in time, allowing the situation to show her if this was truly what she wanted in a relationship. Michelle realized she could not change her boyfriend; she could only take responsibility for herself.

Michelle discovered that she felt burdened in her thoughts and emotions. She was stuck in her own past pattern of fearing guilt about hurting someone else's feelings. She became a victim of her own fears.

The opposite of the "poor me, victim consciousness" is taking action and responsibility for what you want in life. The choice is to turn the situation into an opportunity to grow and learn or wallow in a victim consciousness.

Did Michelle take the responsibility and stand up for her truth? Yes, she did; and because she resolved the underlying conflict within herself, her self-esteem was boosted as well as her motivation to keep her food intake balanced.

Like a River Flowing Freely to the Sea

The following four steps will help you with the challenge to accept more self-responsibility for your life.

(1) *Begin by simply writing the following statement in your journal fifteen times times daily until it happens: "Please, Higher Power show me how to accept responsibility. Thank you."*

(2) *Be aware that answers can come in many ways. Journal about them when they appear in contemplation or your daily life.*

(3) *Contemplate the answers. Journal the highest spiritual insights from your contemplations.*

(4) *Repeat these three steps as often as necessary, until you attain results. Remember, accepting self-responsibility is one way to love yourself more.*

Planting Seeds of Love and Acceptance

This one is simple since the previous techniques have prepared the ground. Now is the time to plant seeds as you persevere and trust your process. The following fable illustrates how a lack of perseverance with patience can be a downfall.

A farmer was too eager for harvest and wanted to help his crops grow. In the middle of the night he went outside and pulled on the new shoots, compromising the health of his crop. In other words, he tried to "push the river."

This attitude of trying to push the river is as error ridden as trying to hurry a harvest and trying to rush to your goals. You can't hasten the goal of shaping your body. Everything happens in good time, so connect with patience. Be aware your own process has its own season and flow, which can lead to harvesting self-esteem and acceptance of your body image.

Plant seeds by writing the following positive statement fifteen times a day for four weeks: "I love and approve of myself." New sprouts of inner self-esteem link to higher consciousness. With a higher state of awareness comes a degree of perception and clarity beyond description.

Freedom from Illusion

A woman named Rebecca has two sisters. One sister is older than Rebecca and one is younger. Both sisters are large women. Rebecca says, "Even my aunts and grandmother are large women. I'm the only one in my family who is tiny."

Rebecca never talks about her weight because it isn't a problem to her. She feels there are other areas of her life that need attention, such as stress at work or stress with her spouse.

You might think that Rebecca is tiny because of what she says and believes. She has no anguish about her size or weight. In fact, she also says that her breasts are perfect. Rebecca is a size fourteen.

Rebecca is free in this area of her life—free of the illusion that she has to worry about her weight. She is free to be who she is, free to be happy with herself.

Reconciling the Conflicting Images of Woman

The book *Return of the Great Goddess* edited by Burleigh Muten scans the past hundred years for the archeological discoveries of more than one thousand artifacts of female icons. These icons, dating from circa 30,000 to 9000 B.C., confirm the sociological relevance of the Great Goddess. For twenty thousand years, the Great Goddess was acknowledged in myth and revered in religious imagination. The results of many archeological digs found coal, bone, and stone females with great egg-shaped bellies, breasts, and buttocks. All showed the fullness of the creative impulse as manifested in the human female form.

It is an art to develop healthy self-esteem in today's world of denigration of the normal feminine form. Each person on an individualized level can resolve these social prejudices.

When you choose to resolve the constraining social roles about women, you learn to let go of the staid, conventional, socially limiting restrictions of what-it-is-to-be-a-woman. You then enter the unknown, an often misunderstood, scary time. Yet, the unknown can be a time of great discovery and personal affirmation an exciting, dynamic time when you never felt so fully alive.

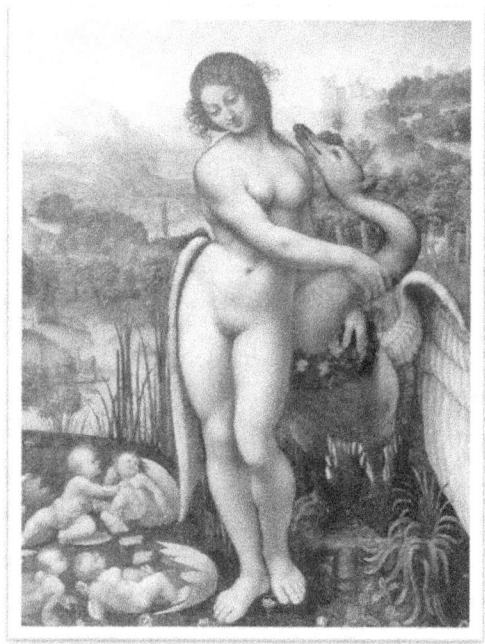

Visit a Museum Technique

The introverted fear of female fat creeps along, infiltrating our culture in as much the same way as a cold war or hate campaign might. This cultural brainwashing can easily get mistranslated into hate against our female bodies. By merely exposing ourselves to cultural beliefs, often we unknowingly allow more of the prejudices (than we'd like to accept) to interject themselves into our psyches and ultimately the fabric of our lives.

My purpose here is to open up different, wider viewpoints so that you can be more aware of how you might respond alternatively when you let go of reacting subconsciously to the beauty myths in culture today.

I began a quest to find full-figured models in history to counter the petite myth and bought a book called *Myths of Greece and Rome*, by Bryan

Holme. I was fascinated by the illustrations, many of which portrayed the female form in lush flesh and soft, flowing lines. One called "Leda and the Swan" by Leonardo da Vinci shows the fullness of the female body in all its beauty as Leda caresses the swan. These pictures soothe my eyes into accepting a more alluring, voluptuous female form.

A feeling of peacefulness envelops me while I view this picture. I feel completeness as I view the true spirit of womanhood embodied in flesh. How refreshing.

Check out any similar book from the library or visit a museum where paintings of the Old Masters are shown. Even good prints of their work will do to help you reestablish a healthy regard for the feminine form (like Rebecca has).

You, too, can develop a healthy self-esteem, free from the constraints of the pressures of our culture. Freeing yourself from false images ultimately leads to the path of empowerment.

What Is Empowerment?

The view of empowerment according to Hippocrates, the father of medicine, is that nothing else produces joys, delights, laughter, grief, and despondency but the brain. Yet in Persian culture, the legendary Persian physician Avicenna(A.D. 980-1037) said the imagination not only acts on one's own body but also other's bodies at great distances. (Persian philosophy believes that thoughts are real and can reach out to influence realms beyond this one.)

I say take the best of both worlds; use your mind and imagination to influence your reality and change your world. Empowerment begins with cutting through the illusions. Yet, most of us need structure and form. You may have been out of control with your eating in the past. Or you may have been so in control that you were overly controlling of everything. Either scenario is out of balance with the natural flow of the universe.

Empowerment is finding what balance means in your life by taking responsibility for your own thoughts, feelings, and actions.

Tools to Help You Empower Yourself

The following technique will help increase your self-esteem and love for your true Self (as in self-caring, not selfish). When you love yourself, then you can truly give to others from the space of an open heart. Holding an open heart with higher consciousness leads to weight balance success.

Empowerment Technique

(1) Close your eyes and look upward to the insight area of your brain. Conceive of a beautiful sound and then a favorite color.

(2) Gently remember a time when you had an experience of valuing what was inside of you as true riches. Be aware that your heart is open now. How is this for you? How do you feel when your heart is open? Write this down in your journal.

Truth is freedom. When you choose to accept truth as what is and start taking steps toward where you want to go, you will achieve success. Be present, sincere, and trust your process.

Centering with Beauty and Stillness

We, as women, dream and walk our path of fullness and beauty. I have found that many spiritual answers, such as how to center and find stillness, are found by being aware of practical, down to earth matters.

You may think of traveling far in order to meet a diet guru and receive enlightenment. Yet the temple of true knowledge is within. Remember, nothing outside of you gives freedom. Only the journey within nourishes freedom. The following parable illustrates this principle of valuing the journey within.

> *In ancient times, at the beginning of the cosmos and the universes, God decided that Soul was so precious It needed to be hidden somewhere safe. So God hid It in the heart of all humans because no one would think to look for it there.*

The operative word here is "think." Intellectualizing removes you from the heart center. Centering in the beauty of the heart is where all true motivation exists.

Breathing Free as a New Baby's Breath

Through active participation, learn how your breath can help you get a second wind, gain motivation, or renew your purpose. Try this from the unique point of view of recognizing yourself as the spiritual being that you are. As a spiritual being, you have one experience after another. All you need to do is take one step deeper into your experiences, let go of old feelings and thoughts, and be aware. You were born with the ability to use your energies in free flowing ways. You were born to breathe freely, enjoy life and make the most of it.

A Breathing Exercise for Feeling Free

Wherever you are, whenever you feel tense all over, close your eyes and imagine your favorite place on earth. As you inhale, see this safe place. And you exhale, see yourself completely relaxed in this place. Smell the air.

Hear the sounds around you. Reach out and touch something near you and describe the feeling to yourself.

Feel your breath enter your nose, flow down your windpipe and into your chest. Let your abdomen expand with the energy of your energy of your breath. Feel this life process as a mystery that renews you constantly without effort. Simply be aware of your breath. To relax and touch base with feeling free, practice this technique at least once a day.

Making Freedom Happen by (Fill-in-the-Blank) Technique

In the following exercise, just let the first thing you think of pop into your mind. No second-guessing! Then write your answers to the questions in your journal. This exercise can also be shared and done with a close friend. Prepare to be surprised by the wisdom that's revealed.

(1) Remember the most favorite activity you ever experienced. Close your eyes for a minute and recall the episode and expect perfect memory. Let the images and sensations associated with this experience flow into your mind. Describe the event by writing the details, beginning with the words, "I was .....".

(2) Gently remember the most loving feelings you ever experienced. Close your eyes and allow the memory to come to mind. It might have revolved around someone you loved, a beloved pet, or an activity? Close your eyes and remember what your heart felt like when you loved. After opening your eyes, describe how it was for you in writing, starting with the words, "I remember loving . . ."

(3) Close your eyes and remember joyfully and successfully accomplishing something after a time of learning and practicing. Write about what you accomplished and the feelings that accompanied your success. Begin with "I accomplished ...." or "When I accomplished plished ____ I felt . . . I heard . . . I remember seeing . . ."

(4) Remember a time when you were in trouble. How did you figure a way out of it? Remember other ways you may have used your creative power to get free of trouble at other times in your life. Write about your memories.

What unique outlook helped you overcome adversity? What did you say and do? You can use this memory exercise anytime you need to tap your creative depths and become more free from the troubles you perceive are binding you.

The Choice of Where to Go Is Always Determined by You

Many techniques in this book give you ways to strengthen yourself to meet the challenges of life and the situations in which you find yourself now. These techniques can help you choose new and different ways to reach and sustain your peak, bringing good health, weight balance success, happiness, and prosperity into your life or not. It's your choice. It's a matter of understanding where you are now and choosing to move beyond the present by placing your attention and focusing your efforts on where you want to be.

Understanding the Mystery and Paradigm of Cycles

Knowing how cycles work in your life is a precious pearl of truth. Like the pearl, it's also a symbol of the deep mysteries of life. You can learn a great deal by studying the cycles of nature that affect individuals, family units, nation groups, and races.

The fluctuating cycles of human life work within the parameters of universal laws. The cycles of birth and death, day and night, sleeping and waking, the four seasons of the year, the four periods of human drama (birth, growth, youth, and old age) are some of the most common human cycles.

Human life cycles can be diminished through ignorance of the universal laws. For example, longevity can be destroyed through vice and debauchery, leading to a downgraded state of health and diminished success in life. Anyone who is low in mental or physical health is at greater risk to succumbing to vice, a complication of the downward spiral.

Successfully rejuvenating the body and living healthily to an advanced age relies on proper nutrition (sometimes by supplementing with a regimen of vitamins and minerals), proper exercise, and good self-esteem. If you alter your diet or activity level, your aging process will change along with your weight balance. By halting or reversing the aging of glands (especially the pituitary gland), you'll begin to feel your cycles changing toward youth again.

To have youth and weight balance success, you must have empowerment and imagination, using both to secure a place in this world. It's all a matter of being clear on what direction you choose and focusing your attention and efforts on which way you want to go.

Understanding Your Personal Cycles Technique

Try the following exercise to better *Understand Your Personal Cycles*. Answer all the questions, then ask, "How can I understand the cycle I am in right now? What could strengthen my awareness and help me choose to ascend, wherever I am in my cycle?"

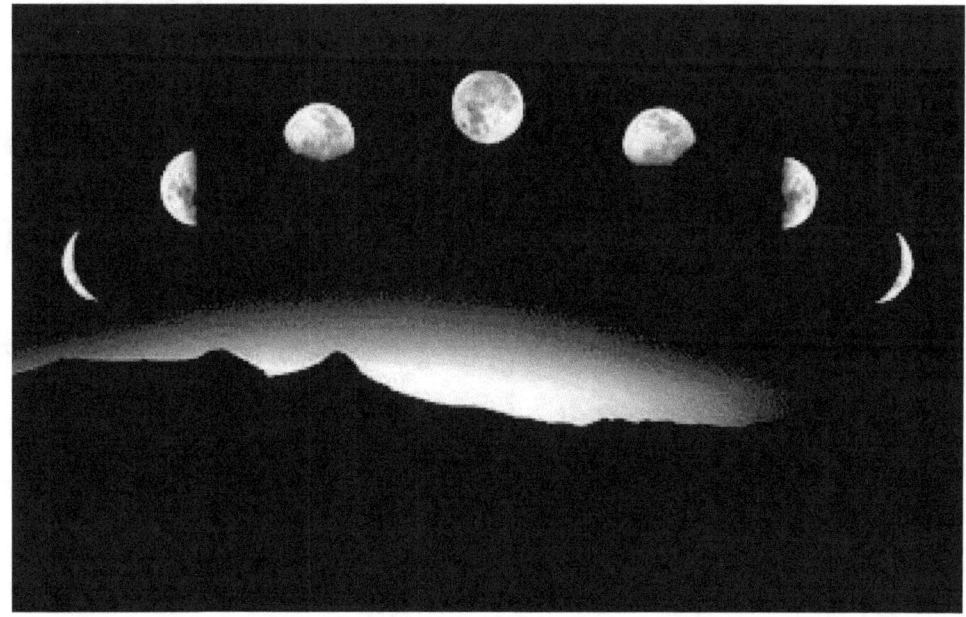

Understanding Your Personal Cycles

(1) Follow the timeline and mark a red "X" on where you are now.

Birth and Growth

1-2-3-4-5-6
*　　7-8-9-10-11-12*
*　　　13-14-15-16-17-18*
*　　　　19-20-21-22-23-24 (4 cycles of 6 years each)*

Youth

25-26-27-28-29-30
*　　31-32-33-34-35-36*
*　　　37-38-39-40-41-42*
*　　　　43-44-45-46-47-48*
*　　　　　49-50-51-52-53-54*
*　　　　　　55-56-57-58-59-60 (6 cycles of 6 years each)*

Old Age

61-62-63-64-65-66
*　　67-68-69-70-71-72*
*　　　73-74-75-76-77-78*
*　　　　79-80-81-82-83-84*
*　　　　　85-86-87-88-89-90*
*　　　　　　91-92-93-94-95-96 (6 cycles, 6 years each)*

(2) Now write a list of significant life events in your journal. Be sure to write the date and how old you were at the time.

(3) Take a yellow highlighting pen and put an "X" on the timeline where a significant event occurred, such as getting married, the birth of a child, deaths, graduations, a residential move, and different diets. Notice the cycles. Mark the major turning points in your life. Ask yourself about your possible life patterns. Do you see a pattern of two-, three-, four-, six-, or twelve-year cycles? This doesn't have to be exact, just approximate. Trust what you see as your cycle of change.

(4) Ask God or Your Higher Power for insight and wisdom on what there is for you to learn about your cycles.

(5) Take notes about the insights you receive. There's no right or wrong way to do this exercise.

Now that you know where you are in your cycles, you can see that taking one step at a time starting now can bring you to the top of this cycle in the best health and weight balance. Start good habits now and you can build them into the cycles that follow as shown in the above timeline.

Knowledge of cycles can help with your awareness of life and nutrition, keeping you growing on the positive side of the loop. All this renews body, mind, and spirit for a longer, happier, more fulfilled life.

What Is Diet Success?

My answer to this question comes from more than forty-three years of struggling with disordered eating and over seventeen years of clinical work with others *plus* fifteen years of counseling in choosing nutritionally dense foods for excellent health.

> *Diet success is a choice you make daily by being willing to keep taking the steps outlined in this book. Releasing doubts, anger, cynicism, and hostility for the personal experience of what it truly means to be free insures that you'll never be the same again.*

Through reading this book, you've found ways to continually love, encourage, and trust yourself on the path of a healthy eating style. Practicing these principles daily is a habit, a discipline, but above all else, an art form.

Life Beyond Diet Success

This book has given you a taste of how much more life has to offer through its keys to accessing the wealth of your experiences. Maybe you've glimpsed insights and a vision of the personal freedom that can be yours if you continue to evolve in consciousness by (1) asking questions, (2) taking steps forward after receiving the answers, and (3) finding support systems that continue to help you evolve even more.

The Cornerstone in the Foundation of Your Success

I believe trust in yourself is *the* major cornerstone in the foundation of your success. With honesty and trust, you can continue your process of unfoldment, gaining greater spiritual insights and new revelations as discoveries on this journey of life reveal the richness of you. For more on the journey of discovery that waits beyond maintaining the new you, turn to Chapter 26.

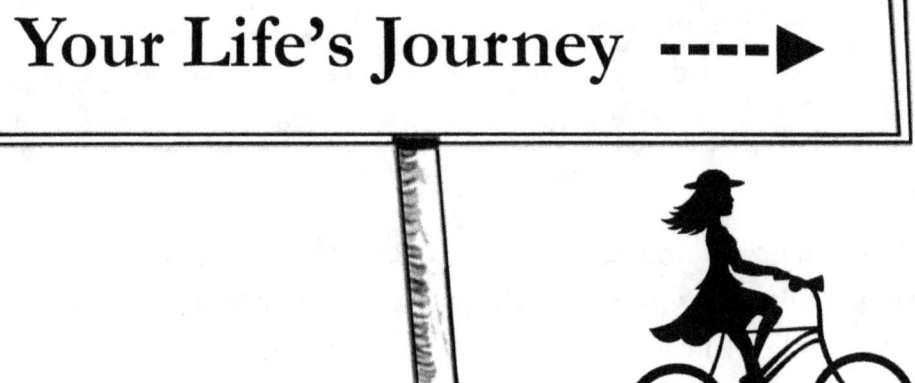

Chapter 26

Your Journey Beyond

Living a Life of Health, Balance, and Freedom – Now and in the Future

Can you connect with the present day feeling that there's more to life? From your experiences throughout this book, I hope you've not only seen but also proven to yourself that there's much more than you previously expected.

Think about your state of mind at the beginning of this book. At that time you might have connected with the concept that life isn't giving you enough. In your quest to get enough, you may have struggled for more control over food through dieting, bingeing, or purging. Or you might have indulged in excessive shopping or overconsumption in any form. These are natural recourses to turn to (and act out) in an effort to fill the void we perceive in our lives.

> *When you choose to poke the spiritual fire within (as you have done by reading and practicing the techniques throughout this book), you always gain much more—more health and more freedom to be who you've always wanted to be.*

Keys for Maintaining the New You

The keys for maintaining the new you are more attitudinal than anything else. First and foremost, know that you are a shining essence of Divine Spirit—Soul.

Souls who shine brightest find ways to give back to the world from the essence of their new selves through their work and creatively through what they have to offer the world. Once you've incorporated what you've received from Divine Spirit, the natural course of an aware Soul is to serve others. The ways in which you choose to serve the world through your work and your creativity also help you grow further in mastery of the principles found in this book.

The Six Steps of Mastery for Making Your Dreams Come True

Your strength as Soul is awesome, considering you use the creativity, potential, and mastery of Soul and the Holy Spirit to realize and live your dreams. What are the six steps to mastery? Let's review the reciprocal relationship that occurs between you and Divine Spirit when you decide to transform your life and manifest your dreams.

The first thing is to (1) *ask* for what you want to receive. Divine Spirit then opens opportunities so that (2) you can *take action*. Taking action is *the* sign Spirit needs before giving you more opportunities, and (3) a *grateful heart* keeps you open to receive more. When Spirit gives you even more, it's time for (4) *imagining* even more of your dream and (5) *surrendering* the outcome to Spirit by allowing It to work on Its timetable. Last comes (6) time to *rest and review* through contemplation. Remember to be grateful by thanking your Higher Power, Divine Spirit, and God daily (blessings flow moreeasily to a grateful heart). Then you (with the assistance of your Higher Power) can start the cycle all over again.

The rest of this chapter is devoted to exploring what it takes to live your dreams. Let's begin by checking in with your purpose statement and your present state of being. The power to experience and manifest your dreams is not in yesterday or tomorrow, but only in today because Soul lives in the present moment.

Checking In with Your Current Purpose Statement Technique

Please restate your current purpose statement.

My purpose is _____.

Has your purpose statement changed since the beginning of the book? What part of it changed? Maybe your purpose statement changed many times throughout this book. The changes may be subtle or conspicuous.

Regarding the subtle changes: What can you do to honor the shifts of awareness that you have experienced already? The subtlest changes are the ones that best help you maintain your balance so moving forward becomes effortless. The knowing, aware Soul learns to pause, acknowledge, and value these changes. Pat yourself on the back if you picked out subtle changes in your progress and purpose statement. Chronicle these changes in your journal.

If you can't find subtle or obvious changes, please take heart. Often the harder we try at something, the worse it gets. Actually trying too hard can reverse your effort with a pile up of forced energy, like a car pile up on a major highway. Be willing to let go and flow into what's next for your purpose. Expending the effort to do this is ultimately worth it. We'll explore how to fine tune a future purpose statement later in this chapter.

Visualization: Fuel for Your Body in Your New Future

Hold on to your seats; this is your captain speaking. We're going for the ride of our lives. We are now landing in a country unlike any you've ever known. Some things may appear familiar, yet be prepared for the unusual. The natives are friendly, gentle, and calm with an imperceptible glow about them that you will love and want to make your own.

As you step off the plane, walk down a plush carpet thick with rose petals strewn by our native hosts. The perfume of the flowers is aromatic. Imagine a tall blonde woman or a man with curly, brown hair approaches and offers you a soma drink. Your escort then leads you to a private patio where others are seated at round tables, talking and laughing together.

As you sip your drink, it gently wipes out all memory of processed foods of any kind. You lean over to ask other guests, "Have you ever tasted or experienced anything like this before?"

"No," they answer. You'd like to have a private supply of this in your home.

Soft flute music wafts through the air as the musicians arrive. They manifest as beings of shimmering light. Their faces glow with great light while you're in their presence. Listening to the flute feels so light and blissful. It's like no other feeling you've ever had. In fact, you want this feeling to last forever.

As you continue sipping the soma drink, you feel the wind caress your arms and face like the stroking of a thousand velvet fingertips. Your escort invites several others to join you for dinner. The menu is illuminated under the glass tabletop. It's made of a filmy airy material that changes as as you read it. The waiter explains that the menu responds to your brain waves. It is activated by and aligned to your individual body chemistry via sensors in your chair. The dishes are named to excite you, as if your body, mind, and spirit are responding in a symphony of harmony.

You glance at the others and smile, wondering, what could this lead to in my life? An answer will come. You know the answer will come to you, either in your dreams or waking dreams.

Using Dream Time for Your Future Endeavors

Throughout this book I've used stories from dreams and other sources to help prompt you to gain awareness and a sense of adventure. Dream time can become a part of your life that is effortless. You can use it to get answers about everything from what foods are right for your body today to what course of action is best for your life tomorrow.

When I first started writing my dreams, I was hostile and often frustrated. I wanted answers right now. Yet for years the answers eluded me. All the while I had many exciting times in my dreams.

Some people might look at these exciting dreams as nightmares, but now I see them as challenges that filled my life with mysteries waiting to be solved. It took a few years of working with dreams and the assistance of my Higher Power before they began to take on an adventurous quality though. By choosing to see my dream experiences in this way, I learned how to ask good questions to get answers about my future. Sound easy? It is. Here's how.

Mocking Up Desire for Dreams of the Future

The first thing you need is desire. Mock up a strong desire.

If you can't do that, then remember a time when you felt excited. Get into that exciting memory and let it just pop into your mind. Relive the memory as best you can. Be there now. Describe it to yourself out loud in a little story. Get into the feelings and fully experience the excitement surrounding that memory.

Ask yourself, "Where do I feel this excitement in my body?" No second-guessing! Let the first thing pop into your mind.

Then ask, "What color is this excitement? What shape is this excitement?" Let the answers pop into your mind, even if they don't make sense. Do it even though you might feel silly. These feelings are okay. Go through them and go with them.

If you still feel a part of yourself wants you to stop, see it for what it is. That judging part of you will usually find fault with everything. If you find yourself thinking, "Oh, that's not going to work," then stop and take a few deep breaths. Ask your Higher Power to help you adjust the negative reaction right now.

Then take this tangible memory of excitement and say out loud "I want to remember my dreams of the future." Say it with passion and write it in your journal. Keep your journal by your bed and use it to record what you dream.

The Prime Obstacle to Recording Your Dreams

If you say, "Oh, I'll write it down later," you'll discover that the dream often disappears when you're ready to record it. As soon as you make a new habit (such as writing down your future dreams), remember to mock up desire for the results that you seek. As the new behavior becomes automatic, you'll continue to follow through with it. The more you practice it, the easier it becomes until it is as automatic as breathing. Then the subconscious takes over with little effort.

> *Remember, if you think you can, you can! If you think you can't, you can't. Either way you are right. That's the power of the mind.*

Choose to train your mind to think you can and it will happen.

Keys to Using Dream Time for Your Future Advantage

Use your dream time for your future advantage by *first* training yourself to effortlessly remember your dreams. *Second,* learn to record your dreams when you first become conscious, upon awakening each morning. *Third,* after several weeks begin to write questions you want answered in your dream journal. This works best if you ask one question at a time and wait for as long as it takes to receive the answer.

Asking too many questions at once can overwhelm you and lead to confusing insights. Feel free to keep asking the same question for weeks. I often ask a question for months because some core questions need that much time to reveal their answers to you. Other insights may come within a few days. I choose to be surprised and amused by the process, instead of trying to dictate or control it in any way.

The Wisdom of Your Inner Voice Found in Dreams

Use the above "dream time asking technique" to find what foods are good for your body. Or alter the questions to find out answers about your future and your life (as I did in the questions that follow in the parentheses). Expect to be surprised by the answers!

(1) What foods do I need to eat today? (What direction do I need to go with my life?)

(2) What is best for my body? (What is best for my future?)

(3) Show me what to add to my food plan. (Show me what priorities to add to my life.)

(4) What food can I learn to let go of eating? (Which activities can I release or say "no" to?)

(5) Show me what to do for balanced eating. (Show me what to do for a future of health, freedom, and love.)

Feel free to ask to be shown more than you need to know. Be sure to thank your Higher Power for helping you with these insights.

Keys to Discovering and Understanding Your Small Inner Voice

> *Prepare yourself to be open to the prompting of Divine Spirit through your small inner voice by exploring the following questions.*

Write down the answers to these questions in your journal after contemplating upon them with your Higher Power.

(1) What abilities do I need to develop to understand my inner voice?

(2) What new strength do I want to take form that I can apply to understanding my small inner voice?

Consciously Listening to Your Inner Voice to Find the Next Step

One way to learn to listen to your inner voice is to journal both your waking dreams and sleeping ones. Jot down clues or symbols as they appear in your dreams or life each day.

When I wrote the first question from the above exercise in my journal, I woke up the next morning and heard my inner voice say, "Explore the love of learning."

I was tempted to minimize what I heard by simply forgetting. My actions clearly illustrated that in my grogginess (that state between waking and sleeping) I was beginning to forget how precious the gift of awareness is. I almost seemed willing to compromise my quest for inner truth for the habit of mental laziness.

Instead, I chose to combat the laziness I felt. I asked, "What new strength do I want to take form as I explore the love of learning?"

I decided one way to get the answer to this question on a cellular level was by writing a core statement fifteen times every day. I wrote it until it eventually manifested in my life. It turned out to be an effective exercise for me to overcome a lazy brain. The statement I wrote fifteen times a day that I needed to know with my whole heart was I am appreciated.

Further into the process I asked in my journal, "What value can I receive from this experience?" My small inner voice whispered, "Freedom."

Freedom implies full knowledge of you. Freedom, like love, can not be erased. Both are states of higher consciousness. Moments of giving and receiving love, like freedom, live in your heart forever.

Warnings from Your Small Inner Voice

Your small inner voice may remind or warn you about ways the negative habits of the mind will try to trip you on your journey to greater awareness, as my mind attempted to do in the above example.

Instead of becoming caught up in a *feedback loop* of blame, shame or retribution against yourself, choose to value what you've learned from the experience. Let go of any self-punishing thoughts or emotions that revolve around your initial reactions to the challenges that face you. When you find yourself starting to spin into a feedback loop, write answers to the following questions in your journal.

(1) What emotions have I navigated so far?

(2) What feelings am I willing to take charge of?

(3) How will I do it and continue to accept the keys of freedom (from my Higher Power and my small inner voice) as they are given to me?

Keeping Your Connection Open

Throughout this book, I asked you to interact with the material by engaging in writing techniques, visualizations and exercises. From the process of reading and experiencing this book, you've grown strong and flexible; emotionally, physically and mentally. This chapter explores what it means to develop that same level of strength and flexibility spiritually, in preparation of your next adventure.

To keep your spiritual connection open, try practicing the techniques given in this chapter for five, ten, or twenty minutes a day. It's easy and brief. You may not be aware of changes right away, but that's not important. What *is* important is to trust and keep your connection to Divine Spirit open, to become stronger spiritually by developing "spiritual muscle" in as much the same way that you develop physical muscle to stay fit.

The Spiritual Quality of Doing without Doing

Have you ever found yourself engaged in a long involved process for work? Many times we daydream as we work by routine or habit and enter into another state of consciousness. Could you remember every part of the task? No. You put your body in motion and then daydreamed while you did it.

Could you remember all the motions you did? No. Entering this zone of "doing without concentrating on what you're doing" is an altered state of consciousness. What's important is that the job was completed. You did it well and didn't have to remember every detail every step of the way. Contemplate upon the concept of doing without doing. Ask to understand its true spiritual significance. Journal the insights that you receive.

Learning by Doing It for Yourself

Have you ever had the experience of wanting to learn how to do an activity and feeling frustrated when someone else tried to do it for you?

I once asked a friend to help me learn to use a newsletter computer program. I was excited and eager to learn and I had some basic MacWrite experience. He sat down in front of his computer and I sat to his right, watching as he showed me how to do it.

As he gave me one term after another to remember, I began to feel frustrated and fearful that I'd never retain it all. My body slumped and I felt my mind wanting to drift off in a daydream. This can happen to anyone who's trying to learn something new when they're *just* not getting it.

I stopped him, leaned back, took a deep breath, and said, "I need to actually do this myself. Could I sit where you're sitting and do it while you explain it to me?" That one action changed everything. When I touched the keyboard, looked at the monitor screen and became actively involved with the material, I started to get it.

If I hadn't known to check with my small inner voice for that intuitive flash of insight, I'd have given up. I probably would have had a less-than-rewarding experience trying to make a newsletter. Yet I learned and mastered the skills to operate a computer and the software by listening inwardly, getting a subtle nudge to move in a certain direction, and then acting upon it with a sense of mastery.

Life is structured in this way. You might start by reading this book, seeing your life reflected in its examples. Yet soon you're ready to interact and get hands-on experience through the techniques, visualizations, and exercises. This is *the way* of learning by doing.

As you learn to appreciate and regularly contact your spiritual intuition (your small inner voice), the more aware you'll become. Eventually it will become effortless and natural for you to recognize and take the next step on your journey of freedom.

Let go of things that impede your progress and direct your attention toward that which assists you. It will make your life more balanced and bring more joy and ease to every day.

Being Practical

One of my patients was blocked and struggling with the issue of taking the next step toward being responsible for keeping herself balanced in all areas of her life.

"I just can't seem to get this," she said.

Finally I asked her to close her eyes, relax and breathe. "Place you inner attention on the center of your forehead where insight occurs in your brain. Now connect with your Higher Power as you know it. Say inwardly, 'Higher Power, I surrender this problem.' Now imagine a beautiful sound, a loving feeling, and a favorite color."

She did this for several minutes. When she opened her eyes, the struggle was gone and she felt better, more open to taking her next step. Later on I shared this story with a colleague. I asked, "Why did it take me so long to put my attention on my Higher Power, which prompted me to remind my patient to reconnect with her Higher Power and surrender the situation?"

My colleague didn't have an answer, but she smiled. She understood how we sometimes forget to put our attention on our Higher Power when we feel blocked or are struggling with an issue, situation, attitude, or belief.

She related that once she worked with a client who came to the first session in a panic and who paced the office the entire time she talked. Soon my colleague remembered an exercise for the patient to try to connect with her Higher Power. This one involved closing her eyes and singing the word "HU" softly (pronounced like the word *hue)*.

Spirit, your Higher Power, and God will work in your life—at the office, at home, anywhere. You will receive the protection and comfort you need if you remember to stay connected to your spiritual resources. Remembering is the key: the sooner, the better.

> *"HU is an ancient name for God,"*

She explained. "Sing it in a long, drawn-out way, like this," she suggested. "HU-U-U-U-U." Within a few moments, the client calmed down enough to sit while she conversed.

Take Time to Rest and Review

Sometimes we're in a hurry to get on with life. When I read a book, I often plunge through it like a thirsty traveler in a desert with no water for five miles. For five metaphorical miles, I'll push myself to get to the water at the next oasis, push myself to read as fast as I can to see what's next.

I do this in life too, pushing myself to finish one project so I can move on to the next one. When is it the time to relax and enjoy the present moment? The answer to this question is why I created the *Rest and Review Celebration* technique.

Reviewing how far you've come is a way to validate and honor your process. A time of rest, review, and celebration invites the honored guest of insight. When the guest of honor finally arrives, you'll find that it is *you!* Later you will honor the gifts you have received on your quest.

One Way to Do the Rest and Review Celebration Technique

Think of each step that you've taken along the way like a dear friend you haven't talked to in a month. It's time to reconnect. In other words, it's time to invite, acknowledge, and treat every step you've taken in this process as the honored guests that they are.

Make an "honored guest list" of your steps so far in your journey of balanced eating. List them all, big or small, grand or minute, flashy or not. All are important; be sure to slight none of them.

How do you prepare? Decide on a date and time. Since this is a rest and review, maybe you'll wear lounging clothes to your celebration. Set the scene in a unique way that makes it special for you. Maybe you'll light scented candles. This *Rest and Review Celebration* is one way to crisply delineate and put closure on the completion of this cycle.

When you started reading this book, you met the antithesis of its principles when you faced problems and obstacles along the way. When you used the techniques in the book, you grew and transformed to become even greater than you ever imagined you'd be.

Now we're at the final step: synthesis. Synthesis is pulling together all the steps you've taken and reflecting on what you've learned. Synthesis happens most naturally when you take time to do the following technique.

Visualize arriving at your celebration and turning on the lights. As you enter the space devoted to the celebration, be aware of the moment when you light the room (or light your scented candles). As light fills the room, capture the moment in your memory by putting your attention upon it. Ask yourself to be aware of catching insights as you turn the light on each step you've taken in your journey throughout this book.

Take time to welcome and acknowledge everyone on your "honored guest list." As you review the chronology of steps you've taken in your journey of balanced eating, take time to feel gratitude for the hidden gifts each step has brought to you. Recognize how the steps took you beyond your problems and stretched you into a greater awareness. Chronicle your realizations and gratitude in your journal.

Now it's time to celebrate. Close your eyes and write down the biggest three things you've learned from your journey; those things you're most grateful for having learned. Take time to reflect as you rest. Close your celebration by singing HU with gratitude and a few moments of quiet reflection.

Resting and reviewing is a way to renew you. Soon enough, more challenges will enter your life. Prepare yourself to stay open so that the spiritual awareness and creativity from Divine Spirit keeps coming.

Contemplation

Daily contemplation is a form of renewal, a mini-time of rest and review. The contemplative techniques in this book can be adapted to fit your ever-changing needs. Choose one time of each day to devote to a daily contemplation period so you can sustain the results of your spiritual intuition.

Each contemplation period starts with closing your eyes. Then look upward to the center of your forehead as you connect with your Higher Power. You may have a favorite sound or word you can chant or sing for five to ten minutes. Then fall into silence for a few more minutes and enjoy the peace.

If thoughts interrupt you during this peaceful quiet time, focus on a natural sound within earshot for a few minutes. Since all sounds are of of God, enjoy the sound as you release whatever is bothering you. Allow bothersome thoughts to glide on the air currents and dissipate as if they were as insubstantial as clouds.

Contemplate on the Delights of Success

Close your eyes and focus your attention upward to the center of your forehead. Take a minute to contemplate upon the delights of the weight balance success you've attained, now living beyond the reach of the coercive desire for certain foods, beyond societal influences and its superficial limitations.

In regards to contemplating on the delights of success, do you remember a time when you felt you were doing completely what God wanted you to do? Is there a feeling in your heart that goes with this awareness? Share this bliss with someone you can trust or write about it in your journal. You can also ask to experience more of this bliss in the future.

The Purpose of Life

The purpose of life is learning how to metaphorically make lemons into lemonade while maintaining a loving, grateful heart. Growth brings more knowledge about the art of turning stumbling blocks of life into stepping stones. This growth and its resulting knowledge can lead you to connect with your personal mission for this lifetime. It's simply heaven on earth when you can vitalize your purpose for being here with joyful, productive living while turning your dreams into reality.

Remember life is either repeating itself (in cycles of feedback loops) or renewing itself (by taking you to newer, higher levels in realizing your mission in life and making your dreams come true). The choice is always ultimately yours.

Designing a New Purpose Focused for the Future

When designing a new purpose statement, try to incorporate what you received in your dreams of the future. We'll also focus on using projection. The type of projection I'm speaking about here is not how many people interpret projection (which is guessing what another person may be thinking or the motive behind their actions). Instead let's explore a more positive interpretation of the term projection.

You can use the practice of instant projection (reaching a higher state of consciousness while projecting yourself into future possibilities) when you combine your new purpose statement with a deepened understanding of and a proficiency with the techniques outlined in this chapter. By honing in on your new purpose and using your creative imagination, you can invite your Higher Power and the spiritual forces of the universe to enhance your future in a positive way.

Soul Is in Control

At this point you know that Soul is *in control* in phenomenal ways. It's what you've always wanted. You're in control of being responsible for getting more answers and more awareness. You, as Soul, were in control when cleaning the negative programming out your mind. It took discipline and constant testing, yet it was a labor of love filled with excitement and joy. Every day you choose to connect with Soul being in control, you grow freer.

Techniques to Give You Experiences of the Heart

Many only dream of the techniques outlined in this book. Some merely read about them without understanding or experiencing them. However, to know a thing with your heart, mind and body, you need to experience it with your whole self on a cellular level (which is the key to its success).

It also takes effort to remember to continue to surrender to your Higher Power, one step at a time. It takes a day to day evolving consciousness to stay open to awareness, to have the flexibility to make attitude shifts, as life reveals new adventures beyond your current success.

The greatest adventure is just beginning. This can be a spiritually golden time for discovering your true purpose, potential, and mission in life, if you so choose.

Putting It All Together: The Ongoing Journey Beyond the New You

Once you've chosen a new purpose, you can adapt the techniques in this book toward the new goals you want to achieve. Any exercise, visualization or technique in this book can be modified so that you can use it over and over again.

Pick up this book and start reading with a new purpose in mind. Concepts may jump out which are pertinent to your new purpose. Use colored highlighting pens to bring attention to the parts that are most meaningful to your new purpose or goals. Date the entries. Choose a different highlighting color when you reread certain sections with a different purpose or goal in mind. Keep reviewing the exercises in this book with a sense of fun and excitement.

You're writing the story of your adventures beyond weight balance success now. It's all up to you. Right now is a great time to start making your dreams come true by making your life a conscious choice.

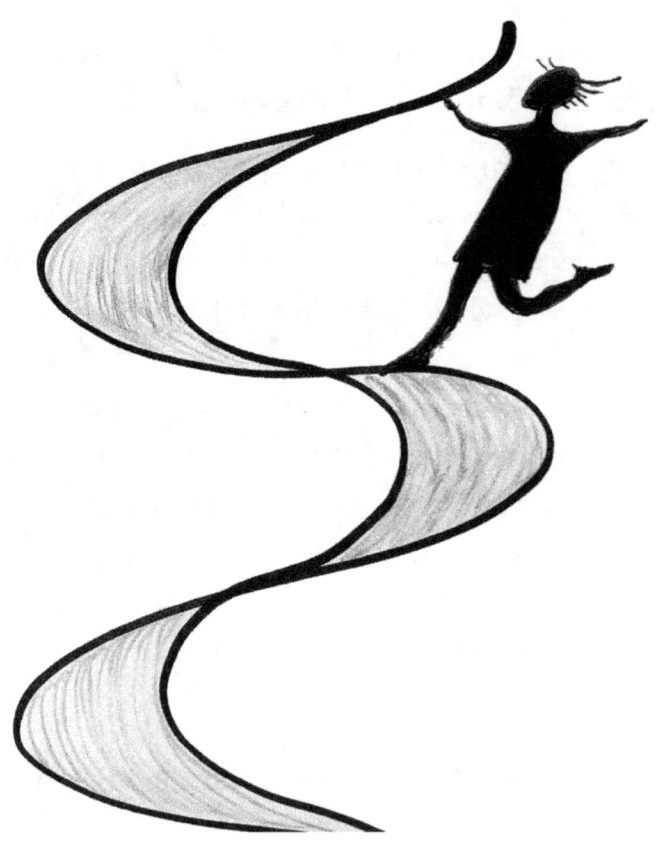

Chapter 27

Epilogue

When I wrote *Cut the Guilt,* I distilled the harvest of my personal struggles and my patients' struggles with eating into learning adventures for others. And yet, there are those who still hunger for this truth.

Recently I took my oldest daughter shopping at the Orlando Premium Outlet Mall. As lunchtime approached, we stepped into the food court for a bite to eat. My hunger died however when I saw the selection of food from which I could choose. My daughter ordered a submarine sandwich for herself and two bottles of water, one for each of us.

I sat and looked around in amazement at all the people, their plates piled high with fast foods of all kinds. Most had sodas in their hands.

I asked my daughter, "I wonder what I could eat here?"

She said, "What about the juice place? Or there's Japanese food."

Previously I had investigated all the food selections and found none adequate for my metabolic type. I realized I'd had a similar problem at breakfast when my daughter served some carbohydrate-based treats I normally don't eat. I could have tried to make do with what was available at lunch and say nothing. However, it was time for me to speak up.

I shared with my daughter that the protein portion sizes were not sufficient and I needed nutrient-rich vegetables for sustenance. Something like baked fish, meat and steamed vegetables would help me last until supper. I explained that I felt sluggish, sleepy, and unmotivated when I ate a diet predominately based on carbohydrates. (candida grows wild with carbs.)

Later, my daughter and I shopped for groceries. We picked out a fresh fish selection and her favorite vegetable for supper. That evening we prepared a metabolically balanced meal that left both of us feeling wonderful.

Since I've personally cultivated this sensitivity, I find it a gift that

I can routinely check how I feel, how my body feels, in relation to what I've eaten. This is what I teach to everyone who walks into my office. The path of weight balance freedom is simply *choosing to be conscious.*

By the following the first section of *Cut the Guilt, The Metabolic Typing Diet, The Food Allergy Cure, and The Body "Knows" Diet,* bodily aches and pains, emotional irritability, anxiety, and even the depression that most people feel when eating the wrong foods can be alleviated.

Before you achieve weight balance, you'll experience dramatic positive changes in the quality of your life and freedom from mood swings and food cravings. This system of weight balance has kindled within me a deep appreciation for the process. I constantly experience a profound satisfaction with my practice as I teach these techniques and exercises to more people every day.

Everyone can experience this freedom in body, mind and spirit.

> *The golden key to a healthy, balanced weight you can sustain and appreciate for the rest of your life is in your hands.*

Your Golden Key

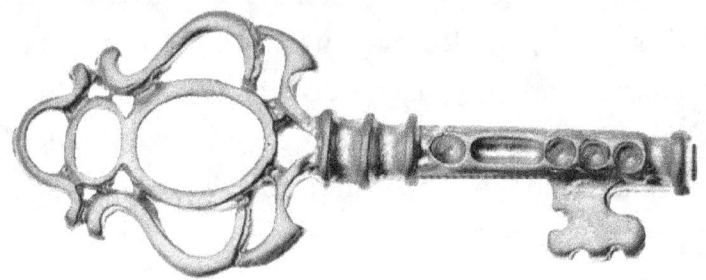

Recommended Reading

Agras, W.S., Crow, S.J, Halmi, K.A., Mitchell, J.E. Wilson, G.T., & Kraemer, H.C. (2000). Outcome predictors for cognitive behavior treatment of bulimia nervosa: Data from a multisite study, *American Journal of Psychiatry,* 157, 1302-1308.

Baer, Jean. *How to be an Assertive (Not Aggressive) Woman in Life, in Love, and on The Job* (Penguin Books USA, Inc., New York, 1976).

Bradshaw, John. *Homecoming: Reclaiming and Championing Your Inner Child* (Bantam Books, New York, 1992).

Braverman, Eric R., M.D., *The Edge Effect* (Sterling Publishing Co., Inc. New York 2004)

Brown, Molly Young. *Growing Whole: Self Realization on an Endangered Planet* (HarperCollins, New York, 1993).

Bulfinch, Thomas. *Myths of Greece and Rome* (Penguin Books USA, Inc., New York, 1979).

Burns, David D., M..D. *The Feeling Good Handbook* (Penguin Books USA, Inc., New York, 1990).

Carson, Rachel. *Silent Spring* (Fawcett Books, Greenwich, 1962).

Cloud, Dr. Henry and Dr. John Townsend. *Boundaries: When to say Yes, When to say No to take Control of Your Life* (Zondervan Publishing House, Grand Rapids, 1992).

Ecstatic Dance. Written by Gabrielle Roth. Directed by Michelle Miller (videocassette, Sounds True, Boulder, 2000).

Food for Thought: Daily Meditations for Dieters and Overeaters (HarperCollins, New York, 1985).

Gold, Mark, M.D., Chief of Addiction Medicine U. of Florida, & McKnight Brain Institute.

Hildebrandt T, Shiovitz R, Afano L, Greif R. Defining image body deception and its role in peer based social comparison theories of body dissatisfaction. *Body Image.* Sept 2008; 5(3): 299-306.

Klemp, Harold. *The Book of Eck Parables;* Volume 2 (Eckankar, Minneapolis, 1988).

Klemp, Harold. *The Book of Eck Parables;* Volume 3 (Eckankar, Minneapolis, 1991).

Klemp, Harold. *Cloak of Consciousness* (Eckankar, Minneapolis, 1991).

Klemp, Harold. *Journey of Soul* (Eckankar, Minneapolis, 1988).

Kubler-Ross, Elisabeth. *On Death and Dying* (Macmillan Publishing Co., Inc., New York, 1969).

Leuner, Hanscarl, M.D., Guided Affective Imagery (GAI) (Jan. 1969) A Method of Intensive Psychotherapy. American Journal of Psychotherapy, Vol.XXIII, No 1, pgs. 4-22 Two.not2.org /psychosynthsis, *The Evolution of Consciousness.*

National Institute for Clinical Excellence (2004) *Eating Disorders: Core interventions in the treatment of anorexia nervosa, bulimia nervosa and related eating disorders.* Clinical guideline 9. London: National Collaborating Centre for Mental Health.

Newberg, Andrew, M.D. & Waldman, Mark Robert, *How God changes the Brain,* Center for Spirituality & mind at U. of Pennsylvania

Schwartz, Jason, P., **Fit into Your Genes** (Fiction Publishing, Inc. Ft. Pierce, Florida (2011).

Stice, E., &Shaw, H.E. (2012). Role of body dissatisfaction in the onset and maintenance of eating pathology: A Synthesis of research findings. *Journal of Psychosomatic Research,* 53, 985-993.

Strober, M., & Johnson, C. (2012). The need for complex ideas in anorexia nervosa:Why biology, environment, and psyche all matter, why clinical benchmarks are needed for managing weight correction. *International Journal of Eating Disorders,* 45. 155-178.

Sutherland, Caroline, M. Sutherland. *The Body "Knows" Diet* (Sutherland Communications, Inc.Washington, 2005).

Wallace, L.M., & von Ranson, K.M. (2012) Perceptions and use of empirically-supported psychotherapies among eating disorder professionals. *Behavior Research and Therapy,* 50 215-222.

Waller, G., Stringer, H. & Meyer, C. (2012) The therapeutic alliance in the early part of cognitive-behavioral therapy for eating disorders. *Journal of Consulting and Clinical Psychology,* 80, 171-175.

References

Introduction

1. *The invalid separation of effects of nature and nurture: Lessons from animal experimentation.* Pages163-192 Intelligence, Heredity, and Environment. R.J. Sternberg and E.L. Grigorenko, eds. New York: Cambridge University Press. Wahlsten, Gottlieb.

2. *The Journal of Clinical Investigation,*Volume 118 Number 10 October 2008, page 3244. Obesity makes for a big headline.

3. Rexford Ahima (an expert in CNS regulation of body weight and energy balance at the University of Pennsylvania).*The Journal of Clinical Investigation* Volume 118 Number 10 October 2008, p. 3244.

An Overview

1. Berthoud HR, Lenard NR, Shin AC (2   011). Food reward, hyperphagia, and obesity. *Am. J. Physiol.* Regul. Integr. Comp. Physiol. 300, R1266–R1277.

Chapter 1   Never Before—But Forever More

1.Raisa B. Deber, PhD; Nancy Kraetschmer, MSc; Jane Irvine, DPhil. What Role Do Patients Wish to Play in Treatment Decision Making? *Arch Intern Med.* 1996;156(13):1414-1420.

2 .William H.Frey. 1985: 147.*Crying: T he Mystery of T ears*by William H. Frey, Ph.D. with Muriel Langset124h. Minneapolis: Winston Press.

3. Fehm-Wolfsdorf, G., Scheible, E., Zenz, H., Born, J., Fehm, H.L., Taste thresholds in man are differentially influenced by hydrocortisone and dexamethasone. *Psychoneuroendocrinology* 14 (6), 433-440. 1989.

Elissa Epel, Rachel Lapidus, Bruce McEwen, Kelly Brownell. Stress may add bite to appetite in women: a laboratory study of stress-induced cortisol and eating behavior. *Psychoneuroendocrinology* 26 (2001) 37-49.

4. K. Elfhag, C. Erlanson-Albertsson. Sweet and fat taste preference in obesity have different associations with personality and eating behavior. *Physiology* & *Behavior* Volume 88, Issues 1-2, 15 June 2006, Pages 61-66.

5. Tom P. Heath, Jan K. Melichar, David J. Nutt, and Lucy F. Donaldson. Human Taste Thresholds Are Modulated by Serotonin and Noradrenaline. *The Journal of Neuroscience*, December 6, 2006, 26(49): 12664-126714.

6. Mary K. Serdula, MD, MPH; Laura Kettel Khan, PhD; William H. Dietz, MD, PhD. 2003 Weight Loss Counseling Revisited. *JAMA*. 2003; 289:1747- 50.

7. Robert Berkow, M.D., Ed., *The Merck Manual of Diagnosis and Therapy*, 13th ed. (Radway, New Jersey: Merck Sharp & Dohme Research Laboratories, 1977) 1177-1180.

8. Hirsch, AR. 1997 *Dr. Hirsch's Guide To Scentsantional Weight Loss*. Rockport, MA: Element Books, 1997.

9. Frank M. Sacks, M.D., George A. Bray, M.D., Vincent J. Carey, Ph.D., Steven R. Smith, M.D., Donna H. Ryan, M.D., Stephen D. Anton, Ph.D., Katherine McManus, M.S., R.D., Catherine M. Champagne, Ph.D., Louise M. Bishop, M.S., R.D., Nancy Laranjo, B.A., Meryl S. Leboff, M.D., Jennifer C. Rood, Ph.D., Lilian de Jonge, Ph.D., Frank L. Greenway, M.D., Catherine M. Loria, Ph.D., Eva Obarzanek, Ph.D., and Donald A. Williamson, Ph.D. Comparison of Weight-Loss Diets with Different Compositions of Fat, Protein, and Carbohydrates. *N Engl J Med*. 2009 February 26;360(9):859-873.

10. Richard J. Johnson, Santos E. Perez-Pozo, Yuri Y. Sautin, Jacek Manitius, Laura Gabriela Sanchez-Lozada, Daniel I. Feig, Mohamed Shafiu, Mark Segal, Richard J. Glassock, Michiko Shimada, Carlos Roncal and Takahiko Nakagawa. Hypothesis: Could Excessive Fructose Intake and Uric Acid Cause Type 2 Diabetes? *Endocrine Reviews* 30 (1): 96-116.

11. Ong, Z. Y., and B. S. Muhlhausler. "Maternal "junk-food" feeding of rat dams alters food choices and development of the mesolimbic reward pathway in the offspring." *The FASEB Journal* 25.7 (2011): 2167-2179.

Chapter 2   Where We Are Today—and How We Got Here

1. "Obesity is epidemic in America. About 80 million Americans are obese, 33.4% of adults". *The Journal of Nutritional Biochemistry*, by Richard Atkinsona, Guidelines for the initiation of obesity treatment, This paper was delivered at the 23-25 October 1997 conference, The Determination, Treatment, and Prevention of Obesity," which was sponsored by the Institute of Nutrition, University of North Carolina at Chapel Hill; Department of Nutrition, School of Public Health and School of Medicine, University of North Carolina at Chapel Hill; and School of Medicine, East Carolina

University, in cooperation with the North American Association for the Study of Obesity, the National Institutes of Health, the American Cancer Society, and Eli Lilly & Company. From 2000: *Prevalence and Trends in Obesity Among US Adults,* 1999-2000 Katherine M. Flegal, PhD; Margaret D. Carroll, MS; Cynthia L. Ogden, PhD; Clifford L. Johnson, MSPH JAMA. 2002;288:1723-1727. The age-adjusted prevalence of obesity was 30.5% in 1999-2000 compared with 22.9% in NHANES III (1988- 1994; *P*<.001). The prevalence of overweight also increased during this period from 55.9% to 64.5%.

2. Hirsch, AR. *Dr. Hirsch's Guide To Scentsantional Weight Loss.* Rockport, MA: Element Books, 1997.

3. *Health Affairs,* 28, no. 5 (2009): w822-w831 (Published online 27 July 2009) doi: 10.1377 Ihlthaff.28.5.w822.

4. Youfa Wang, MayA. Beydoun, Lan Liang, Benjamin Caballero and Shiriki K. Kumanyika. *Obesity* (2008)1610,2323-30.

5. Per-A0 keAlbertsson, Rickard K'ohnke, Sinan C. Emek, Jiemel, Jens F. Rehfeld, Hans-ErikA0 Kerlund and Charlotte Erlanson-Albertsson.*Biochem. J.*(2   007) 401, 727-733 (Printed in Great Britain) doi: 10.1042/ BJ20061463.

6. Gene-Jack Wang, Nora D. Volkow, Frank Telangc, Millard Jaynec, Yeming Mac, Kith Pradhand, Wei Zhud, Christopher T. Wonga, Panayotis K. Thanosc, Allan Geliebtere, Anat Biegona and Joanna S. Fowler. Evidence of gender differences in the ability to inhibit brain activation elicited by food stimulation. *PNAS* January 27, 2009 vol. 106 no. 4 1249-1254.

7. Neel, J.V. Diabetes mellitus: a 'thrifty' genotype rendered detrimental by 'progress'? *Am. J. Hu,. Genet.* 12, 353-362 (1962).

8. Schwartz, M. W. et al. Is the energy homeostasis system inherently biased toward weight gain? *Diabetes* 52, 232-238 (2003).

9. Katie Wynne, Sarah Stanley, Barbara McGowan, Steven Bloom, Appetite Control. *Journal of Endocrinology* (2005) 184, 291-318.

10. USDA's Economic Research Service. Pyramid recommendation based on a sample diet of 2,200 calories. Kantor, Linda Scott. A Dietary Assessment of the U.S. Food Supply: Comparing Per Capita Food Consumption with Food Guide Pyramid Serving Recommendations. *Agricultural Economic Report 72. U.S. Department of Agriculture, Economic Research Service,* December 1998.

11. J R Soc Med. 1997 July; 90 (7): 397-399. *A syllabus for evolutionary medicine.* B G Charlton Department of Psychology, University of Newcastle upon Tyne, England.

12. Andreas Lindqvist, Annemie Baelemans and Charlotte Erlanson-Albertsson. Effects of sucrose, glucose and fructose on peripheral and central appetite signals. *Regulatory Peptides.* Volume 150, Issues 1-3, 9 October 2008, 26-32.

13. Susann Bluher, Christos S Mantzoros. Leptin in humans: lessons from translational research. *Am J Clin Nutr* March 2009 vol. 89 no. 3 991S-997S.

14. *When unhealthy foods hijack overeaters' brains.* April 20, 2009 By Lauran Neergaard, AP Medical Writer.

15. *Junk Food and the American Waistline* by Mark Roberts. 3. 3, 2010 1128 Royal Palm Beach Blvd., Suite 138, Royal Palm Beach, FL 33411.

16. Deborah A. Cohen. Neurophysiological Pathways to Obesity Below Awareness and Beyond Individual Control. *Diabetes* 57:1-5, 2008.

Chapter 3   A Healthy Look at Real Health and True Beauty

1. Grad, Frank P. The   Preamble of the Constitution of the World Health Organization. *Bull. World Health Organ.* 2002, vol.80, n.12, pp.981.

2. Hirsch, AR. *Dr. Hirsch's Guide To Scentsantional Weight Loss.* Rockport, MA: Element Books, 1997.

3. *The Healthy Mind, Healthy Body Handbook* by David S Sobel, M.D. and Robert Ornstein, Ph.D. ISBN: 0965104001 Los Altos, CA: DRX, 1996.

Chapter 4   Eat to Live, Don't Live to Eat

1. Snyder, C. R.; Lopez, Shane J. (2007). *Positive Psychology.* Sage Publications, Inc. pp. 147. ISBN 076192633X.

2. Penrose, L.S. (1931). Freud's Theory of Instinct and Other Psycho-Biological Theories. *Int. J. Psycho-Anal.*, 12:87-97.

3. Most people feel full about 10 minutes after they begin eating, but for those who are obese, it may take almost twice as long for their brains to get the message, according to researchers at the University of Florida's Evelyn F. and William L. McKnight Brain Institute. February 2003 issue of *Psychiatry Annals*.

4. Hirsch, AR. *Dr. Hirsch's Guide To Scentsantional Weight Loss.* Rockport, MA: Element Books, 1997.

Chapter 5   A Brief Overview of Topics In *Cut the Guilt*—Using Biology

1. Nishizawa, S., Benkelfat, C., Young, S., Leyton, M., Mzengeza, S.,de Mon–tigny, C., Blier, P. & Diksic, M. Women have a lower 5-HT synthesis rate than men, suggests that women may have impaired 5-HT function. (1997) *Proc. Natl. Acad.Sci.* USA 94, 5308-5313.

2. Takeda, J Terao, Y Nakaya, Ken-ichi Miyamoto, Yoshinobu Baba, Hiroshi Chuman, Ryuji Kaji, Tetsuro Ohmori, and Kazuhito Rokutan. Stress control and human nutrition tokushima-u.ac.jp [PDF]E. *The Journal of Medical Investigation* Vol. 51 139-145, August 2004.

3. Simopoulos AP. The importance of the ratio of omega-omega-3 essential fatty acids. *Biomed Pharmacother.* 2002; 56: 365-379.

4. Francois Lesperanceacde, Pierre Julienf, Nancy Frasure-Smithabcde. Major depression is associated with lower omega -3 fatty acid levels in patients with recent acute coronary syndromes. *Biological Psychiatry*; Volume 55, Issue 9, Pages 891-896 (1 May 2004).

5. *Overcoming Thyroid Disorders*, by David Brownstein, M.D. Medical Alternatives Press, Inc.; 2nd edition (April 2002).

6. Jean Mayer, *USDA Human Nutrition Research on Aging* at Tufts University, Boston, Mass.

7. M. D. Delva. Vitamin B12 replacement. To B12 or not to B12? *Canadian Family Physician* 1997 May;43:917-922.

Chapter 6   Balancing Omega-3 and Omega-6 Essential Fatty Acids

1. French P, Stanton C, Lawless F., O'Riordan EG, Monahan FJ, Caffrey PJ and Moloney AP. Fatty acid composition, including conjugated linoleic acid, of intramuscular fat from steers offered grazed grass, grass silage, or concentrate-based diets. 2000 *J. Anim. Sci.* 78:2849-2855.

Mandell IB, Buchanan-Smith JG, Campbell CP. Effects of forage vs grain feeding on carcass characteristics, fatty acid composition, and beef quality in Limousin-cross steers when time on feed is controlled. *J Anim Sci* 1998; 76:2619-2630.

2. DA Pan, AJ Hulbert, LH Storlien. Supplement: n-3 Fatty Acids: Recommendations for Therapeutics and Prevention. *Journal of Clinical Nutrition,* Vol. 83, No. 6, S1499-1504S, June 2006.

3. David A. Pan, A. J. Hulbert and L. H. Storlien. Nutrition Dietary Fats, Membrane Phospholipids and Obesity. *Journal of Nutrition*, 1994-Am Soc.

4. Maroon J, Bost J. Omega-3 Fatty acids (fish oil) as an anti-inflammatory: an alternative to nonsteroidal anti-inflammatory drugs for discogenic pain. *Surg Neurol* 2006;65:326-331.

5. Calder P. N-3 Polyunsaturated fatty acids, inflammation and autoimmune diseases. *Am J Clin Nutr* 2006;89:S 1505-1519.

6. Montori VM, Farmer A, Wolan PC, et al. Fish oil supplementation in type 2 diabetes: A quantitative systemic review. *Diabetes Care* 2000; 23; 1407-45.

7. Shima Jazayeri, Mehdi Tehrani-Doost, Seyed A. Keshavarz, Mostafa Hosseini, Abolghassem Djazayery, Homayoun Amini, Mahmoud Jalali and Malcolm Peet. Conclusions: In the present 8 week trial EPA and fluoxetine [the name of the drug sold as Prozac] had equal therapeutic effects in major depressive disorder. *Australian and New Zealand Journal of Psychiatry* 2008, Vol. 42, No. 3, 192-198.

8. Freeman MP, Hibbeln JR, Wisner KL, et al. Omega -3 fatty acids: evidence basis for treatment and future research in psychiatry *J Clin Psychiatry*. 2006;67(12):1954-1967. Erratum in: *J Clin Psychiatry*. 2007; 68(2):338.

9. Parker G, Gibson NA, Brotchie H, Heruc G, Rees AM, Hadzi- Pavlovic D. Omega-3 fatty acids and mood disorders. *Am J Psychiatry*. 2006;163 (6):969-978.

10. Raeder MB, Steen VM, Vollset SE, Bjelland I. Associations between cod liver oil use and symptoms of depression: The Hordaland Health Study. *J Affect. Disord.* 2006 Dec 18.

11. Frangou S, Lewis M, McCrone P. Efficacy of ethyleicosapentaenoic acid in bipolar depression: randomised double-blind placebo-controlled study. *Br J Psychiatry*. 2006 Jan;188:46-50.

12. Bruinsma KA, Taren DL. Dieting, essential fatty acid intake, and depression. *Nutr Rev*. 2000 Apr;58(4):98-108.

13. Osher Y, Belmaker RH, Nemets B. Clinical trials of PUFAs in depression: State of the art. *World J Biol Psychiatry*. 2006;7(4):223-30.

14. Appleton KM, Hayward RC, Gunnell D, et al. Effects of n-3 long-chain polyunsaturated fatty acids on depressed mood: systematic review of published trials. *Am J Clin Nutr*. 2006 Dec;84(6):1308-16.

15. Keck PE, Jr., Mintz J, McElroy SL, et al. Double-blind, randomized, placebo-controlled trials of ethyleicosapentanoate in the treatment of bipolar depression and rapid cycling bipolar disorder. *Biol Psychiatry*. 2006 Nov 1;60(9):1020-1022.

16. van Strater AC, Bouvy PF. Omega-3 fatty acids in the treatment of affective disorders: an overview of the literature. *Tijdschr Psychiatr.* 2007;49(2):85-94.

17. Freeman MP, Hibbeln JR, Wisner KL, et al. Omega-3 fatty acids: evidence basis for treatment and future research in psychiatry. *J Clin Psychiatry.* 2006 Dec; 67(12):1954-1967.

18. AP Simopoulos. Human requirement for N-3 polyunsaturated fatty acids. *Poultry Science,* Vol. 79, Issue 7, 961-970.

19. Calabrese JR, et al. Fish oils and bipolar disorder. *Archives of Gen Psychiatry* 1999; 56:413-414.

Hibbeln JR. Fish consumption and major depression. *The Lancet* 1998; 351:1213 (correspondence).

20. Kalmijn S, et al. Dietary fat intake and the risk of incident dementia in the Rotterdam Study. *Annals of Neurology* 1997; 42(5):776-782. & Yehuda S, et al. Yehuda, S., S. Rabinovitz, R.L. Carasso, and D.I. Mostofsky. "Essential fatty acid preparation improves Alzheimer's patients' quality of life." *Int J Neurosci* 87:141-149 (1996).

21. Stevens L, Zhang W, Peck L, et al. EFA Supplementation in children with inattention, hyperactivity, and other disruptive behaviors. *Lipids* 2003; 38:1007-1021.

22. DiGiacomo RA, et al. Fish oil Dietary Supplementation in Patients with Raynaud's Phenomenon: A Double-Blind, Controlled, Prospective Study. *Amer J Med* 1989; 86:158-164.

23. Conner WE. Importance of n-3 fatty acids in health and disease. *Amer J Clin Nutr* 2000; 71(Suppl.):171S-175S.

24. Simopoulos AP. Omega-3 fatty acids in health and disease and in growth and development. *Am J Clin Nutr* 1991; 54:438-463.

25. Eaton, et al., op cit, 1996. *Back* To *Our Ancestor's Diet-A Healthy Move.* Ken Edwards, DC, DACBN, CCN William J. Rice, DC, DACBN, CCN, FACCN.

26. Lecture by Mark Gold, M.D., a Dizney Eminent Scholar and Distin-guished Professor at the University of Florida, College of Medicine's Brain Institute and Chairman of the Department of Psychiatry. His research has led to changes in the treatment of opiate and cocaine addictions and of obesity. Over the past decade, Dr. Gold has pioneered the hypothesis of hedonic overeating or pathological attachment to food as an addiction and overeating as a substance dependence disorder that causes obesity.

27. Source: Economic Research Service, USDA. *Food Review* Vol. 23, Issue 2 Structural Change in the U.S. Food Industry. Gregory K. Price.

28. J. M. Leheska, L. D. Thompson, J. C. Howe, E. Hentges, J. Boyce, J. C. Brooks, B. Shriver, L. Hoover and M. F. Miller. Effects of conventional and grass-feeding systems on the nutrient composition of beef. *J. Anim Sci.* 2008. 86:3575-3585.

29. M. H. Gillis, S. K. Duckett and J. R. Sackmann. Effects of supplemental rumen-protected conjugated linoleic acid or corn oil on fatty acid composition of adipose tissues in beef cattle. *J. Animal Sci* 80 (5):1202-1211.

30. Eaton SB, Konner M. Paleolithic nutrition. A consideration of its nature and current implications. *New Engl J Med.* 1985; 312:283-289.

31. Simopoulos AP. New products from the agri-food industry: The return of n-3 fatty acids into the food supply. *Lipids.*1999;34 (suppl): S297-S301.

32. Simopoulos AP. Omega-3 fatty acids in health and disease and in growth and development. *Am J Clin Nutr.*1991;54:438-463.

33. Simopoulos AP. Genetic variation and evolutionary aspects of diet. In: Papas A, editors. *Antioxidants in Nutrition and Health.* Boca Raton: CRC Press, 1999. p. 65-88.

34. Simopoulos AP. Evolutionary aspects of omega-3 fatty acids in the food supply. *Prostaglandins Leukot Essent Fatty Acids.*1999;60:421-29.

35. Eaton SB, Eaton SB III, Sinclair AJ, Cordain L, Mann NJ. Dietary intake of long-chain polyunsaturated fatty acids during the Paleolithic. *World Rev Nutr Diet.* 1998;83:12-23.

36. Hunter JE. Omega-3 fatty acids from vegetable oils. In: Galli C, Simopoulos AP, eds. *Biological Effects and Nutritional Essentiality. Series A: Life Sciences.* New York: Plenum Press, 1989. vol. 171,43-55.

37. Raper NR, Cronin FJ, Exler J. Omega-3 fatty acid content of the US food supply. *J Am College Nutr.* 1992;11:304.

38. Ledger HP. Body composition as a basis for a comparative study of some East African animals. *Symp Zool Soc London.*1968;21:289-310.

39. Crawford MA. Fatty acid ratios in free-living and domestic animals. *Lancet.* 1968; i: 1329-1333.

40. Crawford MA, Gale MM, Woodford MH. Linoleic acid and linolenic acid elongation products in muscle tissue of Syncerus caffer and other ruminant species. *Biochem J.* 1969;115: 25-27.

41. Simopoulos AP, Norman HA, Gillaspy JE, Duke JA. Common purslane: A source of omega-3 fatty acids and antioxidants. *J Am College Nutr.* 1992;11:374-382.

Chapter 7   Our Body's Survival Mechanism Needs Tweaking

1. Richard Well, MEd., CDE, Melissa Conrad Stoppler, M.D. *Medicine-Net.com*, June 1, 2010.

2. Menshikova EF, Ritov VB, Fairfull L, et al. Effects of exercise on mitochondrial content and function in aging human skeletal muscle. *J Gerontol: Bio Sci* 2006; 61:534-540 & *Professionalization of Exercise Physiologyonline* ISSN 1099-5862 Vol. 6 No 9 September 2003 Limitation of Maximal Oxygen Consumption: The Holy Grail of Exercise Physiology or Fool's Gold? Joe Warpeha, CSCS, EPC.

3. wwwmedicinenet.com/script/main/art.asp? article key=80256.

4. Soo, Chee. 1979. The Toa Of Long Life, The Chinese Art of Ch'ing Ming. London and New York: Gordon and Cremonesi Publishers.

5. Linda Turner, Wolfgang Linden, Candace Marshall. Electrodermal Activity at Acupuncture Points Differentiates Patients with Current Pain from Pain-Free Controls *Applied Psychophysiology and Biofeedback* March 2013, Volume 38, Issue 1, pp 71-80.

Hyvärinen J, Karlsson M. Low-resistance skin points that may coincide with acupuncture loci. *Journal Med Biol.* 1977 Apr;55(2):88-94.

6. J.Reginster, R.Deroisy, L.Rovati, R.Lee, E.Lejeune, O.Bruyere, G.Giacovelli, Y.Henrotin, J.Dacre, C.Gossett. Long-term effects of glucosamine sulphate on osteoarthritis progression: a randomised, placebo-controlled clinical trial. *The Lancet,* Volume 357, Issue 9252, Pages 251-256.

7. *Prolo Your Pain Away!* Hauser, Ross, Hauser, Marion. Beulah Press, 2002.

Chapter 8   Optimize Your Body's Metabolism

1. Lowe, John C., Comparison of Cynomel and Hypo Support Formula: Their Physiological Effects. *Thyroid Science* 01/2009; 4:1-11.

2. Syed N. Huda, Sally M. Grantham-McGregor, Khan M. Rahman and Andrew Tomkins. Biochemical Hypothyroidism Secondary to Iodine Deficiency Is Associated with Poor School Achievement and Cognition in Bangladeshi Children. *Journal of Nutrition.* 1999;129:980-987.

3. S Bargagna, D Dinetti, A Pinchera, M Marcheschi, L Montanelli, S Presciuttini, and L Chiovato. School attainments in children with congenital hypothyroidism detected by neonatal screening and treated early in life. *European Journal of Endocrinology,* Vol. 140, Issue 5, 407-413.

4. Michael Bauer, Peter C. Whybrow, Bauer M, Heinz A, Whybrow PC. Thyroid Hormone, Neural Tissue and Mood Modulation Thyroid hormones, serotonin and mood: of synergy and significance in the adult brain. *World J Biol Psychiatry* (2001) 2, 59-69.

5. SDI/Verispan, VONA, Full year 2008. 2008 Top 200 generic drugs by total prescriptions. *www.drugtopics.com*. Number 4 is Levothyroxine. Levothyroxine, is a synthetic form of (thyroxine).

6. *Overcoming Thyroid Disorders,* by David Brownstein, M.D. Medical Alternatives Press, Inc.; 2nd edition (April 2002).

7. Estrogen reduces the efficiency of thyroid hormones, so the female body compensates by producing more thyroid hormone than males do. Women who take birth control pills may trigger a borderline low thyroid due the higher levels of estrogen from birth control pills. *An interview with Dr. Ray Peat* by Mary Shomon, Nov. 2000.

8. Crofton KM et al. Short-term in vivo exposure to the water contaminant triclosan: Evidence for disruption of thyroxine. Environ Toxicol Pharmacol 24 (2007) 194-197. Aiello A, Larson E, Levy S. Consumer Antibacterial Soaps: Effective or Just Risky? *Clinical Infectious Diseases*. 2007;45: S137-147.

9. McClellan, K. and R. U. Halden (2010). Pharmaceuticals and personal care products in archived U.S. biosolids from the 2001 EPA national sewage sludge survey. *Water Research* 44(2): 658-668.

10. J Lee, D Brownstein, A McAllister, D Zava. Excess cortisol blocks T4 to T3 conversion - *Endocrine Reviews* 2/2002, 23(1):38-89.

11. Petur Magnusson and Gregers Sorensen. Treatment of Hyperthyroidism with Methylthiouracil (pages 263- 282). *Acta Medica Scandinavica* Volume 125, Issue 3, pages 263-82, Jan./Dec. 1946.

12. Kapandji I.A. *The Physiology of the Joints.*Vol. 1. Churchill Livingstone. 1982.

13. Grade 4 muscles indicate a minor impairment that will cause abnormalities in structural stability, gait, and athletic performance. Yet many physical therapists, orthopedists, neurologists, and physiatrists consider a grade 4 muscle weaknesses relatively unimportant and may overlook it. (Chart on following page).

5	Normal (N)	Holds test position against maximal resistance
4+	Good + (G+)	Holds test position against moderate to strong pressure
4	Good (G+)	Holds test position against moderate resistance
4-	Good - (G-)	Holds test position against slight to moderate pressure
3+	Fair + (F+)	Holds test position against slight resistance
3	Fair (F)	Holds test position against gravity
3-	Fair - (F-)	Gradual release from test position
2+	Poor + (P+)	Moves through partial range of motion against gravity
2	Poor (P)	Moves through full range of motion with gravity eliminated
2-	Poor - (P-)	Moves through partial range of motion with gravity eliminated
1	Trace (T)	No visible movement–palpable tendon contraction
0	0	No palpable or observable muscle contraction

14. Mandl, L.R., Endocrine and autoimmune aspects of the health history of John F. Kennedy. *Annals of Internal Medicine.* 2009;151: 350-354

15. *The New York Times,* November 17, 2002. In J.F.K. File, Hidden Illness, Pain and Pills. Altman, I, Purdum, T.

16. Barnes, B.O. and Galton, L.: *Hypothyroidism: The Unsuspected Illness.* New York, Harper and Row Publishers, 1976.

17. *Could Your Thyroid Be Causing Your Symptoms?* By Mary Shomon, About.com Guide Updated June 19, 2006. Ken Woliner, M.D., http: //thyroid. about.com /cs/ testsforthyroid/a/isityourthyroid htm.

18. Lowe, J.C.: Comparison of electronic thermometers with Galinstanin glass thermometers. *Thyroid Science,* 4(3):CLS1-9, 2009.

19. *Menstruating women must take their temperatures on the 2nd, 3rd and 4th days of their periods only.* Thyroiduk.org.uk/tuk/pages/diagnosis/barnes html.

20. AP Report: *Tons of released drugs taint U.S. water.* The Associated Press. Published: April 19, 2009.

21. Jeff Donn, Martha Mendoza and Justin Pritchard. Reference to the chemicals found: *Tap Water Testing AP*: Drugs found in drinking water Updated 9/12/2008 2:02 PM. Associated Press.

22. Surks, M.I., Ortiz, E., Daniels, G.H., Sawin, C.T., Col, N.F., Franklyn, J.A., Hershman, J.M., Burman, K.D., Denke, M.A., Gorman, C., Cooper, R.S. & Weissman, N.J. (2004) Subclinical thyroid disease: scientific review and guidelines for diagnosis and management. *JAMA,* 291, 228-238.

23. *Iodine: Why You Need It, Why You Can't Live Without It*, 2nd Edition David Brownstein, MD Medical Alternatives Press, Michigan, 2006, p.77-78.

24. Kelly FC. Iodine in medicine and pharmacy since its discovery ±1811- 1961. *Proc R Soc Med*, 1961; 54:831-836.

25. Wolff J and Chaikoff IL. Plasma inorganic iodide as a homeostatic regulator of thyroid function. *J Biol Chem*, 1948; 174:555 564.

26. Wolff J. Iodide goiter and the pharmacologic effects of excess iodide. *Am J Med,* 1969; 47:101-124.

27. Abraham GE, Flechas JD, Hakala JC. Othoiodosupplementation: Iodine sufficiency of the whole human body. *The Original Internist*, 2002; 9(4):30-41.

28. Abraham GE. The safe and effective implementation of orthoiodo–supplementation in medical practice. *The Original Internist*, 2004; 11(1):17-36.

29. Abraham GE. The concept of orthoiodosupplementation and its clinical implications. *The Original Internist*, 2004; 11(2):29-38.

30. A. Girard, S.B. Andrus, D.M. Hegsted, Excretion of labeled thyroxine in the presence of cholesterol-cholic acid supplements, *Metabolism*, Volume 15, Issue 8, August 1966, Pages 714-719.

31. For more information on the role of iodine as it pertains to your health, I suggest the book, *Iodine: Why You Need It, Why You Can't Live Without It*, by David Brownstein, M.D.

32. A. P. Weetman. Whose Thyroid Hormone Replacement is it Anyway? *Clin Endocrinol*. 2006; 64(3):231-233.

33. Gay J. Canaris, MD, MSPH; Neil R. Manowitz, PhD; Gilbert Mayor, MD; E. Chester Ridgway, MD. The Colorado Thyroid Disease Prevalence Study. *Arch Intern Med*. 2000;160:526-534.

34. A. Elisabeth Hak, MD, MSc; Huibert A.P. Pols, MD, PhD; Theo J. Visser, MD, PhD; Hemmo A. Drexhage, MD, PhD; Albert Hofman, MD, PhD; and Jacqueline C.M. Witteman, PhD. Subclinical Hypothyroidism Is an Independent Risk Factor for Atherosclerosis and Myocardial Infarction in Elderly Women:The Rotterdam Study. *Annals of Internal Medicine*, February 15, 2000; vol.123 no.4: 270-278.

35. *Thyroid Power: 10 Steps to Total Health* by Richard Shames M.D. and Karilee Shames, Ph.D., R.N. Harper Collins Publishers, June 01, 2002.

36. Utiger RD. Therapy of hypothyroidism-when are changes needed? *New England Journal of Medicine* 1990;323:126-127.

Bunevičius, Robertas, et al. "Effects of thyroxine as compared with thyroxine plus triiodothyronine in patients with hypothyroidism." *New England Journal of Medicine* 340.6 (1999): 424-429.

Smith SR. Desiccated thyroid preparations. Obsolete therapy. *ArchIntern Med* 1984;144:926-927.

Rees-Jones RW, Rolla AR, Larsen PR. Hormonal content of thyroid replacement preparations. *JAMA* 1980;243:549-550.

Alan R. Gaby, MD. Sub-laboratory Hypothyroidism and the Empirical use of Armour Thyroid. *Alternative Medicine Review*, Volume 9, Number 2, 2004, pages 157-179.

37. Bunevicius Robertas, Jakubonien Neli, Jurkevicius Renaldas, Cernicat Jurate, Lašas Liudvikas, Prange Arthur. Thyroxine vs thyroxine plus triiodo-thyronine in treatment of hypothyroidism after thyroidectomy for Graves' disease. *Endocrine*, Vol. 18, Number 2, 129-133, DOI: 10.1385 ENDO:18:2:129.

38. Ridha Arem, MD: *The Thyroid Solution* [p. 285] (1999). Ridha Arem, M.D., is Associate Professor of Medicine in the Division of Endocrinology and Metabolism at Baylor College of Medicine in Houston, Texas. He is also Chief of Endocrinology and Metabolism at Ben Taub General Hospital in Houston.

39. (Reference chart below.)

Drug	Thyroid Tablets USP (Armour® Thyroid)	Liotrix Tablets USP (Thyrolar®)	Liothronine Tablets, USP (Cytomel®)	Levothyroxine Tablets, USP (Unithroid®, Levoxyl®, Levothroid®, Synthroid®)
Approx. Dose Equivalent	¼ grain (15 mg)	¼		25 mcg (.025 mg)
Approx. Dose Equivalent	½ grain (30 mg)	½	12.5 mcg	50 mcg (.05 mg)
Approx. Dose Equivalent	1 grain (60 mg)	1	25 mcg	100 mcg (.01 mg)
Approx. Dose Equivalent	1 ½ grains (90 mg)	1 ½	37.5 mcg	150 mcg (.015 mg)
Approx. Dose Equivalent	2 grains (120 mg)	2	50 mcg	200 mcg (.02 mg)
Approx. Dose Equivalent	3 grains (180 mg)	3	75 mcg	300 mcg (.03 mg)

Chapter 9   Over Stressed and Overweight

1. Nicki Weiss is an internationally recognized Certified Professional Sales Management Coach, Master Trainer, and workshop leader. nicki@saleswise.ca

2. Feero, William. "Magnetic Field Management" In Proceedings of the *Scientific Workshop on the Health Effects of Electric and Magnetic Fields on Workers*, edited by Bierbaum, P. and Peters, J., pp-pp. National Institute for Occupational Safety and Health. Cincinnati, OH. 1991.

International Commission on Non-Ionizing Radiation Protection. "Guide-lines for Limiting Exposure to Static Magnetic Fields." *Health Physics.* Vol. 96, No. 4. 2009.

National Research Council, Committee on the Possible Effects of Electromagnetic Fields on Biologic Systems. *Possible Health Effects of Exposure to Residential Electric and Magnetic Fields.* National Academy Press. Washington, DC. 1997.

World Health Organization. *Extremely Low Frequency Fields.* Environmental Health Criteria Monograph No. 238. Geneva. 2007.

Kheifets, Leeka. The Precautionary Principle and EMF. *Journal of Risk Research.* Vol.4 No. 2. 2001.

National Institutes for Environmental Health. EMF *Questions and Answers: Electric and Magnetic Fields Associated with Use of Electric Power.* Research Triangle Park, NC. 2002.

National Grid. "Calculating and measuring fields from power lines" EMFs. info: *Electric and Magnetic Fields.* www.emfs.info/Sources of EMFs/ Overhead power-lines/Calculating/

PPL Electric Utilities Corporation. *Magnetic Field Management.* 2004.

Chang, G. and Jenning, C. *Magnetic Field Survey at PG&E Photovoltaic Sites.* Pacific Gas and Electric Company Research and Development Department. 8-94.

3. PJ Kulkosky. *Satiation: from gut to brain,* 1998 Oxford University Press, USA.

4. Drug interactions with 5-HTP (5-hydroxytryptophan) and tryptophan are classified as serious with the following medications. *furazolidone, isocarboxazid, linezolid, methylene blue, moclobemide, pargyline, and tranylcypromine.* Please consult your clinician.

5. Wilson, J. L. (2007). *Adrenal Fatigue: The 21ˢᵗ Century Stress Syndrome.* Petaluma, CA: Smart.

6. Note for California Residents: California State health law requires that the testing of any specimen collected or mailed from California be sent with a written order from a health care professional licensed in California to order laboratory tests. This includes the following disciplines: M.D.; D.C.;LAc; R.D.; D.O.; N.P.; and Pharmacists (R.PH). As of September 2002 (Senate Bill 577), such lab tests may be ordered by complementary or alternative health care practitioners "not providing services that require medical training." If you are a California resident and would still like to order online, please visit: www. canaryclub.org or www. virginiahopkinstestkits.com These sites will help you order online, with a licensed physician, in the state of California.

Note for New York Residents: New York State health law prohibits the testing of specimens collected in or mailed from New York, and prohibits the transmission of data from the laboratory to NY physicians or residents. Therefore, direct receipt of lab results for NY residents is not presently possible.

7. http://www.genovadiagnostics.com/

8. http://diagnostechs.com/Home.aspx

9. http://www.zrtlab.com/ 1-866-600-1636

10. Torres, S., & Nowson, C. (2007). Relationship between stress, eating behaior, and obesity. *Nutrition,* 23 (11-12), 887-894.

11. Adam TC, Epel ES. *Physiol Behav.* 2007 Jul 24;91(4):449-458.

12. Nieuwenhuizen AG, Rutters F. The hypothalamic-pituitaryadrenal-axis in the regulation of energy balance. *Physiol Behav.* 2008 May 23;94(2):169-177.

13. Kissebah AH, Krakower G. Regional adiposity and morbidity. *Physiol Rev* 1994;74:761-811. Lapidus L, Bengtsson T, Hallstrom T, Bjorntorp P.

Distribution of adipose tissue and risk of cardiovascular disease and death: a 12-year follow-up of participants in the population study of women in Gothenburg, Sweden. *BMJ* 1984;289:1257-1261.

14. Lee BK, Glass TA, McAtee MJ, Wand GS, Bandeen-Roche K,Bolla KI, Schwartz BS. Associations of salivary cortisol with cognitive function in the Baltimore memory study.*Arch Gen Psychiatry.* 2007Jul;64(7):810-18.

Chapter 10   To B12 or Not to B12—That Is the Question

1. Lindenbaum J, Healton EB, Savage DG, et al. Neuropsychiatric disorders caused by cobalamin [B12] deficiency in the absence of anemia or macrocytosis. *New England Journal of Medicine* 318, 26:1720-8, 1988.

2. Strachan RW, Henderson JG. Psychiatric syndromes due to avitaminosis B12 with normal blood and marrow. *Quart J Med* 34, 135: 303-317, 1965.

3. Suter PM, Golner BB, Goldin BR, Morrow ED, Russell RM. Reversal of protein-bound vitamin B12 malabsorption with antibiotics in atrophic gastritis. *Gastroenterology* 1991; 101:1039-1045.

4. Stefan P. Marcuard, MD. Letters: Omeprazole and Vitamin B12. *Annals of Internal Medicine*, July 1, 1994 vol.121:1:74.

5. Holtmann G., Kriebel R., Singer M.V.; Mental stress and gastric acid secretion: do personality traits influence the response? *Dig Dis Sci.* 1990 Aug; 35(8):998-1007.

6. Jean Mayer, *USDA Human Nutrition Research on Aging* at Tufts University, Boston, Mass.

7. Ken Fujioka, MD, Follow-up of Nutritional and Metabolic Problems After Bariatric Surgery. *Diabetes Care* 28:481-484, 2005.

8. *Low, Subnormal, or Suboptimal Vitamin B12 "Epidemic" Related Medical Journal Articles (152 articles that follow are listed as reference 8)*

1. Bradford GS, Taylor CT. Omeprazole and vitamin B12 deficiency. *Ann Pharmacother.* 1999 May;33(5):641-643.

2. Marcuard SP, Albernaz L, Khazanie PG. Omeprazole therapy causes malabsorption of cyanocobalamin (vitamin B12). *Ann Intern Med.* 1994 Feb 1;120(3):211-215.

3. Durand C, Mary S, Brazo P, Dollfus S. Psychiatric manifestations of vitamin B12 deficiency: a case report. *Encephale;* 2003 Nov- Dec;29 (6): 560-565.

4. Malouf M, Grimley EJ, Areosa SA. Folic acid with or without vitamin B12 for cognition and dementia. *Cochrane Database Syst Rev.* 2003; (4): CD004514.

5. Termanini B, Gibril F, Sutliff V E, Yu F, Venzon DJ, Jensen RT. Effect of longterm gastric acid suppressive therapy on serum vitamin B12 levels in patients with Zollinger-Ellison syndrome. *Am J Med* 1998 May; 104(5):422-430.

6. Ruscin JM, Page RL 2nd, Valuck RJ. Vitamin B12 deficiency associated with histamine (2)-receptor antagonists and a protonpump inhibitor. *Ann Pharmacother*, 2002 May;36(5):812-816.

7. Bellou A, Aimone-Gastin I, De Korwin JD, Bronowicki JP, Moneret-Vautrin A, Nicolas JP, Bigard MA, Gueant JL. Cobalamin deficiency with megaloblastic anaemia in one patient under long-term omeprazole therapy. *J Intern Med* 1996 Sep;240(3):161-164.

8. Andres E, Perrin AE, Kraemer JP, Goichot B, Demengeat C, Ruellan A, Grunenberger F, Constantinesco A, Schlienger JL. Anemia caused by vitamin B 12 deficiency in subjects aged over 75 years: new hypotheses. A study of 20 cases. *Rev Med Interne*. 2000 Nov; 21(11):946-954.

9. Force RW, Nahata MC. Effect of histamine H2-receptor antagonists on vitamin B12 absorption. *Ann Pharmacother*. 1992Oct;26(10):1283-1286.

10. Andres E, Loukili NH, Noel E, Kaltenbach G, Abdelgheni MB, Perrin AE, Noblet-Dick M, Maloisel F, Schlienger JL, Blickle JF. Vitamin B12 (cobalamin) deficiency in elderly patients. *CMAJ*. 2004 Aug 3; 171 (3): 251-259. Review.

11. Saltzman JR, Kemp JA, Golner BB, Pedrosa MC, Dallal GE, Russell RM. Effect of hypochlorhydria due to omeprazole treatment or atrophic gastritis on protein-bound vitamin B12 absorption. *J Am Coll Nutr*. 1994 Dec; 13(6):584-591.

12. Schenk BE, Kuipers EJ, Klinkenberg-Knol EC, Bloemena EC, Sandell M, Nelis GF, Snel P, Festen HP, Meuwissen SG. Atrophic gastritis during long-term omeprazole therapy affects serum vitamin B12 levels. *Aliment Pharmacol Ther*. 1999 Oct;13(10):1343-1346.

13. Andres E, Affenberger S, Vinzio S, Kurtz JE, Noel E, Kaltenbach G, Maloisel F, Schlienger JL, Blickle JF. Food cobalamin malabsorption in elderly patients: clinical manifestations and treatment. *Am J Med*. 2005 Oct; 118(10):1154-1159.

14. Seal EC, Metz J, Flicker L, Melny J. A randomized, double-blind, placebo-controlled study of oral vitamin B12 supplementation in older patients with subnormal or borderline serum vitamin B12 concentrations. *J Am Geriatr Soc*. 2002 Jan;50 (1):146-151.

15. Kaltenbach G, Andres E, Barnier-Figue G, Noblet-Dick M, Noel E, Vogel T, Perrin AE, Berthel M. Low vitamin B12 levels in elderly patients cured within one week by oral cobalamin therapy. *Presse Med*. 2005 Mar 12; 34(5): 358-62.

16. Lindstedt G. Nitrous oxide can cause cobalamin deficiency. Vitamin B12 is a simple and cheap remedy. *Lakartidningen*. 1999 Nov 3;96(44): 4801-4805.

17. Loew D, Wanitschke R, Schroedter A. Studies on vitamin B12 status in the elderly—prophylactic and therapeutic consequences. *Int J Vitam Nutr Res.* 1999 May;69(3):228-233.

18. Petchkrua W, Little JW, Burns SP, Stiens SA, James JJ. Vitamin B12 deficiency in spinal cord injury: a retrospective study. *J Spinal Cord Med.* 2003 Summer; 26(2):116-121.

19. O'Gorman P, Holmes D, Ramanan AV, Bose-Haider B, Lewis MJ, Will A. Dietary vitamin B12 deficiency in an adolescent white boy. *J Clin Pathol.* 2002 Jun;55(6): 475-476.

20. Grasbeck R. Imerslund-Grasbeck syndrome (selective vitamin B12 malabsorption with proteinuria). Orphanet. *J Rare Dis.* 2006 May19;1:17.

21. Carmel R. Nutritional vitamin-B12 deficiency. Possible contributory role of subtle vitamin B12 malabsorption. *Ann Intern Med.* 1978 May; 88(5): 647-649.

22. Teplitsky V, Huminer D, Zoldan J, Pitlik S, Shohat M, Mittelman, M. Hereditary partial transcobalamin II deficiency with neurologic, mental and hematologic abnormalities in children and adults. *Isr Med Assoc J.* 2003 Dec;5(12):868-872.

23. Andres E, Noel E, Kaltenbach G, Perrin AE, Vinzio S, Goichot B, Schlienger JL, Blickle JF. Vitamin B12 deficiency with normal Schilling test or non-dissociation of vitamin B12 and its carrier proteins in elderly patients. A study of 60 patients. *Rev Med Interne.* 2003 Apr;24(4): 218-223.

24. Koop H. Review article: metabolic consequences of long-term inhibition of acid secretion by omeprazole. *Aliment Pharmacol Ther.* 1992 Aug;6(4): 399-406. Review.

25. Ray JG, Cole DE, Boss SC. An Ontario-wide study of vitamin B12, serum folate, and red cell folate levels in relation to plasma homocysteine: is a preventable public health issue on the rise?. *Clin Biochem.* 2000 Jul; 33(5):337-343.

26. Wolters M, Strohle A, Hahn A. Age-associated changes in the metabolism of vitamin B12 and folic acid: prevalence, aetiopathogenesis and pathophysiological consequences. *Z Gerontol Geriatr.* 2004 Apr; 37(2): 109-135.

27. Kaltenbach G, Noblet-Dick M, Andres E, Barnier-Figue G, Noel E, Vogel T, Perrin AE, Martin-Hunyadi C, Berthel M, Kuntzmann F. Early response to oral cobalamin therapy in older patients with vitamin B12 deficiency. *Ann Med Interne* (Paris). 2003 Mar;154(2):91-95.

28. Misra UK, Kalita J, Das A. Vitamin B12 deficiency neurological syn-dromes: a clinical, MRI and electrodiagnostic study. *Electromyogr Clin Neurophysiol.* 2003 Jan-Feb;43(1):57-64.

29. Dagnelie PC. Nutrition and health potential health benefits and risks of vegetarianism and limited consumption of meat in the Netherlands. *Ned Tijdschr Geneeskd.* 2003 Jul 5;147(27):1308-13.

30. Mattsson N, Kilander A, Bjornsson E. Helicobacter pylori can in rare cases be the cause of iron and vitamin B12 deficiency. No increased risk of iron and vitamin B 12 deficiency due to proton pump inhibitors. *Lakartidningen.* 2004 Jun 3;101(23):2014-2025.

31. Kaptan K, Beyan C, Ural AU, Cetin T, Avcu F, Gulsen M, Finci R, Yalcin A. Helicobacter pylori is it a novel causative agent in Vitamin B12 deficiency? *Arch Intern Med.* 2000 May 8;160(9):1349-1353.

32. Chesner IM, Montgomery RD. Small bowel contamination and vitamin B12 deficiency in the elderly. *J Clin Gastroenterol.* 1986 Aug; 8(4):447-450.

33. Park S, Johnson MA. What is an adequate dose of oral vitamin B12 in older people with poor vitamin B12 status? *Nutr Rev.* 2006 Aug; 64 (8):373-378.

34. Aguirre Errasti C, Barreiro Garcia G, Canovas Fernandez A, Alonso Alonso JJ, de la Prieta Lopez R. Study of cobalamin deficiency in gastrectomized and aged subjects. *Rev Clin Esp.* 2001 Feb;201(2):75-80.

35. Oh R, Brown DL.Vitamin B12 deficiency. *Am Fam Physician.* 2003 Mar 1;67(5):979-986 and 993-994.

Bopp-Kistler I, Ruegger-Frey B, Grob D, Six P. Vitamin B12 deficiency in geriatrics. Schweiz Rundsch *Med Prax.* 1999 Nov 4;88(45): 1867-1875.

36. Herrmann W, Obeid R, Schorr H, Geisel J. Functional vitamin B12 deficiency and determination of holotranscobalamin in populations at risk. *Clin Chem Lab Med.* 2003 Nov;41(11):1478-88.

37. Malouf R, Areosa Sastre A. Vitamin B12 for cognition. *Cochrane Database Syst Rev.* 2003;(3):CD004326

38. Vrethem M, Mattsson E, Hebelka H, Leerbeck K, Osterberg A, Landtblom AM, Balla B, Nilsson H, Hultgren M, Brattstrom L, Kagedal B. Increased plasma homocysteine levels without signs of vitamin B12 deficiency in patients with multiple sclerosis assessed by blood and cerebrospinal fluid homocysteine and methylmalonic acid. *Mult Scler.* 2003 Jun;9(3):239-245.

39. Maamar M, Tazi-Mezalek Z, Harmouche H, Ammouri W, Zahlane M, Adnaoui M, Aouni M, Mohattane A, Maaouni A. Neurological manifestations of vitamin B12 deficiency: a retrospective study of 26 cases. *Rev Med Interne.* 2006 Jun;27(6):442-7. Epub 2006 Feb 28.

40. Lerner V, Kanevsky M. Acute dementia with delirium due to vitamin B12 deficiency: a case report. *Int J Psychiatry Med.* 2002;32(2) :215-220.

41. Lechner K, Fodinger M, Grisold W, Puspok A, Sillaber C. VitaminB12 deficiency. New data on an old theme. *Wien Klin Wochenschr.*2005 Sep; 117(17):579-591.

42. Eussen SJ, de Groot LC, Clarke R, Schneede J, Ueland PM, Hoefnagels WH, van Staveren WA. Oral cyanocobalamin supplementation in older people with vitamin B12 deficiency: a dose-finding trial. *Arch Intern Med.* 2005 May 23; 165(10): 1167-1172.

43. Bondeson E, Meisel T, Eggertsen R. A simple health control for the elderly. Screening for vitamin B12 deficiency and thyroid disease. *Lakartidningen.* 1997 Nov 19;94(47):4329-4332. Swedish.

44. Carmel R, Green R, Rosenblatt DS, Watkins D. Update on cobalamin, folate, and homocysteine. *Hematology Am Soc* Hematol Educ Program. 2003;:62-81.

45. Abd-el-Gawa G, Abrahamsson K, Norlen L, Hjalmas K, Hanson E. Vitamin B12 and folate after 5-12 years of continent ileal urostomy (Kock reservoir) in children and adolescents. *Eur Urol.* 2002 Feb; 41(2):199-205.

46. Muller P, Fischer H, Sorger D. Vitamin B12-level in serum of diabetics receiving long-term buformin therapy. *Z Gesamte Inn Med.* 1981 Mar 15;36(6):226-228

47. Petavy-Catala C, Fontes V, Gironet N, Huttenberger B, Lorette G, Vaillant L. Clinical manifestations of the mouth revealing Vitamin B12 deficiency before the onset of anemia *Ann Dermatol Venereol.* 2003 Feb;130 (2 Pt 1):191-194.

48. Baik HW, Russell RM. Vitamin B12 deficiency in the elderly. *Annu Rev Nutr.* 1999;19:357-377.

49. Romieu I, Trenga C. Diet and obstructive lung diseases. *Epidemiol Rev.* 2001;23(2):268-287.

50. Salom IL, Silvis SE, Doscherholmen A. Effect of cimetidine on the absorption of vitamin B12. *Scand J Gastroenterol.* 1982 Jan;17(1):129-131.

51. Wiersinga WJ, de Rooij SE, Huijmans JG, Fischer C, Hoekstra JB. Diagnosis of vitamin B12 deficiency revised. *Ned Tijdschr Geneeskd.* 2005 Dec 10;149(50):2789-2794.

52. Aimone-Gastin I, Pierson H, Jeandel C, Bronowicki JP, Plenat F, Lambert D, Nabet-Belleville F, Gueant JL. Prospective evaluation of protein bound vitamin B12 (cobalamin) malabsorption in the elderly using trout flesh labeled in vivo with 57 Co-cobalamin. *Gut.* 1997 Oct;41(4):475-479.

53. Aaron S, Kumar S, Vijayan J, Jacob J, Alexander M, Gnanamuthu C. Clinical and laboratory features and response to treatment in patients presenting with vitamin B12 deficiency-related neurological syndromes. *Neurol India.* 2005 Mar;53(1):55-58; discussion 59.

54. Mawer EB, Davies M. Vitamin D nutrition and bone disease in adults. *Rev Endocr Metab Disord.* 2001 Apr;2(2):153-164.

55. Figlin E, Chetrit A, Shahar A, Shpilberg O, Zivelin A, Rosenberg N, Brok-Simoni F, Gadoth N, Sela BA, Seligsohn U. High prevalences of vitamin B12 and folic acid deficiency in elderly subjects in Israel. *Br J Haematol.* 2003 Nov; 123(4):696-701.

56. Lane LA, Rojas-Fernandez C. Treatment of vitamin B12 deficiency anemia: oral versus parenteral therapy. *Ann Pharmacother.* 2002 Jul-Aug; 36(7-8): 1268-72.

57. Peracchi M, Bamonti Catena F, Pomati M, De Franceschi M, Scalabrino G. Human cobalamin deficiency: alterations in serum tumour necrosis factor-alpha and epidermal growth factor. *Eur J Haematol.* 2001 Aug; 67(2):123-127.

58. Remacha AF, Souto JC, Ramila E, Perea G, Sarda MP, Fontcuberta J. Enhanced risk of thrombotic disease in patients with acquired vitamin B12 and/or folate deficiency: role of hyperhomocysteinemia. *Ann Hematol.* 2002 Nov;81 (11):616-621. Epub 2002 Nov 9.

59. Abyad A. Prevalence of vitamin B12 deficiency among demented patients and cognitive recovery with cobalamin replacement. *J Nutr Health Aging.* 2002;6(4):254-260.

60. Carmel R. Cobalamin, the stomach, and aging. *Am J Clin Nutr.* 1997 Oct; 66(4):750-759.

61. Andres E, Kaltenbach G, Noblet-Dick M, Noel E, Vinzio S, Perrin AE, Berthel M, Blickle JF. Hematological response to short-term oral cyanocobalamin therapy for the treatment of cobalamin deficiencies in elderly patients. *J Nutr Health Aging.* 2006 JanFeb;10(1):3-6.

62. Avcu N, Avcu F, Beyan C, Ural AU, Kaptan K, Ozyurt M, Nevruz O, Yalcin A. The relationship between gastric-oral Helicobacter pylori and oral hygiene in patients with vitamin B12-deficiency anemia. *Oral Surg Oral Med* Oral Pathol Oral Radiol Endod. 2001 Aug;92(2):166-169.

63. Moore A, Ryan J, Watts M, Pillay I, Clinch D, Lyons D. Orthostatic tolerance in older patients with vitamin B12 deficiency before and after vitamin B12 replacement. *Clin Auton Res.* 2004 Apr;14(2): 67-71.

64. Suzuki DM, Alagiakrishnan K, Masaki KH, Okada A, Carethers M. Patient acceptance of intranasal cobalamin gel for vitamin B12 replacement therapy. *Hawaii Med J.* 2006 Nov;65(11):311-314.

65. Beitzke M, Pfister P, Fortin J, Skrabal F. Autonomic dysfunction and hemodynamics in vitamin B12 deficiency. *Auton Neurosci.* 2002 Apr 18;97 (1): 45-54.

66. Serin E, Gumurdulu Y, Ozer B, Kayaselcuk F, Yilmaz U, Kocak R. Impact of Helicobacter pylori on the development of vitamin B12 deficiency in the absence of gastric atrophy. *Helicobacter.* 2002 Dec;7(6):337-41.

67. Dahele A, Ghosh S. Vitamin B12 deficiency in untreated celiac disease. *Am J Gastroenterol.* 2001 Mar; 96(3):745-750.

68. Meertens L, Solano L. Vitamin B12, folic acid and mental function in the elderly. *Invest Clin.* 2005 Mar;46(1):53-63.

69. Braham-Jmili N, Ltaief A, Ghorbel H, Omri H, Mahjoub T, Braham Y, Bahri F, Jemni L, Hedhili A, Kortas M. Apport of serum vitamin B12 determination in the diagnosis of deficiency: about 95 cases. *Tunis Med.* 2004 Apr;82(4):350-357.

70. Adachi S, Kawamoto T, Otsuka M, Todoroki T, Fukao K. Enteral vitamin B12 supplements reverse postgastrectomy B12 deficiency. *Ann Surg.* 2000 Aug; 232(2):199-201.

71. Takasaki Y, Moriuchi Y, Tsushima H, Ikeda E, Koura S, Taguchi J, Fuku–shima T, Tomonaga M, Ikeda S. Effectiveness of oral vitamin B12 therapy for pernicious anemia and vitamin B12 deficiency anemia. *Rinsho Ketsueki.* 2002 Mar;43(3):165-169.

72. ter Heide H, Hendriks HJ, Heijmans H, Menheere PP, Spaapen LJ, Bakker JA, Forget PP. Are children with cystic fibrosis who are treated with a proton-pump inhibitor at risk for vitamin B12 deficiency? *J Pediatr Gastroenterol Nutr.* 2001 Sep;33(3):342-345.

73. Lucas MH, Elgazzar AH. Detection of protein bound vitamin B12 malabsorption. A case report and review of the literature. *Clin Nucl Med.* 1994 Nov;19(11):1001-1003.

74. Cordingley FT, Crawford GP. Giardia infection causes vitamin B12 deficiency. *Aust N Z J Med.* 1986 Feb;16(1):78-79.

75. Rogers LM, Boy E, Miller JW, Green R, Rodriguez M, Chew F, Allen LH. Predictors of cobalamin deficiency in Guatemalan school children: diet, Helicobacter pylori, or bacterial overgrowth? *J Pediatr Gastroenterol Nutr.* 2003 Jan;36(1):27-36.

76. Hvas AM, Buhl H, Laursen NB, Hesse B, Berglund L, Nexo E. The effect of recombinant human intrinsic factor on the uptake of vitamin B12 in patients with evident vitamin B12 deficiency. *Haematologica.*2006 Jun; 91(6):805-808. Epub 2006 May 16.

77. Valuck RJ, Ruscin JM. A case-control study on adverse effects: H2 blocker or proton pump inhibitor use and risk of vitamin B12 deficiency in older adults. *J Clin Epidemiol.* 2004 Apr;57(4):422-428.

78. Watts DT. Vitamin B12 replacement therapy: how much is enough? *Wis Med J.* 1994 May;93(5):203-205.

79. Andres E, Perrin AE, Demangeat C, Kurtz JE, Vinzio S, Grunenberger F, Goichot B, Schlienger JL. The syndrome of food-cobalamin malabsorption revisited in a department of internal medicine. A monocentric cohort study of 80 patients. *Eur J Intern Med.* 2003 Jul; 14(4):221-226.

80. Gimsing P, Hippe E, Helleberg-Rasmussen I, Moesgaard M, Nielsen JL, Bastrup-Madsen P, Berlin R, Hansen T. Cobalamin forms in plasma and tissue during treatment of vitamin B12 deficiency. *Scand J Haematol.* 1982 Oct;29 (4):311-18.

81. Mitchell SL, Rockwood K. The association between antiulcer medication and initiation of cobalamin replacement in older persons. *J Clin Epidemiol.* 2001 May; 54(5):531-534.

82. Billion S, Tribout B, Cadet E, Queinnec C, Rochette J, Wheatley P, Bataille P. Hyperhomocysteinaemia, folate and vitamin B12 in unsupplemented haemodialysis patients: effect of oral therapy with folic acid and vitamin B12. *Nephrol Dial Transplant.* 2002 Mar;17(3):455-461.

83. Dickey W. Low serum vitamin B12 is common in coeliac disease and is not due to autoimmune gastritis. *Eur J Gastroenterol Hepatol.*2002 Apr; 14(4):425-47.

84. Coppen A, Bolander-Gouaille C. Treatment of depression: time to consider folic acid and vitamin B12. *J Psychopharmacol.* 2005 Jan;19(1):59-65.

85. Stabler SP, Allen RH. Vitamin B12 deficiency as a worldwide problem. *Annu Rev Nutr.* 2004;24:299-326.

86. Lindgren A, Bagge E, Cederblad A, Nilsson O, Persson H, Kilander AF. Schilling and protein-bound cobalamin absorption tests are poor instruments for diagnosing cobalamin malabsorption. *J Intern Med.* 1997 Jun;241(6):477-484.

87. Herrmann W. The importance of hyperhomocysteinemia as a risk factor for diseases: an overview. *Clin Chem Lab Med.* 2001 Aug;39(8):666-674.

88. Nilsson M, Norberg B, Hultdin J, Sandstrom H, Westman G, Lokk J. Medical intelligence in Sweden. Vitamin B12: oral compared with parenteral? *Postgrad Med J.* 2005 Mar;81(953):191-193.

89. Bolaman Z, Kadikoylu G, Yukselen V, Yavasoglu I, Barutca S, Senturk T. Oral versus intramuscular cobalamin treatment in megaloblastic anemia: a single-center, prospective, randomized, open-label study. *Clin Ther.* 2003 Dec;25(12):3124-3134.

90. Thompson WG, Freedman ML. Vitamin B12 and geriatrics: unanswered questions. *Acta Haematol.* 1989; 82(4):169-174.

91. Dharmarajan TS, Norkus EP. Approaches to vitamin B12 deficiency. Early treatment may prevent devastating complications. *Postgrad Med.* 2001 Jul; 110(1): 99-105; quiz 106.

92. Robinson M, White FJ, Cleary MA, Wraith E, Lam WK, Walter JH. Increased risk of vitamin B12 deficiency in patients with phenylketonuria on an unrestricted or relaxed diet. *J Pediatr.* 2000 Apr;136(4):545-547.

93. Donaldson MS. Metabolic vitamin B12 status on a mostly raw vegan diet with follow-up using tablets, nutritional yeast, or probiotic supplements. *Ann Nutr Metab.* 2000;44(5-6):229-234.

94. Gessler NN, Alekseeva NV, Bykhovskii VIa. Change in tryptamine metabolism in vitamin B12 deficiency. *Vopr Med Khim.* 1994 Jan- Feb;40(1): 47-49.

95. Silver H. Vitamin B12 levels are low in hospitalized psychiatric patients. *Isr J Psychiatry Relat Sci.* 2000;37(1):41-45.

96. Yakout H, Bissada NK.Intermediate effects of the ileocaecal urinary reservoir (Charleston pouch 1) on serum vitamin B12 concentrations: can vitamin B12 deficiency be prevented? *BJU Int.*2003 May;91(7): 653-5; discussion 655-656.

97. Moretti R, Torre P, Antonello RM, Cattaruzza T, Cazzato G, Bava A. Vitamin B12 and folate depletion in cognition: a review. *Neurol India.* 2004 Sep;52(3):310-318.

98. Sharabi A, Cohen E, Sulkes J, Garty M. Replacement therapy for vitamin B12 deficiency: comparison between the sublingual and oral route. *Br J Clin Pharmacol.* 2003 Dec;56(6):635-638.

Campbell CD, Ganesh J, Ficicioglu C. Two newborns with nutritional vitamin B12 deficiency: challenges in newborn screening for vitamin B12 deficiency. *Haematologica.* 2005 Dec;90(12 Suppl):ECR45.

Oosterhuis WP, Niessen RW, Bossuyt PM, Sanders GT, Sturk A. Diagnostic value of the mean corpuscular volume in the detection of vitamin B12 deficiency. *Scand J Clin Lab Invest.* 2000 Feb;60(1):9-18.

99. Schneede J. Prerequisites for establishing general recommendations for diagnosis and treatment of vitamin B12 dficiency and cost-utility evaluation of these guidelines. *Scand J Clin Lab Invest.* 2003;63(5):369-375.

100. Puri V, Chaudhry N, Goel S, Gulati P, Nehru R, Chowdhury D. Vitamin B12 deficiency: a clinical and electrophysiological profile. *Electromyogr Clin Neurophysiol.* 2005 Jul-Aug;45(5):273-284.

101. Campbell AK, Miller JW, Green R, Haan MN, Allen LH. Plasma vitamin B12 concentrations in an elderly latino population are predicted by serum gastrin concentrations and crystalline vitamin B-12 intake.*J Nutr.*2003 Sep;133(9):2770-2776.

102. Chui CH, Lau FY, Wong R, Soo OY, Lam CK, Lee PW, Leung HK, So CK, Tsoi WC, Tang N, Lam WK, Cheng G. Vitamin B12 deficiency-need for a new guideline. *Nutrition.* 2001 NovDec;17(11-12):917-920.

103. Dommisse J. Subtle vitamin-B12 deficiency and psychiatry: a largely unnoticed but devastating relationship? *Med Hypotheses.* 1991 Feb; 34(2): 131-140.

104. van Walraven CG, Naylor CD. Use of vitamin B12 injections among elderly patients by primary care practitioners in Ontario. *CMAJ.* 1999 Jul 27; 161(2):146-149.

105. Loukili NH, Andres E. Vitamin B12 in the adult: of metabolism and deficiencies. *Ann Endocrinol* (Paris). 2003 Nov;64(5 Pt 1):376-382.

106. Girard P, Lebrun C, Peyrade F, Brunetto JL, Chatel M. Orthostatic hypotension revealing vitamin B12 deficiency. *Rev Neurol* (Paris). 1998 May; 154(4):342-344.

107. Dutta SK. Vitamin B12 malabsorption and omeprazole therapy. *J Am Coll Nutr.* 1994 Dec;13(6):544-5. & *J Am Coll Nutr.* 1995 Jun;14(3):218.

108. Gumurdulu Y, Serin E, Ozer B, Aydin M, Yapar AF, Kayaselcuk F, Yilmaz U, Boyacioglu S. The impact of B12 treatment on gastric emptying time in patients with Helicobacter pylori infection. *J Clin Gastroenterol.* 2003 Sep;37(3):230-233.

110. Al-Momen AK. Unusual presentation of vitamin B12 deficiency. *Ann Saudi Med.* 1993 May;13(3):226-230.

111. Tomczykiewicz K, Tutaj A, Janda R. Neurological disorders of vitamin B12 deficiency. *Neurol Neurochir Pol.* 1998 NovDec;32 (6):1473-1484

112. Collins JE, Rolles CJ, Sutton H, Ackery D. Vitamin B12 absorption after necrotizing enterocolitis. *Arch Dis Child.* 1984 Aug;59 (8):731-734.

113. Iseki T. Vitamin B12 and transcobalamin in chronic myeloproliferative disorders. *Rinsho Byori.* 1993 Dec;41 (12): 1310-1321.

114. Gruener DM, Kunkel EJ, Snyderman DA, Infante MR, Rodgers C, Field HL. Dietary vitamin B12 deficiency in a patient with multiple sclerosis. *Gen Hosp Psychiatry.* 1994 May;16(3):224-228.

115. Andres E, Federici L. Vitamin B12 deficiency in patients receiving metformin clinical data. *Arch Intern Med.* 2007 Apr 9;167(7):729; author reply 730-31.

116. Bandy LC, Clarke-Pearson DL, Creasman WT. Vitamin B12 deficiency following therapy in gynecologic oncology. *Gynecol Oncol*.1984 Mar; 17(3):370-374.

117. Sabatino D, Kosuri S, Remollino A, Shotter B. Cobalamin deficiency presenting with cutaneous hyperpigmentation: a report of two siblings. *Pediatr Hematol Oncol*. 1998 Sep-Oct;15(5):447-450.

118. Akdal G, Yener GG, Ada E, Halmagyi GM. Eye movement disorders in vitamin B12 deficiency: two new cases and a review of the literature. *Eur J Neurol*. 2007 Oct;14(10):1170-1172.

119. Yamamura Y. Studies on experimentally induced vitamin B12 deficiency. II. Vitamin B12 content in blood, bone marrow and various tissues of guinea pigs fed on diet deficient in hematopoietic vitamins. *Naika Hokan*. 1966 Jan;13(1):15-21.

120. McLoughlin JL, Cantrill RC. Vitamin B12 deficiency alters the distribution of membrane proteins on linear sucrose gradients in the fruit bat brain. *Neurosci Lett*. 1984 Aug 24;49(1-2):175-180.

121. Venkataraman S, Biswas DK, Johnson BC. Effect of propionate on the induction of vitamin B12 deficiency in chicks and rats. *J Nutr*.1967 Oct;93(2):131-134.

122. Lin SH, Sourial NA, Lu KC, Hsueh EJ. Imerslund-Grasbeck syndrome in a Chinese family with distinct skin lesions refractory to vitamin B12. *J Clin Pathol*. 1994 Oct;47(10):956-958.

123. Lavy NW. Omeprazole and vitamin B12. *Ann Intern Med*. 1994 Jul 1;121(1):74.

124. Volkov L. The master key effect of vitamin B12 in treatment of malignancy A potential therapy? *Med Hypotheses*. 2007 Jul 17.

125. Yamamura Y. Studies on experimentally induced vitamin B12 deficiency. Manifestations observed on bodily growth, hematological findings and other pathological symptoms. *Naika Hokan*. 1966 Jan; 13(1):1-14.

126. Tomkin GH. Metformin and B 12 malabsorption. *Ann Intern Med*. 1972 Apr;76(4):668.

127. Sudo K, Tashiro K. Cerebral white matter lesions associated with vitamin B12 deficiency. *Neurology*. 1998 Jul;51(1):325-326.

128. Nusbaum MR, Kiser WR, Ellis D, Runkle G, Kugler J P. Vitamin B12 deficiency. *J Fam Pract*. 1993 Apr;36 (4):373; author reply 373, 377.

129. Pacala JT. Vitamin B12 deficiency. *J Fam Pract*. 1993 Apr; 36(4):373; author reply 373, 377.

130. Britt RP, Harper CM. Vitamin-B12 deficiency in Asian immigrants. *Lancet*. 1976 Oct 9;2(7989):799.

131. Mayall M. Vitamin B12 deficiency and nitrous oxide. *Lancet.*1999 May 1;353(9163):1529.

132. Goh K. Vitamin B12 deficiency in an 18p-patient. *Arch PatholLab Med.* 1981 Mar;105(3):164.

133. Nyberg W. Diphyllobothrium latum and human nutrition, with particular reference to vitamin B12 deficiency. *Proc Nutr Soc.* 1963;22:8-14.

134. Harris R. The EEG in anesthetized juvenile baboons during an experi–mental investigation of vitamin B12 deficiency. *Electroencephalogr Clin Neurophysiol.* 1969 Sep;27(7):671.

135. Bial AK. Review: Limited evidence from 2 randomised controlled trials suggests that oral and intramuscular vitamin B12 have similar effectiveness for vitamin B12 deficiency. *Evid Based Med.* 2006 Feb;11(1):9.

136. Fatterpaker P, Lavate WV, Mulgaonkat AG, Noronha JM, Rege DV, Tipnis HP, Sreenivasan A. Experimental production of vitamin B12 deficiency in rats and mice on a maize-groundnut-meal diet. *Br J Nutr.* 1959;13:439-447.

137. Labenz J, Stolte M. Vision and hearing disorders with omeprazole: the facts. *Leber Magen Darm.* 1995 Jan;25(1):6-8, 11.

138. Becker DE, Smith SE, Loosli JK. Vitamin B12 and Cobalt Deficiency in Sheep. *Science.* 1949 Jul 15;110(2846):71-72.

139. Kaptan K, Beyan C, Ifran. Helicobacter pylori and vitamin B12 deficiency. *Haematologica.* 2006 Dec; 91(12 Suppl):ELT10. A.

140. Fitzgerald MA. Drug-induced vitamin B12 deficiency. *Nurse Pract.* 2007 Sep;32(9):6-7.

141. Pristoupilova K, Slavikova V. Coenzyme forms of vitamin B12 and their physiologic significance. *Cas Lek Cesk.* 1984 Nov 30;123 (48):1457-60.

142. Dale FH. Ability of the Bobwhite to Grow and Reproduce without a Dietary Source of Vitamin B12. *Science.*1955 May 6;121(3149):675-676.

143. Other factors related to vitamin B12. *Biochem J.* 1955 Feb 19;59 (337th Meeting):xxvii KON SK.

144. Buhs RP, Newstead EG, Trenner NR. An analog of vitamin B12. *Science.* 1951 Jun 1;113(2944):625-6.

145. Heaton JM. Vitamin B12 and the eye. *Proc Nutr Soc.*1960;19:100-05.

146. Whitmarsh JM, Albans JW, Wright RD. Vitamin B12 in sewage. *Biochem J.* 1955 May 14;60(340th Meeting):xxvii.

147. Rickes EL, Brink NG, Koniuszy FR, Wood TR, Folkers K. Crystalline Vitamin B12. *Science*. 1948 Apr 16;107(2781):396-397.

148. Wright MH. Thymidine and Vitamin B12. *Science*. 1949 Sep 9; 110 (2854): 257-8.

149. Caballero MR, Lukawska J, Lee TH, Dugue P. Allergy to B12: two cases of successful desensitization with cyanocobalamin. *Allergy*. 2007 Sep 5.

151. Horwitt MK, Liebert E, Kreisler O, Wittman P. Studies of Vitamin Deficiency. *Science*. 1946 Nov 1;104(2705):407-408.

152. King JD. Dietary deficiency, nerve lesions and the dental tissues. *J Physiol*. 1936 Oct 16;88(1):62-77.

9. H. L. Newbold. Vitamin B12: Placebo or neglected therapeutic tool? Original Research Article. *Medical Hypotheses,* Volume 28, Issue 3, March 1989, Pages 155-164.

10. Frank J. Heck. Proper Use Of Iron, Liver Extract, Vitamin B12, And Folic Acid In Anemias. *J Am Med Assoc*. 1952;148(10):783-8.

11. Anemia caused by vitamin B 12 deficiency in subjects aged over 75 years: new hypotheses. A study of 20 cases *Rev Med Interne*. 2000 Nov; 21(11):946-954. French.

12. Andres E, Loukili NH, Noel E, Kaltenbach G, Abdelgheni MB, Perrin AE, Noblet-Dick M, Maloisel F, Schlienger JL, Blickle JF. Vitamin B12 (cobalamin) deficiency in elderly patients. Review *CMAJ*. 2004 Aug 3;171(3):251-259.

13. Andres E, Affenberger S, Vinzio S, Kurtz JE, Noel E, Kaltenbach G, Maloisel F, Schlienger JL, Blickle JF. *Am J Med*. 2005 Oct; 118 (10):1154-9. Food-cobalamin malabsorption in elderly patients: clinical manifestations and treatment.

14. Loew D, Wanitschke R, Schroedter A. Studies on vitamin B12 status in the elderly-prophylactic and therapeutic consequences. *Int J Vitam Nutr Res*. 1999 May;69(3):228-233.

15. Dharmarajan TS, Adiga GU, Norkus EP. Vitamin B12 deficiency. Recognizing subtle symptoms in older adults. *Geriatrics*. 2003 Mar;58(3):30-4, 37-8.

16. Wolters M, Strehle A, Hahn A. Age-associated changes in the metabolism of vitamin B(12) and folic acid: prevalence, aetiopathogenesis and pathophysiological consequences. *Z Gerontol Geriatr*. 2004 Apr;37(2):109-135.

17. Kaltenbach G, Noblet-Dick M, Andres E, Barnier-Figue G, Noel E, Vogel T, Perrin AE, Martin-Hunyadi C, Berthel M, Kuntzmann F. Early response to oral cobalamin therapy in older patients with vitamin B12 deficiency. *Ann Med Interne* (Paris). 2003 Mar;154(2):91-95

18. Bopp-Kistler I, Ruegger-Frey B,Grob D, Six P. Vitamin B12 deficiency in geriatrics. *Praxis* (Bern 1994). 1999 Nov 4; 88(45):1867-1875.

19. Eussen SJ, de Groot LC, Clarke R, Schneede J, Ueland PM, Hoefnagels WH, van Staveren WA. Oral cyanocobalamin supplementation in older people with vitamin B12 deficiency: a dose-finding trial. *Arch Intern Med.* 2005 May 23;165(10):1167-1172.

20. Vitamin B12 deficiency in the elderly. *Annu Rev Nutr.* 1999;19:357-77. Review.

21. August, 2007 *Journal of the American Geriatrics Society* reported that Long-term use of H2 blockers, including Axid, Pepcid, Tagamet, and Zantac, increases the risk of mental decline in later life because this interferes with the absorption of vitamin B12, which is important for mental function.

Chapter 11   Ladies, Meet Progesterone, the Hormone Your Body Loves

1. Michael Lam, M.D., M.P.H., A.B.A.A.M., *Estrogen Dominance (The Silent Epidemic)*, drlam.com/articles/Estrogen_Dominance.asp.

2. Tapiero H, Ba GN, et al. Estrogens and environmental estrogens. *Biomed Pharmacother.* 2002 Feb;56(1):36-44. Review.

3. Bradlow HL, Davis DL, Lin G, et al. Effects of pesticides on the ratio of 16 alpha/2-hydroxyestrone: a biologic marker of breast cancer risk. *Environ Health Perspect.* 1995;103(Suppl 7):147-150.

4. Zimmerman P.A.;Francis G.L.; Poth M. Hormon-containing cosmetics   may cause signs of early sexual development *Military medicine* Y.1995, vol. 160, No. 12, pages 628-30.

5. Cesario, S. K. and Hughes, L.A. (2007), Precocious Puberty: A Comprehensive Review of Literature. *Journal of Obstetric, Gynecologic, & Neonatal Nursing*, 36: 263-274.

6. Chandra M. Tiwary, MBBS, MRCP, DCH, MA, MBA, MPH. Premature Sexual Development in Children Following the Use of Estrogen or Placenta-Containing Hair Products. *Clin Pediatr* Dec.1998 vol.37 no.12 733-39.

7. A. M. Api, Toxicological profile of diethylphthalate: a vehicle for fragrance and cosmetic ingredients. *Food and Chemical Toxicology.* Volume 39, Issue 2, February 2001, Pages 97-108.

8. P.D. Darbre, BSc, PhD. Environmental oestrogens, cosmetics and breast cancer. *Clinical Endocrinology & Metabolism,* Volume 20, Issue 1, Pages 121-143. March 2006.

9. Personal conversations with David Zava, Ph.D. in endocrinology, specializing in breast cancer, co-author of *What Your Doctor May Not Tell You About Breast Cancer.* Warner Books, 2002.

10. Mayes JS, Watson GH. Direct effects of sex steroid hormones on adipose tissues and obesity. *Obes Rev.* 2004 Nov; 5(4): 197-216. Review.

11. Note for California Residents: California State health law requires that the testing of any specimen collected or mailed from California be sent with a written order from a health care professional licensed in California to order laboratory tests. This includes the following disciplines: M.D.; D.C.; LAc; R.D.; D.O.; N.P.; and Pharmacists (R.PH). As of September 2002 (Senate Bill 577), such lab tests may be ordered by complementary or alternative health care practitioners "not providing services that require medical training." If you are a California resident and would still like to order online contact: www.canaryclub.org or www.virginiahopkins–testkits.com. These sites will help you order online, with a licensed physician, in the state of California.

Note for New York Residents: New York State health law prohibits the testing of specimens collected in or mailed from New York, and prohibits the transmission of data from the laboratory to NY physicians or residents. Therefore, direct receipt of lab results for NY residents is not currently possible.

12. Yang TS, Tsan SR, Chang SP, Ng RT. Efficacy and safety of estriol replacement therapy for climacteric women. *Zhonghua Yi Xue Za Zhi* (Taipei). 1995 May;55(5):386-91.

13. Tzingounis VA, Aksu MF, Greenblatt RB. Estriol in the management of the menopause. *JAMA.* 1978 Apr 21;239(16):1638-41.

14. Lee, R. John, The Estrogen Question: Guidelines for supplementing safely and effectively, John R. Lee, M.D *Medical Letter Issue* 1998 November.

15. Lee, R. John, Zava, David, Ropkins, Virginia. *What Your Doctor May Not Tell You About Breast Cancer.* Warner Books, 2002.

16. Lee, R. John, The Estrogen Question: Guidelines for supplementing safely and effectively, John R. Lee, M.D Medical Letter Issue 1998 November.

17. Campagnoli C.; Pregnancy, progesterone and progestins in relation to breast cancer risk.; *J Steroid Biochem Mol Biol.* 2005 Dec;97(5):441-50).

Chapter 12   A Sweet Tooth Can Be a Bitter Pill to Swallow

1. Jacob Teitelbaum, M.D., *U.S. Adults Eat 150 Pounds of Sugar Per Year.* United Press International, November 1, 2010.

2. According to figures from the most recent *Federal Continuing Survey of Food Intakes by Individuals* (1994-1996).

3. Foster-Powell K,Rolt SRA,Brand-Miller JC. International table of glycemic index and glycemic load values: 2002. *The American Journal of Clinical Nutrition.* 2002. 76(1):5-56.

Reiser S. Randler RB, Gardner LB, Rallfrisch JG, Michaelis OE, Prather ES. Isocaloric exchange of dietary starch and sucrose in humans. *The American Journal of Clinical Nutrition.*1979.32:2206-16.

Hallfrisch J, Ellwood KC, Michealis OE, Reiser S, O'dorisio TM, Prather ES. Effects of Dietary Fructose on Plasma Glucose and Hormone Responses in Normal and Hyperinsulinemic Men. *Journal of Nutrition.* 1983. 113:1819-1826.

Brand JC, Nicholson PL, Thorburn AW, Truswell AS. Food processing and the glycemic index. *The American Journal of Clinical Nutrition.* 1985. 42:1192-1196.

4. Hoebel BG, Avena NM, Bocarsly ME, et al. Natural addiction: a behavioral and circuit model based on sugar addiction in rats. *J Addict Med.* 2009; 3: 33- 41.

5. Avena NM, Rada P, Hoebel BG. Evidence for sugar addiction: behavioral and neurochemical effects of intermittent, excessive sugar intake. *Neurosci Biobehav Rev.* 2008;32:20 -39.

6. Wang GJ, Volkow ND, Thanos PK,et al. Imaging of brain dopamine pathways: Implications for understanding obesity. *J Addict Med.* 2009;3:8 -18.

7. Lam RW, Levitan RD, Tam EM, Yatham LN, Lamoureux S, ZisAP. L-tryptophan augmentation of light therapy in patients with seasonal affective disorder. *Can J Psychiatry* 1997;42:303-306.

8. Calapai G, Crupi A, Firenzuoli F, et al. Serotonin, norepinephrine and dopamine involvement in the antidepressant action of Hypericum perforatum. *Pharmacopsychiatry* 2001;34:45-49.

9. Kaehler ST, Sinner C, Chatterjee SS, et al. Hyperforin enhances the extracellar concentrations of catecholamines, serotonin and glutamate in the rat locus coeruleus. *Neurosci Lett* 1999;262:199-202.

10. Mucuna pruriens in Parkinson's disease: a double blind clinical and pharmacological study. *J Neurol Neurosurg Psychiatry.* 2004 Dec; 75 (12): 1672-1677.

11. Manyam BV, Dhanasekaran M, Hare TA. Neuroprotective effects of the antiparkinson drug Mucuna pruriens. *Phytother Res.* 2004 Sep;18(9): 706-712. Department of Neurology, Health Science Center College of Medicine, Temple, TX 76508.

12. Arno K. Kumagai. Glucose transport in brain and retina: implications in the management and complications of diabetes. *Diabetesl Metabolism Research and Reviews.* Volume 15, Issue 4, pages 261-273, July/August 1999.

Chapter 13   Light Up Your Health

1. Teodor T. Postolache, MD; Thomas A. Wehr, MD; Richard L. Doty, PhD; Leo Sher, MD; Erick H. Turner, MD; John J. Bartko, PhD; Norman E. Rosenthal, MD. Patients With Seasonal Affective Disorder Have Lower Odor Detection Thresholds Than Control Subjects. *Arch Gen Psychiatry*/Vol. 59, Dec 2002; 1119-1122.

2. Rosenthal NE, Sack DA, Gillin JC, Lewy AJ, Goodwin FK, Davenport Y, et al. Seasonal affective disorder: a description of the syndrome and prelimnary findings with light therapy. *Arch Gen Psychiatry* 1984; 41:72-80.

3. Lam RW, Levitan RD. Pathopshyiology of seasonal affective disorder: a review. *Journal of Psychiatry & Neuroscience* 2000;25:469-79.

4. Schwartz PJ, Murphy DL, Wehr TA, Garcia-Borreguero D, Oren DA, Moul, et al. Effects of metachlorophenylpiperazine infusions in patients with seasonal affective disorder and healthy control subjects. Diurnal responses and nocturnal regulatory mechanisms. *Arch Gen Psychiatry* 1997;54:375-385.

5. Skwerer RG, Jacobsen FM, Duncan CC, Kelly KA, Sack DA, Tamarkin L, et al. Neurobiology of seasonal affective disorder and phototherapy. *J Biol Rhythnms* 1988;3:135-154.

6. Calapai G, Crupi A, Firenzuoli F, et al. Serotonin, norepinephrine and dopamine involvement in the antidepressant action of Hypericum perforatum. *Pharmacopsychiatry* 2001;34:45-49.

7. Kaehler ST, Sinner C, Chatterjee SS, et al. Hyperforin enhances the extracellular concentrations of catecholamines, serotonin and glutamate in the rat locus coeruleus. *Neurosci Lett* 1999;262:199-202.

8. Seasonal pattern specifier. In: *Diagnostic and Statistical Manual of Mental Disorders* DSM-IV-TR. 4th ed. Arlington, Va.: American Psychiatric Association; 2000.

9. Ravindran AV, et al. Complementary and alternative medicine treatments. Canadian Network for Mood and Anxiety Treatments (CANMAT) clinical guidelines for the management of major depressive disorder in adults. *Journal of Affective Disorders*. 2009;117:S54.

10. Sarris J, et al. Kava and St. John's Wort: Current evidence for use in mood and anxiety disorders. *Journal of Alternative and Complementary Medicine*. 2009;15:827.

11. Hall-Flavin DK (expert opinion). *Mayo Clinic*, Rochester Minn. 10-31-09.

12. Rosen LN, Targum SD, Terman M, et al. Prevalence of seasonal affective disorder at four latitudes. *Psychiatry Res* 1990;31: 131-144.

13. Magnusson A, Stefanson JG. Prevalence of seasonal affective disorder in Iceland. *Archives of General Psychiatry* 1993; 50: 941-946.

14. Magnusson A, Axelsson J. The prevalence of seasonal affective disorder is low among descendants of Icelandic emigrants in Canada. *Archives of General Psychiatry* 1993; 50: 947-951.

15. Markku Timonen, Juuso Nissila, Anu Liettu, Jari Jokelainen, Heidi Jurvelin, Antti Aunio, Pirkko Räsänen, Timo Takala-University of Oulu, Institute of Health Sciences. Can transcranial brain-targeted bright light treatment via ear canals be effective in relieving symptoms in seasonal affective disorder? A pilot study. *Medical hypotheses*, 2012 Apr ;78 (4):511-522 296809.

16. Lam RW, Levitan RD, Tam EM, Yatham LN, Lamoureux S, ZisAP. L-tryptophan augmentation of light therapy in patients with seasonal affective disorder. *Can J Psychiatry* 1997;42:303-6.

17. Calapai G, Crupi A, Firenzuoli F, et al. Serotonin, norepinephrine and dopamine involvement in the antidepressant action of Hypericum perforatum. *Pharmacopsychiatry* 2001;34:45-49.

18. Kaehler ST, Sinner C, Chatterjee SS, et al. Hyperforin enhances the extracellular concentrations of catecholamines, serotonin and glutamate in the rat locus coeruleus. *Neurosci Lett* 1999;262: 199-202.

19. Katzenschlager R, Evans A, Manson A, Patsalos PN, Ratnaraj N, Watt H, et al. Mucuna pruriens in Parkinsons disease: a double blind clinical and pharmacological study. *J Neurol Neurosurg Psychiatry* 2004;75: 1672-1677.

20. Manyam BV, Dhanasekaran M, Hare TA. Neuroprotective effects of the antiparkinson drug Mucuna pruriens. *Phytother Res.* 2004 Sep;18(9):706-712. Department of Neurology, Health Science Center College of Medicine, Temple, TX 76508.

21. L Lundt. Modafinil treatment in patients with seasonal affective disorder winter depression: an open-label pilot study. *J Affect Disord*. Volume 81, Issue 2, Pages 173-178 (August 2004).

RH Howland. Pharmacotherapy for Psychotropic Drug-Related Weight Gain. *Journal of Psychosocial Nursing & Mental Health Services* Volume 46. Issue 7: 15-18.

Dackis CA, Kampman KM, Lynch KG, Pettinati HM, O'Brien CP: A double-blind, placebo-controlled trial of modafinil for cocaine dependence. *Neuropsychopharmacology* 2005;30:205- 211.

22. Peter J. Morgan, Alexander W. Rossa, Julian G. Mercera and Perry Barretta. What can we learn from seasonal animals about the regulation of energy balance? *Progress in Brain Research* Volume 153, 2006, Pages 325-337.

23. Thompson C. Melatonin and seasonal affective disorder. In: Miles A, Philbrick DRS, Thompson C, eds. *Melatonin Clinical Perspectives*. Oxford University Press, Oxford 1988; 228-42.

Chapter 14   Putting the Pieces Together

1. David M. Marks, Manan J. Shah, Ashwin A. Patkar, Prakash S. Masand, Geun-Young Park and Chi-Un Pae. Serotonin-Norepinephrine Reuptake Inhibitors for PainControl: Premise and Promise, *Current Neuropharmacology, 2009, 7, 331-336.*

Jung, Alan C., Thomas Staiger, and Mark Sullivan. The efficacy of selective serotonin reuptake inhibitors for the management of chronic pain. *Journal of General Internal Medicine* 12.6 (1997): 384-389.

Barkin, Robert L., and Jan Fawcett. The management challenges of chronic pain: the role of antidepressants. *American Journal of Therapeutics* 7.1 (2000): 31.

Bolay, Hayrunnisa, and Michael A. Moskowitz. Mechanisms of pain modulation in chronic syndromes. *Neurology* 59.5 suppl 2 (2002): S2-S7.

Iyengar, Smriti, et al. Efficacy of duloxetine, a potent and balanced serotonin-norepinephrine reuptake inhibitor in persistent pain models in rats. *Journal of Pharmacology and Experimental Therapeutics,* 311.2 (2004): 576-584.

2. Michael Bauer, Peter C. Whybrow. Thyroid Hormone, Neural Tissue and Mood Modulation *World J Biol Psychiatry* (2001) 2, 59-69.

Bauer M, Heinz A, Whybrow PC . Thyroid hormones, serotonin and mood: of synergy and significance in the adult brain. *Mol Psychiatry*. 2002;7(2):140-56.

Chapter 15   New Research

1. Cummings DE, Weigle DS, Frayo RS, Breen PA, Ma MK, Dellinger EP, and Purnell JQ. Plasma ghrelin levels after diet-induced weight loss or gastric bypass surgery. *N Engl J Med* 346: 1623-1630, 2002.

2. Katie Wynne, Sarah Stanley, Barbara McGowan and Steve Bloom. Appetite control. *Journal of Endocrinology* (2005) 184, 291-318.

3. Bluher S, Mantzoros CS. Leptin in humans: lessons from translational research. *Am J Clin Nutr.* 2009 Mar;89 (3):991S-997S.

4. *U.S. Centers for Disease Control and Prevention* in September, 2009.

5. B. Baranowska, M. Radzikowska, E. Wasilewska-Dziubinska, K. Roguski, M. Borowiec. Disturbed release of gastrointestinal peptides in anorexia nervosa and in obesity. *Diabetes, Obesity and Metabolism*, Volume 2, Issue 2, pages 99-103, Mar. 2000.

R. L. Batterham, C. W. Le Roux, M. A. Cohen, A. J. Park, S. M. Ellis, M. Patterson, G. S. Frost, M. A. Ghatei and S. R. Bloom. Pancreatic polypeptide reduces appetite and food intake in humans. *The Journal of Clinical Endocrinology & Metabolism* Vol. 88, No. 8 3989-3992.

Christian L. Roth, Pablo J. Enriori, Katia Harz, Joachim Woelfle, Michael A. Cowley and Thomas Reinehr. Peptide YY Is a Regulator of Energy Homeostasis in Obese Children before and after Weight Loss. *The Journal of Clinical Endocrinology & Metabolism* Vol. 90, No. 12 6386-6391.

6. Owais B. Chaudhri, PHD, Katie Wynne, PHD and Stephen R. Bloom, MD, DSC. *Diabetes Care* February 2008 vol. 31 no. Supplement 2 S284-S289.

7. Wynne K, Park AJ, Small CJ, Patterson M, Ellis SM, Murphy KG, Wren AM, Frost GS, Meeran K, Ghatei MA, Bloom SR: Subcutaneous oxyntomodulin reduces body weight in overweight and obese subjects: a double-blind, randomized, controlled trial. *Diabetes* 54:2390-2395, 2005.

8. Wynne K, Park AJ, Small CJ, Meeran K, Ghatei MA, Frost GS, Bloom SR: Oxyntomodulin increases energy expenditure in addition to decreasing energy intake in overweight and obese humans: a randomized controlled trial. *Int J Obes* (Lond) 30:1729-1736, 2006.

9. Le Roux CW, Aylwin SJ, Batterham RL, Borg CM, Coyle F, Prasad V, Shurey S,Ghatei MA, Patel AG, Bloom SR: Gut hormone profiles following bariatric surgery favor an anorectic state, facilitate weight loss, and improve metabolic parameters. *Ann Surg* 243:108-114, 2006.

10. Theodore N Pappas. Physiological satiety implications of gastrointestinal antiobesity surgery. *American Journal of Clinical Nutrition*, Vol 55, 571S-572S. 1992.

11. Ritter, R. C. (2004) Gastrointestinal mechanisms of satiation for food. *Physiol. Behav.* 81, 249- 273.

12. Jill A Parnell and Raylene A Reimer. Weight loss during oligofructose supplementation is associated with decreased ghrelin and increased peptide YY in overweight and obese adults. *Am J Clin Nutr* June 2009 vol. 89 no. 6, 1751-1759.

13. Ambikaipakan Balasubramaniam. Clinical potentials of neuropeptide Y family of hormones.*The American Journal of Surgery* Volume 183, Issue 4, Pages 430-434, April 2002.

NR Levens, Zuana O Della. Neuropeptide Y Y5 receptor antagonists as anti-obesity drugs.*Current Opinion in Investigational Drugs* 20034:1198-1204.

Z. Zukowska-Grojec, NeuropeptideY, novel sympathetic stress hormone and more, *Annals of the New York Academy of Sciences*, December 29, 1995.

L.E. Kuo et al., Neuropeptide Y acts directly in the periphery on fat tissue and mediates stress-induced obesity and metabolic syndrome, *NatureMedicine,* published on line July 1, 2007.

Thomas H. Maugh II (July 2, 2007). *Research points to way to eliminate belly fat.* Chicago Tribune.

Kuo LE, Kitlinska JB, Tilan JU, et al. (July 2007). Neuropeptide Y acts directly in the periphery on fat tissue and mediates stress-induced obesity and metabolic syndrome. *Nat. Med.* 13 (7): 803- 811.

GLOSSARY

1. *Born Together—Reared Apart The Landmark Minnesota Study*, Nancy L. Segal, June 2012. Harvard University Press.

2. Hin, Harold, et al. Clinical relevance of low serum vitamin B12 concentrations in older people: the Banbury B12 study. *Age and ageing* 35.4 (2006): 416-422.

www.ingramcontent.com/pod-product-compliance
Lightning Source LLC
Chambersburg PA
CBHW081427170526
45166CB00008B/2117

* 9 7 8 1 4 8 9 5 3 1 7 2 8 *